Novel Immunotherapeutic Approaches to the Treatment of Cancer

Paul D. Rennert
Editor

Novel Immunotherapeutic Approaches to the Treatment of Cancer

Drug Development and Clinical Application

Springer

Editor
Paul D. Rennert
SugarCone Biotech LLC
Holliston, MA, USA

Aleta Biotherapeutics
Natick, MA, USA

ISBN 978-3-319-29825-2 ISBN 978-3-319-29827-6 (eBook)
DOI 10.1007/978-3-319-29827-6

Library of Congress Control Number: 2016939247

Printed on acid-free paper

This Springer imprint is published by Springer Nature
The registered company is Springer International Publishing AG Switzerland

This book is dedicated to the memory of Dr. Holbrook Edwin Kidd Kohrt (1977-2016). Holbrook was born in Scranton, Pennsylvania, and at an early age was found to have sporadic hemophilia (factor VIII). He overcame amazing obstacles and outlived the majority of his hemophiliac cohort, most of whom succumbed to transfusion-related infections, such as HIV/AIDS. Amazingly, Holbrook was able to clear and recover from an HCV infection, then relying on recombinant factor to keep him alive. Early on, he realized the power of the immune system to control such things as infection and cancer. Driven by not only his own personal experiences, but also his desire to help others, Holbrook pursued a career in medicine and translational research. He graduated as valedictorian of his class at Muhlenburg College. He then went on to attend Stanford University Medical School as a Baxter Foundation Scholar, going on to complete residency and fellowship there as well. He was a Howard Hughes Medical Institute Scholar, American Society of Hematology Research Fellow, and Damon Runyon Cancer Research Foundation Clinical Investigator, amongst other numerous awards. He completed his MD and obtained a PhD in tumor immunology and clinical trials design during fellowship. Holbrook worked tirelessly to drive innovation in cancer immunotherapy, publishing widely and impacting deeply, as he was involved with numerous projects that spanned basic, translational, and clinical boundaries. In his short time on earth, he inspired, innovated, and intimately cared for not only patients, but also anyone he touched.

I first met Holbrook in residency when he was finishing medical school at Stanford. We went through oncology fellowship together, and shared the struggles of training and postdoctoral fellowship – spending countless hours in the lab, performing endless experiments, struggling for funding – but ultimately, we shared a passion for science, immunotherapy, and a shared goal of improving lives. During my father's struggle with metastatic colon cancer, Holbrook was there, providing critical support and after-hours anti-emetic prescriptions. He was not only the type of oncologist you wished for if you were a patient, he was the type of physician-scientist you wished for as a colleague, and the type of friend you'd be lucky to have.

In thinking about how one might live a life, I think Holbrook would answer: with passion, compassion, and purpose…and there's no doubt that is exactly how he lived his life. He had written that his mission in life was to "give people more time for them to express their love."

Without a doubt, that is exactly what he accomplished

Russell K. Pachynski, MD
Assistant Professor
Division of Oncology
Washington University

Contents

Introduction

The era of immuno-oncology is upon us, and we have just in a few years moved from hypothesis testing and preclinical modeling to extraordinary and transformative advances in the development of therapeutics for cancer treatment. Diverse classes of therapeutics contributed to the outstanding pace of progress, driven by equally diverse technologies. Monoclonal antibodies continued to demonstrate their importance, with outstanding data coming from clinical trials of antagonist antibodies targeting immune checkpoint targets, high potency depleting antibodies targeting tumor antigens, antibody-drug conjugates, and agonist antibodies, notably to members of the TNF receptor superfamily. Taylor Schreiber reviews this latter class of antibodies that present interesting drug development challenges. Importantly, all of these diverse therapeutics synergize, sometime dramatically, in preclinical models, and in the case of immune checkpoint therapeutics, this has been exploited clinically. Indeed the role of immune checkpoint therapy as a singular and unprecedented backbone for a vast array of combinations has become a dominant theme, as discussed by Arlene Sharpe and colleagues. While the focus until recently has really been on T cell responses to tumors, Russell Pachynski and Holbrook Kohrt remind us that NK cells are potent anti-tumor lymphocytes, and must be brought to bear as we attack cancer cells from multiple angles. Another area ripe for combination with the immune checkpoint antibodies is the so-called onco-vaccines that target tumor antigens. Vaccine development is transforming from a once-neglected backwater into one of the dominant areas of cancer research, driven by a new understanding of the breadth of tumor antigens that can be uncovered, and to which T cells respond. Of note however, many of these novel antigens, or neo-antigens, appear to be patient-specific, raising a new challenge for the field. At the same time novel approaches to adjuvancy are improving vaccine delivery and potency—the complexities and advances in the vaccine field are addressed by Joshua D. Brody.

Antibody technology also contributed antigen-binding domains to chimeric-antigen-receptor bearing T cells, termed CAR-T, a technology that has altered the landscape of acute lymphocytic leukemia care and is making significant inroads into the treatment of several difficult B cell lymphomas. While the treatment of solid tumors with CAR-T cells has lagged behind, advances in gene engineering and gene editing will significantly alter this technology as it develops further, perhaps allowing broader use across tumor types. Gene editing technologies such as CRISPR/Cas9 are poised to become the next disruptive force in biomedicine, impacting cellular therapies but also allowing us to consider direct attacks on tumor cells, as a highly specific gene therapy approach. Thomas Cradick reviews CRISPR and other gene editing and also covers some of the cellular therapies such as CAR-T.

The understanding of the mechanisms underlying diverse therapeutic classes also advanced, notably in expanding our view of the nature of T cell responses in tumors. A close examination of the states of T cell exhaustion and T cell effector function, and the complexities and consequences thereof, has broadened our understanding of T cell fates, as discussed by Lawrence Kane and Greg Delgoffe. Such understanding has provided a foundation for biomarker exploration and may lead to the discovery of novel targets. There are a variety of sources for new targets of course, including the remarkable tumor microenvironment, newly appreciated as a foundational component not only of tumor architecture but also as a key mediator of the immunosuppressive tumor milieu. Christopher Thanos reviews the tumor microenvironment and some of the more interesting targets found therein. Another approach to novel target discovery is to investigate proteins or pathways that share phylogenetic features with validated targets. I take a look at emerging targets within the Ig superfamily as an example of this type of drug discovery. The assessment of novel targets in the context of personalized cancer therapy is discussed by Cokey Nguyen.

Clinical milestones in 2015 included multiple approvals of immune checkpoint inhibitors targeting PD-1 and the first approval of a combination immune checkpoint therapy using the anti-CTLA4 antibody ipilimumab and the anti-PD-1 antibody nivolumab. It is extraordinary to find that this combination is now considered to be the front-line treatment of choice for newly diagnosed metastatic melanoma, especially for patients that do not carry a BRAF mutation. Another anti-PD-1 antibody, pembrolizumab, has also been approved for front-line treatment of metastatic melanoma. These approvals alone show very clearly the pace at which immuno-oncology is supplanting not only chemotherapy and radiotherapy but also targeted drug therapeutics, until very recently the major focus of every biotech and pharmaceutical oncology drug development portfolio. Advanced metastatic melanoma, once considered a lethal and essentially incurable cancer, has become a tractable cancer, at least for those patients who respond to immunotherapeutics.

While the immune checkpoint antibodies and CAR-T cellular therapies clearly captured the public's imagination and investor's attention, we continued to see the advance of "workhorse" antibodies, those directed to tumor biology or tumor targets. Depleting antibodies cemented their place in the anti-tumor armory, as daratumumab and elotuzumab dramatically showed, while antibody-drug conjugates advanced across many indications, and using many diverse drug conjugation technologies. Christopher Thanos and I review just some of the advances in the antibody-drug conjugate development, a field that we predict will expand rapidly in coming years.

This volume is meant to give the reader a flavor of the excitement of this transformative era by taking a broad view of the discovery, drug development, and clinical landscapes. For those of us in the academic, medical, and biopharmaceutical fields the intense pace of progress is energizing, uplifting, and exhausting, as we swing harder and harder for the home runs, those drugs that truly give cancer patients hope for a cure, that most elusive of goals. As we will see, meaningful and lasting clinical responses are real for more and more cancer patients across more and more indications. The singular purpose of the authors of this volume is to continue improving cancer therapy, to give all patients a chance at a cure.

Paul D. Rennert
SugarCone Biotech LLC
Holliston, MA, USA
Aleta Biotherapeutics
Natick, MA, USA

Chapter 1
Enhancing the Efficacy of Checkpoint Blockade Through Combination Therapies

Vikram R. Juneja, Martin W. LaFleur, Robert T. Manguso, and Arlene H. Sharpe

1 Introduction

As the role of the immune system in cancer has become increasingly clear, so too has the potential for therapies that aim to restore the balance in favor of antitumor immunity and away from immunosuppression (Dougan and Dranoff 2009; Vanneman and Dranoff 2012). One of the most exciting therapies to emerge is "checkpoint blockade," in which antibodies are used to disrupt pathways that

V.R. Juneja
Department of Microbiology and Immunobiology, Harvard Medical School, Boston, MA 02115, USA

Evergrande Center for Immunologic Diseases, Harvard Medical School and Brigham and Women's Hospital, Boston, MA, USA

M.W. LaFleur
Department of Microbiology and Immunobiology, Harvard Medical School, Boston, MA 02115, USA

Evergrande Center for Immunologic Diseases, Harvard Medical School and Brigham and Women's Hospital, Boston, MA, USA

Department of Pediatric Oncology, Dana-Farber Cancer Institute, Boston, MA 02115, USA

R.T. Manguso
Department of Pediatric Oncology, Dana-Farber Cancer Institute, Boston, MA 02115, USA

A.H. Sharpe (✉)
Department of Microbiology and Immunobiology, Harvard Medical School, Boston, MA 02115, USA

Evergrande Center for Immunologic Diseases, Harvard Medical School and Brigham and Women's Hospital, Boston, MA, USA

Department of Pathology, Brigham and Women's Hospital, Boston, MA 02115, USA
e-mail: Arlene_Sharpe@hms.harvard.edu

P.D. Rennert (ed.), *Novel Immunotherapeutic Approaches to the Treatment of Cancer*, DOI 10.1007/978-3-319-29827-6_1

suppress T cell responses to tumors (Pardoll 2012; Topalian et al. 2015). This approach has led to some of the most striking clinical trial results in many years, with 20–50 % response rates across a range of cancers and unprecedented durability (Table 1.1). The search is on to find combination therapies with the many other tools in the clinician's toolbox to improve response rates while maintaining the durability of response to checkpoint blockade with acceptable toxicity (Sharma and Allison 2015; Brahmer et al. 2010; Fox et al. 2011). To make this search efficient and practical, there needs to be a rational approach to identify potentially synergistic combinations.

Checkpoint blockade aims to block the interactions between coinhibitory receptors on T cells and their ligands, which can be expressed on many cell types (Table 1.2). Ligation of coinhibitory receptors (e.g., PD-1, CTLA-4, TIM-3, LAG-3, TIGIT) can diminish T cell activation, homing to tissue, and effector function, and can affect the function of suppressive regulatory T cells (Schietinger and Greenberg 2014; Wherry 2011). Under physiologic conditions, these pathways are in place to prevent autoimmunity (T cells attacking self) and tissue damage (resolution of inflammation). However, the upregulation of coinhibitory pathways can prevent effective immunity; such is the case in many cancers (Schietinger and Greenberg 2014; Wherry 2011). Tumor-infiltrating T cells often express multiple coinhibitory receptors on their surface, and tumor cells and other cells in the tumor microenvironment often express their ligands (Ahmadzadeh et al. 2009). Blockade of these interactions in the clinic can have profound effects, though the specific mechanisms underlying these effects remain unclear. An understanding of these mechanisms is critical for the principled combination of checkpoint blockade with other therapies to increase the fraction of patients who respond to therapy.

There is already strong evidence that combining checkpoint blockade agents with each other and with other therapeutic strategies can lead to synergies. Clinical trials studying the combination of antibodies targeting PD-1 and CTLA-4 have shown survival benefits beyond that of either agent alone (Larkin et al. 2015; Wolchok et al. 2013; Postow et al. 2015). Multiple clinical studies of checkpoint blockade in combination with different classes of therapeutics (including other immunotherapies, targeted therapies, vaccines, radiation and chemotherapy) are underway (Table 1.1).

The goal of this chapter is to provide an overview of checkpoint blockade and combination therapy strategies. We first discuss the current understanding of the mechanisms underlying checkpoint blockade, with a focus on the two most clinically relevant pathways to date, the PD-1 and CTLA-4 pathways. We then present an overview of the combinations that are being examined preclinically and clinically. Finally, we explore important questions that need to be addressed to design combination therapies involving checkpoint blockade in a principled manner.

Table 1.1 Selected checkpoint blockade clinical trials

Pathway	Cancer types	Phase	Year	Response rates	Survival
CTLA-4					
Tremelimumab[a]	Metastatic Melanoma (Camacho et al. 2009)	1/2	2009	9.8 % (10 mg/kg) 9.3 % (15 mg/kg)	9.97 months (10 mg/kg) 11.53 months (15 mg/kg)
Tremelimumab	Advanced Melanoma (Kirkwood et al. 2010)	2	2010	6.6 %	10.0 months
Ipilimumab[b,*]	Stage 3 or 4 Melanoma (Hodi et al. 2010)	3	2010	5.7 % (Ipi + gp100) 10.9 % (Ipi) 1.5 % (gp100)	10.0 months (Ipi + gp100) 10.1 months (Ipi) 6.4 months (gp100)
Ipilimumab[*]	Advanced Melanoma with Brain Metastases (Margolin et al. 2012)	2	2012	10 %	13.3 months
Tremelimumab vs. Physician Choice Chemotherapy	Advanced Melanoma (Ribas et al. 2013)	3	2013	10.7 % (Tremel) 9.8 % (Chemo)	12.6 months (Tremel) 10.7 months (Chemo)
Ipilimumab	Metastatic Uveal Melanoma (Zimmer et al. 2015)	2	2015	0.0 %	6.8 months
PD-1					
Nivolumab[c,*]	Metastatic Melanoma, Colorectal, CR-Prostate, NSCLC, RCC (Brahmer et al. 2010)	1	2010	100 % (RCC), 10 % (Melanoma), 7.1 % (Colorectal)	Not evaluated
Nivolumab[*]	Melanoma, NSCLC, Colorectal, RCC, CR-Prostate (Topalian et al. 2012)	1	2012	18 % (NSCLC), 28 % (Melanoma), 27 % (RCC)	Not evaluated
Pembrolizumab[d,*]	Advanced Melanoma (Hamid et al. 2013)	1	2013	38 %	Not reached

(continued)

Table 1.1 (continued)

Pathway	Cancer types	Phase	Year	Response rates	Survival
Nivolumab*	Advanced Melanoma (Topalian et al. 2014)	1	2014	31 %	16.8 months
Pembrolizumab*	Advanced Melanoma (Robert et al. 2014)	1	2014	26 %	Not evaluated
Nivolumab*	Refractory Squamous NSCLC (Rizvi et al. 2015b)	2	2015	14.5 %	8.2 months
Nivolumab**	Relapsed/Refractory Hodgkin's Lymphoma (Ansell et al. 2015)	1	2015	87 %	Not reached
Nivolumab vs. Dacarbazine*	Untreated Metastatic Melanoma (Robert et al. 2015a)	3	2015	40.00 % (Nivo) 13.9 % (Dacarb)	Not reached (Nivo) 10.8 months (Dacarb)
Pembrolizumab* vs. Investigator Choice Chemotherapy	Ipilimumab Refractory Melanoma (Dummer et al. 2015)	2	2015	21 % (Pembro 2 mg/kg), 25 % (Pembro 10 mg/kg), 4 % (Chemo)	Not evaluated
Pembrolizumab**	NSCLC (Garon et al. 2015)	1	2015	19.4 %	Not reached
Pembrolizumab* vs. Ipilimumab*	Advanced Melanoma (Robert et al. 2015b)	3	2015	Pembro (2 wk)-33.7 % Pembro (3 wk)-32.9 % Ipi-11.9 %	Not reached
Nivolumab vs. Docetaxel*	Advanced Squamous NSCLC (Brahmer et al. 2015)	3	2015	20 % (Nivo) 9 % (Doce)	9.2 months (Nivo) 6.0 months (Doce)
Pembrolizumab	Progressive Metastatic Colorectal Cancer (Le et al. 2015a)	2	2015	40 % (MR deficient) 0 % (MR proficient)	Not reached (MR deficient) 5.0 months (MR proficient)

PD-L1					
BMS-936559[e]	Melanoma, NSCLC, Colorectal, Pancreatic, Gastric, Breast, Ovarian, and RCC (Brahmer et al. 2012)	1	2012	17.3 % (Melanoma) 11.8 % (RCC) 10.2 % (NSCLC) 5.9 % (Ovarian)	Not evaluated
MPDL3280A[f,**]	Metastatic bladder (Powles et al. 2014)	1	2014	43 % (IHC2/3)*** 11 % (IHC0/1)***	Not evaluated
LAG-3					
IMP-321[g]	Advanced Renal Cell Carcinoma (Brignone et al. 2009)	1	2009	0 %	Not evaluated
Combination therapies					
IMP-321 + Paclitaxel*	Metastatic Breast Carcinoma (Brignone et al. 2010)	1/2	2010	90 %	Not evaluated
Ipilimumab* + Dacarbazine*	Stage 3 or 4 Melanoma (Robert et al. 2011)	3	2011	15.2 % (Dacarb + Ipi) 10.3 % (Dacarb)	11.2 months (Dacarb + Ipi) 9.1 months (Dacarb)
Ipilimumab* + Fotemustine*	Stage 3 or 4 Melanoma (Di Giacomo et al. 2012)	2	2012	29.1 %	13.3 months
Ipilimumab + Poxviral Vaccine	Metastatic Prostate (Madan et al. 2012)	1	2012	58 %	34.4 months
Tremelimumab + IFNα*	Stage 4 Melanoma (Tarhini et al. 2012)	2	2012	24 %	21 months

(continued)

Table 1.1 (continued)

Pathway	Cancer types	Phase	Year	Response rates	Survival
Ipilimumab* + Nivolumab*	Stage 3 or 4 Melanoma (Wolchok et al. 2013)	1	2013	40.00 %	Not evaluated
Ipilimumab* + Sargramostim*	Metastatic Melanoma (Hodi et al. 2014b)	2	2014	15.5 % (Sargra + Ipi), 14.8 % (Ipi)	17.5 months (Sargra + Ipi) 12.7 months (Ipi)
Pidilizumab[h] + Rituximab*	Relapsed Follicular Lymphoma (Westin et al. 2014)	2	2014	66 %	Not evaluated
Ipilimumab* + Radiation	Stage 4 Melanoma (Twyman-Saint Victor et al. 2015)	1	2015	18 %	10.7 months
Nivolumab + Ipilimumab vs. Ipilimumab	Untreated BRAF WT Advanced Melanoma (Postow et al. 2015)	2	2015	61 % (Nivo + Ipi) 11 % (Ipi)	Not evaluated
Nivolumab + Ipilimumab vs. Nivolumab vs. Ipilimumab	Untreated Melanoma (Larkin et al. 2015)	3	2015	57.6 % (Nivo + Ipi) 43.7 % (Nivo) 19.0 % (Ipi)	Not evaluated

MR mismatch repair
*FDA-Approved
**FDA Breakthrough Status
***IHC0/1: <5 % PD-L1$^+$, IHC2/3: >5 % PD-L1$^+$
[a]Tremelimumab also known as CP-675,206 or Ticilimumab [Human Monoclonal IgG2]
[b]Ipilimumab also known as MDX010, MDX101, or Yervoy [Human Monoclonal IgG1]
[c]Nivolumab also known as MDX-1106, Opdivo, BMS-936558, or ONO-4538 [Human Monoclonal IgG4]
[d]Pembrolizumab also known as MK-3475, Keytruda, Lambrolizumab [Humanized Mouse Monoclonal IgG4]
[e]BMS-936559 [Human Monoclonal Ig G4]
[f]MPDL3280A [Human Monoclonal with Engineered Fc for avoiding ADCC]
[g]IMP-321 [LAG-3 Ig Fusion]
[h]Pidilizumab also known as CT-011 [Humanized Mouse Monoclonal IgG1]

Table 1.2 Costimulatory and coinhibitory pathways under investigation for tumor immunotherapies

Molecule	Expression profile	Role	Ligand	Expression profile
Costimulatory				
CD28	T cells	Priming, cell growth, survival, memory	B7-1 (CD80) B7-2 (CD86) ICOSL (human only)	T cells, B cells, dendritic cells, macrophages, monocytes
ICOS (CD278)	T cells, NKT cells, ILC2	Cell growth, differentiation, effector function, survival, memory	ICOSL	T cells, B cells, dendritic cells, macrophage, monocytes, granulocytes
CD27	T cells, B cells, NK cells	Priming, cell growth, differentiation, effector function, survival, memory	CD70	T cells, B cells
CD137 (4-1BB)	T cells, B cells, macrophages, monocytes, epithelial cells	Cell growth, effector function, survival, memory	CD137L (4-1BBL)	T cells, B cells, macrophages, monocytes, dendritic cells, epithelial cells
			Galectin-9	All cells
OX40	T cells, B cells	Cell growth, differentiation, effector function, survival, memory	OX40L	B cells, dendritic cells, T cells, endothelial cells
CD226	T cells, B cells, NK cells, macrophages, monocytes, stem cells, platelets	Cell growth, differentiation, effector function	CD112	Stem cells, dendritic cells, macrophages, monocytes, endothelial cells, platelets, epithelial cells, T cells, B cells
			CD155	Stem cells, dendritic cells, macrophages, monocytes, endothelial cells, platelets, epithelial cells, T cells, B cells
GITR	T cells, macrophages, monocytes	Cell growth, effector function	GITRL	B cells, macrophages/monocytes, dendritic cells

(continued)

Table 1.2 (continued)

Molecule	Expression profile	Role	Ligand	Expression profile
Coinhibitory				
CTLA-4 (CD152)	T cells, B cells	Cell growth, effector function, survival, memory	B7-1 (CD80) B7-2 (CD86)	T cells, B cells, dendritic cells, macrophages, monocytes
PD-1 (CD279)	T cells, B cells, macrophages, monocytes	Cell growth, effector function, survival, memory	PD-L1 (B7-H1, CD274)	T cells, B cells, dendritic cells, NK cells, macrophages, monocytes, epithelial cells, endothelial cells, stromal cells
			PD-L2 (B7-DC, CD273)	Mainly dendritic cells, macrophages
LAG-3 (CD223)	T cells, NK cells, B cells, dendritic cells	Cell growth, effector function	MHCII	B cells, dendritic cells, macrophages, monocytes, endothelial cells
TIM-3	T cells, dendritic cells, macrophages, monocytes	Cell growth, differentiation, effector function, memory	Galectin-9	All cells
			Phosphatidylserine	All cells
			HMGB1	All cells
TIGIT	T cells, NK cells	Cell growth, effector function	CD112	Stem cells, dendritic cells, macrophages, monocytes, endothelial cells, platelets, epithelial cells, T cells, B cells
			CD155	Stem cells, dendritic cells, macrophages, monocytes, endothelial cells, platelets, epithelial cells, T cells, B cells
BTLA	T cells, B cells, dendritic cells, macrophages, monocytes	Cell growth, effector function, survival, memory	HVEM	T cells, B cells, dendritic cells, NK cells, macrophages, monocytes, epithelial cells
CD200R	Macrophages, monocytes, T cells, NK cells, dendritic cells	Priming, effector function	CD200	B cells, dendritic cells, macrophages, monocytes, endothelial cells
CEACAM1 (CD66a)	T cells, granulocytes, epithelial cells, NK cells	Proliferation, effector function	Not known	Not known
VISTA	Macrophages, monocytes, granulocytes, T cells	Activation, effector function	Not known	Not known

2 Current Understanding of Mechanisms

2.1 *CTLA-4 Blockade*

CTLA-4 (Cytotoxic T Lymphocyte Antigen 4) was the first T cell co-receptor identified as inhibitory, and has a critical role in maintaining immune tolerance (Tivol et al. 1995; Waterhouse et al. 1995; Brunet et al. 1987). CTLA-4 also was the first coinhibitory receptor to show therapeutic promise in mouse models of cancer when blocked with a monoclonal antibody (Leach et al. 1996). Accordingly, CTLA-4 was the first coinhibitory receptor to be targeted in clinical trials and eventually approved for clinical use (Hodi et al. 2010). It is perhaps therefore surprising that the mechanism(s) by which CTLA-4 controls T cell responses remains controversial.

CTLA-4 is inducibly expressed upon activation of naive T cells ($CD4^+FoxP3^-$ and $CD8^+$) and constitutively expressed on suppressive regulatory T cells ($CD4^+FoxP3^+$, Tregs) (Alegre et al. 1996). CTLA-4 has both cell-intrinsic and cell-extrinsic functions (Grosso and Jure-Kunkel 2013). It binds to the same ligands (B7-1 and B7-2) as the costimulatory receptor CD28, but with a higher affinity (van der Merwe et al. 1997; Freeman et al. 1992; Freeman et al. 1993a; Freeman et al. 1993b). CTLA-4 inhibits the activation of naïve T cells and is a critical mediator of Treg cell suppressive function (Wing et al. 2008). CTLA-4 can inhibit T cell activation intrinsically, either by outcompeting CD28 or by recruiting phosphatases to the cytoplasmic domain of CTLA-4 upon ligation, leading to decreased TCR and CD28 signaling (Marengère et al. 1996; Grohmann et al. 2002). CTLA-4 also may inhibit activation of other T cells in a cell extrinsic fashion by leading to downregulation of B7-1 and B7-2 on antigen-presenting cells (APCs), either indirectly (through cytokines such as IL-10) or directly (transendocytosis) (Grohmann et al. 2002; Chen et al. 1998; Qureshi et al. 2011). Whereas other coinhibitory molecules seem to exert their influence primarily at the site of immune response, CTLA-4 is critical for initial activation of T cells in secondary lymphoid organs. Mice that lack CTLA-4 develop a fatal systemic inflammatory phenotype within 2–4 weeks of birth, characterized by uncontrolled T cell expansion (Tivol et al. 1995; Waterhouse et al. 1995). Analogously, humans with heterozygous CTLA-4 mutations have increased susceptibility to severe immune dysregulation (Kuehn et al. 2014; Schubert et al. 2014; Topalian and Sharpe 2014). Therefore, although questions remain about mechanisms, it is clear that CTLA-4 plays a critical role in attenuating T cell responses.

The seminal work demonstrating that CTLA-4 blockade can promote antitumor immune responses in mouse tumor models was performed in James Allison's lab in the mid-1990s (Leach et al. 1996). Since then, the basic science exploring the specific mechanisms underlying this efficacy has proceeded in parallel with the clinical development of antibodies that have a similar effect. Blockade of CTLA-4 on both effector T cells and regulatory T cells is necessary for optimal antitumor immunity, suggesting multiple modes of action (Peggs et al. 2009). In some, but not all mouse models, $CD4^+$ T cells are necessary for therapeutic benefit with CTLA-4 blockade, whereas $CD8^+$ T cells appear to always be necessary

(Hurwitz et al. 1998; van Elsas et al. 1999). This is likely because cytotoxic CD8$^+$ T cells are responsible for killing tumor cells, an important mode of antitumor immunity. Recent reports suggest that depletion of intratumoral regulatory T cells (the highest expressors of CTLA-4) may be a critical part of the therapeutic mechanism (Bulliard et al. 2013; Selby et al. 2013; Simpson et al. 2013).

The relevance of many of these findings to human cancer patients is an active area of investigation. Because of the challenges of obtaining fresh tumor samples from patients, many clinical studies have focused on peripheral blood samples. A recent study of blood samples from patients undergoing anti-CTLA-4 therapy showed an increase in new tumor-reactive T cell clones, but no change in preexisting clones (Kvistborg et al. 2014). This suggests that anti-CTLA-4 has a major effect on T cell priming (i.e., in the lymph nodes). Although studies such as this are informative, the phenotype of tumor-infiltrating lymphocytes (TILs) can differ drastically from peripheral sites (draining lymph node, blood, etc.) (Ahmadzadeh et al. 2009). Investigators are now designing protocols to obtain serial tumor biopsies before and during treatment. Initial studies of this sort show that anti-CTLA-4 increases T cell responses within the tumor (Cooper et al. 2014). In addition, mutational load in tumors prior to therapy has been correlated with response to anti-CTLA-4 in patients, suggesting that this therapy requires an immunogenic tumor (i.e., it can be recognized by T cells) (Snyder et al. 2014).

It is important to note that, while CTLA-4 blockade can induce striking antitumor immunity in some patients, many patients also experience immune-related adverse events (irAEs), generally manifesting as tissue-specific inflammation (Teply and Lipson 2014). This can be managed by administration of immunosuppressive drugs, and temporally or permanently stopping anti-CTLA-4 therapy. A better understanding of the mechanism of action of anti-CTLA-4 antibodies is needed to minimize the associated toxicities and increase the fraction of responding patients.

2.2 *PD-1 Pathway Blockade*

The PD-1 (programmed death 1) pathway plays a critical role in regulating peripheral T cell tolerance and protects healthy tissues from inflammatory tissue damage (Topalian et al. 2015; Flies et al. 2011; Francisco et al. 2010a; Ostrand-Rosenberg et al. 2014). Similarly to CTLA-4, PD-1 is induced on naïve T cells upon activation, and engagement by either of its ligands PD-L1 (B7-H1) or PD-L2 (B7-DC) sends inhibitory signals into T cells (Keir et al. 2008). This can attenuate the initial activation of T cells in the lymphoid organs, or it can diminish effector T cell functions in tissue (Keir et al. 2007). In the setting of an acute viral infection, PD-1 is upregulated on T cells but returns to baseline upon viral clearance (Petrovas et al. 2006). In contrast, in the setting of a chronic infection and cancer, T cells that are continuously exposed to antigen express high levels of PD-1 and eventually become dysfunctional (Wherry 2011). PD-1 is also constitutively expressed on Tregs, and affects their suppressive capacity (Francisco et al. 2010b). Expression of PD-1 ligands dampens the local immune response and controls resolution of inflammation after clearance of microbes. PD-L1 is constitutively expressed on many immune cell types and its expression can be induced on many nonimmune cells (including epithelial cells, vascular endothelial and stromal cells) by pro-inflammatory cytokines (e.g., Type I and II IFNs, TNFα, VEGF) (Keir et al. 2007). PD-L2 is expressed primarily by APCs, induced by many of the same cytokines as PD-L1, but IL-4 and GM-CSF are the most potent stimuli for PD-L2 expression (Francisco et al. 2010b). Tumor cells can express one or both PD-1 ligands, as do many of the other cells in the tumor microenvironment (e.g., fibroblasts, endothelial cells, immune cells) (Flies et al. 2011). Multiple and reinforcing mechanisms drive PD-L1 and PD-L2 expression on tumor cells, including oncogenic signaling (e.g., AKT), amplifications and/or translocations of chromosome 9p24 (which contains PD-L1 and PD-L2), and Epstein Barr Virus latent membrane protein 1 (LMP1). This constitutive expression of PD-L1 is termed "innate immune resistance." In addition, PD-L1 expression can be induced on tumor cells in response to T cells producing immunostimulatory cytokines (such as IFNs) (Spranger et al. 2013). This is termed "adaptive immune resistance," and represents a mechanism by which tumor cells attempt to evade immune mediated antitumor responses (Spranger et al. 2013; Spranger et al. 2015; Taube et al. 2012). Thus, there are multiple means by which PD-1 signaling may contribute to the immunosuppressive tumor environment.

Ligation of PD-1 negatively regulates T cells in several ways. First, engagement of PD-1 diminishes the signals downstream of TCR stimulation, and facilitates the downregulation of the TCR itself, leading to decreased activation and cytokine production (Karwacz et al. 2011; Sheppard et al. 2004). Second, PD-1 ligation can induce genes that impair T cell proliferation and cytokine production (e.g., the transcription factor batf) (Quigley et al. 2010), and can decrease anti-apoptotic gene expression and increase pro-apoptotic gene expression (e.g., bcl-xl), reducing T cell survival (Gibbons et al. 2012; Parry et al. 2005). Third, PD-1 signaling can decrease the production of cytotoxic molecules by T cells, decreasing their killing capacity (Azuma et al. 2008; Barber et al. 2006). Fourth, the PD-1 pathway can promote the induction of regulatory T cells from naïve or Th cells (iTregs), which suppress effector T cells (Francisco et al. 2009). Therefore, PD-1 signaling can modulate T cells in multiple ways that synergize to suppress immune responses.

Many important questions remain about the mechanisms that underlie antitumor immunity induced by PD-1 blockade. As a monotherapy, PD-1 blockade works in ~20–50 % of patients, but we do not understand the molecular nature of an effective antitumor response, nor know how to identify patients who will respond to PD-1 blockade. Furthermore, we do not understand why patients fail to respond to anti-PD-1/PD-L1. This knowledge is needed for rational combination of PD-1 pathway blockade with other therapies to treat patients who do not respond to anti-PD-1 or anti-PD-L1 alone.

Recent work has begun to address these questions. Several papers have noted that PD-1 is more frequently expressed on tumor-specific TILs than on the bulk TIL population, and that the TILs from patients who respond to PD-1 blockade are more clonal prior to therapy than in patients that do not respond (Ahmadzadeh et al. 2009; Gros et al. 2014; Tumeh et al. 2014). TIL clonality is often used as a measure for antigen-specific T cell responses, as T cells proliferate in response to their cognate antigen (e.g., clonal expansion). Similar to CTLA-4 blockade, multiple studies have shown that a higher mutational burden—specifically, non-synonymous mutations—is associated with a better response to PD-1 blockade (Messina et al. 2012; Le et al. 2015a). These nonsynonymous mutations likely give rise to neoantigens and induce tumor-specific T cells. Similarly, multiple studies have shown that response to PD-1 pathway blockade is more frequent in the setting of PD-L1 expression in the tumor microenvironment (on either tumor cells or nontumor cells, or both) (Larkin et al. 2015; Taube et al. 2012; Garon et al. 2015). It is important to note, however, that responses to PD-1 checkpoint blockade can occur even when PD-L1 expression is not observed, and that PD-L1 expression is not needed for response to combined PD-1 and CTLA-4 therapy. It is likely that a high mutation rate and PD-L1 expression are in fact linked, as a high mutation rate correlates with a higher $CD8^+$ T cell infiltration into tumors, which produce cytokines that can lead to increased PD-L1 expression in the tumor (i.e., adaptive immune resistance) (Spranger et al. 2013). Indeed, initial observations support the link between mutation rate and PD-L1 expression, but further work is needed to explore this concept (Le et al. 2015a).

2.3 *Additional Coinhibitory Pathways*

The success of anti-CTLA-4 and anti-PD-1 in the clinic has led to the search for other checkpoint molecules that can be targeted, especially in cases where anti-CTLA-4 or anti-PD-1 immunotherapy has little or no effect. There are many known checkpoint molecules (Table 1.2), and understanding the immunoregulatory roles of these molecules in cancer is an active area of investigation. Therapeutic targeting of several of these molecules has progressed to clinical trials (Shin and Ribas 2015).

One promising target is LAG-3 (lymphocyte-activation gene-3) (Goldberg and Drake 2011). LAG-3 is expressed on effector and regulatory T cells, B cells, NK cells and plasmacytoid dendritic cells, and binds with high affinity to MHCII to negatively regulate T cell responses (Shin and Ribas 2015). Whereas mice deficient in LAG-3 alone or PD-1 alone are generally healthy, mice lacking both LAG-3 and PD-1 develop systemic autoimmunity, highlighting the synergy between these two pathways in controlling T cell tolerance (Okazaki et al. 2011; Woo et al. 2012). T cells in tumors can co-express PD-1 and LAG-3, and combined blockade of PD-1 and LAG-3 in tumor models has a greater therapeutic benefit than blockade of either alone (Woo et al. 2012; Matsuzaki et al. 2010). These findings have given impetus to clinical trials with anti-LAG-3 antibodies (Shin and Ribas 2015).

Another promising target is TIM-3 (T-cell immunoglobulin and mucin-domain containing-3), which is expressed on T cells (Th1 and Tc1 cells) as well as on monocytes, macrophages and dendritic cells (Anderson 2014). TILs that express PD-1 can also express TIM-3; the $CD8^+PD\text{-}1^+TIM\text{-}3^+$ population is thought to be more dysfunctional than the $CD8^+$ $PD\text{-}1^+TIM\text{-}3^-$ population (Fourcade et al. 2010; Sakuishi et al. 2010). TIM-3 binds to galectin 9, HMGB1, and phosphatidylserine

(Chiba et al. 2012; DeKruyff et al. 2010; Zhu et al. 2005). Tumor cells and other cells in the tumor microenvironment, such as myeloid-derived suppressor cells (MDSCs), can express galectin-9 (Compagno et al. 2013). Signals through TIM-3 can lead to T cell death or tolerance (Zhu et al. 2005). In addition to impairing effector T cell function, TIM-3 expression on Tregs may enhance their suppressive capacity (Gautron et al. 2014) and TIM-3 on dendritic cells may decrease their ability to present antigens to stimulate T cells (Nakayama et al. 2009). Thus, TIM-3 may regulate innate and adaptive cells in the tumor microenvironment. Blockade of TIM-3 alone can induce antitumor immunity in some mouse models, and has shown potent synergy with PD-1 blockade (Sakuishi et al. 2010).

Another emerging coinhibitory receptor in cancer immunotherapy is TIGIT (T cell immunoreceptor with Ig and ITIM domains), which is expressed on T cells upon activation, as well as on NK cells (Shin and Ribas 2015). TIGIT shares the ligands CD155 and CD112 with CD226, but TIGIT ligation leads to T cell inhibition while CD226 ligation leads to T cell stimulation (Lozano et al. 2012). A recent study showed that co-blockade of TIGIT and PD-L1 led to tumor regression in a tumor model whereas blockade of either alone had minimal effect, suggesting a synergy between these pathways (Johnston et al. 2014).

3 Combination Therapies Involving Checkpoint Blockade

3.1 Overview of Goals of Rational Combinations with Checkpoint Blockade

The major goal of combining checkpoint blockade with other therapies is to increase the fraction of patients who respond to therapy, while maintaining the durability of response and minimizing the toxicity. In order to analyze the infinite space of potential combination strategies (i.e., therapy, timing, dosing) with a finite set of resources (i.e., money and clinical trials), it is imperative to take a principled approach to testing combinations. It is likely that the optimal combination will differ between different cancers and even between patients with the same clinical diagnosis. Thus, it is critical to gain mechanistic insights into why certain combinations succeed or fail, rather than simply evaluating response. These insights will allow clinicians to confidently choose specific combinations for each patient.

The goals of checkpoint blockade are to either stimulate new antitumor T cells to attack tumors or to relieve suppression of existing antitumor T cells, or both (Fig. 1.1). In cases where there is a lack of clinical response to checkpoint blockade monotherapy, there is likely a failure in one or both of these goals, or it may be that antitumor T cells alone are not sufficient to control the tumor. This may be the case in particularly proliferative tumors, such that the growth rate outcompetes the rate of killing by T cells, in tumors with a relatively low mutation burden so there are few antigens to drive T cell responses, or in tumors that create a particularly suppressive microenvironment. Thus, combining checkpoint blockade with therapies

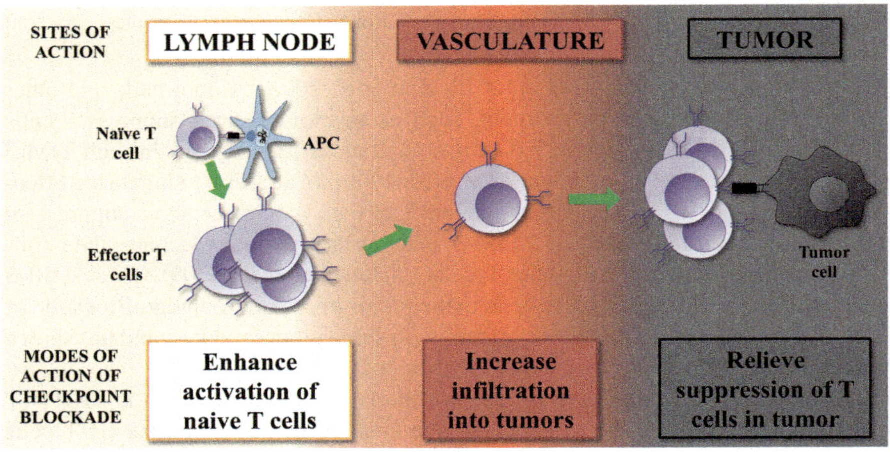

Fig. 1.1 Mechanisms by which checkpoint blockade antibodies may induce antitumor immunity. Checkpoint blockade may enhance the initial activation of naïve T cells by antigen-presenting cells (APCs) in the lymph node, increase the infiltration of activated effector T cells through the vasculature into the tumor, or relieve the suppression of the immune response in the tumor microenvironment

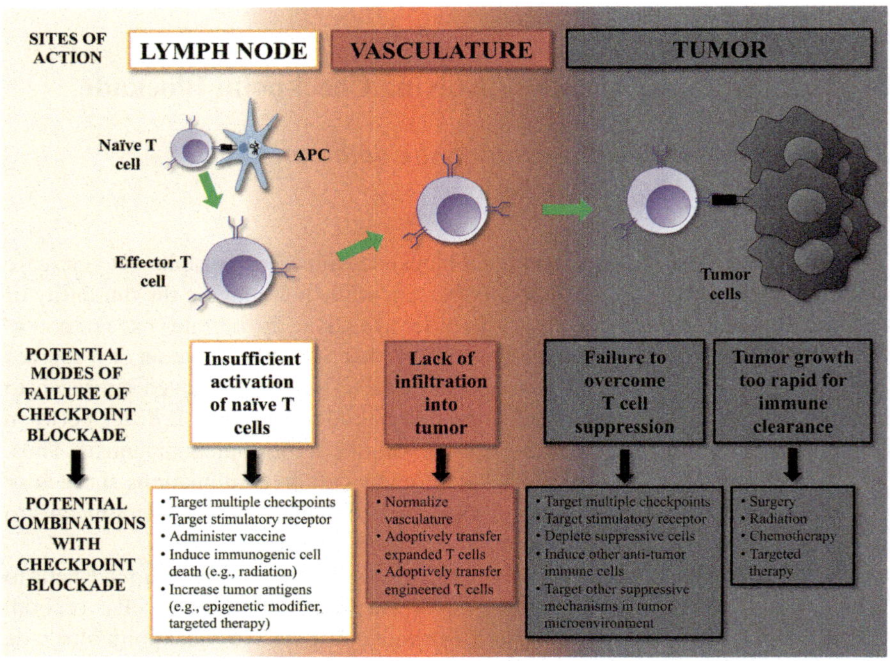

Fig. 1.2 Potential modes of failure for checkpoint blockade monotherapy and combination therapies to overcome failure. Checkpoint blockade monotherapy may be insufficient to induce an effective antitumor immune response due to insufficient activation of naïve T cells in the lymph node, lack of infiltration of effector T cells into the tumor, failure to overcome T cell suppression in the tumor, or a tumor growth rate that outcompetes the immune response. Selected potential combinations to surmount these failure modes are shown

that overcome these three possible failure modes may lead to synergies (Fig. 1.2). Therapies to combine with checkpoint blockade should: (1) increase the number of antitumor T cells (i.e., increase antigenicity of tumor, induce immunogenic cell death), (2) enhance the intrinsic function of antitumor T cells (i.e., block other suppressive pathways, upregulate stimulatory pathways), (3) extrinsically support antitumor T cell responses to tumors (i.e., stimulate other immune cell types that can promote antitumor immunity), and/or (4) simply debulk the tumor to allow the immune response to catch up to tumor growth.

Over the last decade, many studies have examined the effect of therapies not traditionally thought to affect the immune system on immune responses (Table 1.3). Many therapies can affect the immune system including targeted therapies (epigenetic modifiers, antiangiogenic agents, small molecules targeted at specific mutations), radiation therapy, and chemotherapy. These findings suggest that multiple types of cancer therapies have the potential to synergize with checkpoint blockade. In this section, we will discuss the principles behind specific combinations that are being studied, as well as summarize insights gained from preclinical and clinical studies of these combinations.

3.2 *Combining Checkpoint Blockade with Other Immunotherapies*

One approach is to combine checkpoint blockade with other immunotherapies. Multiple immunotherapies (e.g., vaccines, T cell stimulatory agents, T cell transfer) have been extensively studied, and many may target one or more of the three failure modes of checkpoint blockade. However, without understanding the precise mechanisms underlying checkpoint blockade, it is currently difficult to predict whether these therapeutics will be synergistic or redundant, or perhaps even negate one another. Importantly, targeting multiple axes of the immune response may lead to an increased frequency or severity of autoimmune side effects. Thus, careful preclinical evaluation of these combinations is critical.

3.2.1 Targeting Multiple Checkpoint Blockade Agents

In cases where checkpoint blockade monotherapy fails because a single agent is not enough to overcome T cell suppression, it may be beneficial to target multiple checkpoints. This approach may be considered when a large fraction of TILs express multiple coinhibitory receptors or display other features of T cell dysfunction (i.e., diminished proliferation, cytokine production, or cytotoxicity). Not surprisingly, the most extensively studied combination of checkpoint blockade agents is anti-CTLA-4 plus anti-PD-1 antibodies. Preclinical studies show impressive synergies between these two approaches, even in situations where monotherapy has a relatively weak

Table 1.3 Effects of non-immunologic cancer therapies on the immune system

Therapeutic agent	Effect on tumor	Effect on immune system
Chemotherapies		
Anthracyclines (Doxorubicin, Daunorubicin, Idarubicin, etc)	Kills tumor cells by intercalating DNA/RNA	– Causes immunogenic cell death of cancer cells leading to ATP and HMGB1 release that stimulates DCs and increases T cell priming (Fucikova et al. 2011; Ghiringhelli et al. 2009; Ma et al. 2013; Sistigu et al. 2014)
Oxaliplatin (Eloxatin)	Kills tumor cells by crosslinking DNA and inhibiting DNA synthesis	– Causes calreticulin exposure and HMGB1 release by dying tumor cells, which stimulates DCs via TLR4 to prime T cell immunity (Apetoh et al. 2007; Tesniere et al. 2010)
Cyclophosphamide (Endoxan, Cytoxan, Neosar, Procytox, Revimmune, Cycloblastin)	Kills tumor cells by alkylating DNA and inhibiting replication	– Causes immunogenic cell death resulting in calreticulin exposure and HMGB1 release. Selectively depletes Tregs and restores T cell and NK cell effector functions (Ghiringhelli et al. 2004; Ghiringhelli et al. 2007; Lutsiak et al. 2005; Schiavoni et al. 2011)
Gemcitabine (Gemzar)	A nucleoside analog that inhibits DNA replication	– Selectively depletes myeloid-derived suppressor cells and restores T cell and NK cell activity (Suzuki et al. 2005; Vincent et al. 2010)
5-Fluorouracil (Adrucil, Carac, Efudex, Efudix)	A pyrimidine analog that inhibits thymidylate synthase, thus inhibiting DNA replication	– Selectively kills myeloid-derived suppressor cells, reducing inhibition of T cells (Vincent et al. 2010)
Surgery and radiation therapy		
Surgical resection	Debulking of tumor or complete removal of primary tumor mass	– Restores T and B cell antitumor activity; reduces the number of MDSCs (Danna et al. 2004; Salvadori et al. 2000)
Radiotherapy	Kills tumor cells by causing severe DNA damage and eventually cell death. Can be targeted to deliver a higher dose or radiation to tumor than to surrounding tissue	– Causes immunogenic cell death of tumor cells, resulting in HMGB1 release that stimulates DCs via TLR4 to prime T cell immunity (Jing et al. 2015; Soukup and Wang 2015) – Causes DCs to secrete IFN-beta after the sensing of tumor cell DNA by the STING-cGAS pathway (Burnette et al. 2011; Deng et al. 2014; Woo et al. 2014) – Increases TCR repertoire diversity of tumor infiltrating $CD8^+$ T cells (Twyman-Saint Victor et al. 2015)

Small molecule inhibitors		
Vemurafenib (Zelboraf)	Selective inhibitor of the BRAF-V600E mutant	– Increases expression of melanocyte differentiation antigens, decreases melanoma cell expression of IL-6, IL-10 and VEGF, increases clonal expansion of T cells in tumor, and causes an upregulation of PD-L1 on tumor cells (Cooper et al. 2014; Sumimoto et al. 2006; Boni et al. 2010; Cooper et al. 2013a) – Concurrent treatment with PD-1 blockade is synergistic (Cooper et al. 2014)
Imatinib (Gleevec)	Inhibitor of oncogenic tyrosine kinases such as ABL and KIT	– Improves antitumor immunity in gastrointestinal stromal tumors by blocking IDO and increasing NK cell activation (Balachandran et al. 2011; Menard et al. 2009) – Decreases the number and suppressive capacity of Tregs (Larmonier et al. 2008) – Increases B cell production of tumor-specific antibodies (Ozao-Choy et al. 2009)
Sunitinib (Sutent)	Inhibitor of multiple tumor-associated kinases such as PDGFR and VEGFR	– Decreases the numbers of tumor-infiltrating Tregs and MDSCs (Ozao-Choy et al. 2009; Ko et al. 2009) – Decreases PD-1 and CTLA-4 expression on T cells and PD-L1 expression on MDSCs and pDCs (Ozao-Choy et al. 2009) – Blocks STAT3 and promotes in vivo expansion of T cells (Kujawski et al. 2010)
HDAC inhibitors (Vorinostat, Romidepsin)	Block the silencing of gene expression through epigenetic repression. Mechanisms not completely understood	– Suppresses Tregs and MDSCs, leading to enhanced CTL effector function and synergy with PD-1 blockade (Bridle et al. 2013; Kim et al. 2014; Shen et al. 2012)

(continued)

Table 1.3 (continued)

Therapeutic agent	Effect on tumor	Effect on immune system
Biologics		
Trastuzumab (Herclon, Herceptin)	Blocks signaling through HER2	– Increases DC cross-presentation and priming of T cells and synergizes with anti-PD-1 (Stagg et al. 2011; Disis et al. 2009; Park et al. 2010)
Bevacizumab (Avastin)	Inhibits angiogenesis by blocking VEGF	– Increases DC maturation and infiltration of antigen-specific $CD8^+$ T cells (Shrimali et al. 2010; Yang et al. 2009) – Reduces expression of checkpoint pathway molecules including PD-1, CTLA-4, Lag-3, and Tim-3 on T cells and synergizes with PD-1 blockade (Voron et al. 2015)
Cetuximab (Erbitux)	Blocks growth signals through EGFR	– Enhances DC-mediated phagocytosis and priming of T cell responses (Correale et al. 2012) – Increases infiltration of NK cells and ADCC (Marechal et al. 2010) – Increases complement-dependent tumor cell lysis (Dechant et al. 2008; Hsu et al. 2010)

effect (Curran et al. 2010; Duraiswamy et al. 2013; Mangsbo et al. 2010; Spranger et al. 2014). Similarly, clinical combination of anti-CTLA-4 plus anti-PD-1 shows clinical response rates (specifically, durable response rates) above either agent alone, which further supports nonredundant roles for these antibodies (Larkin et al. 2015; Wolchok et al. 2013; Postow et al. 2015). However, this increased efficacy comes at the cost of increased frequency of irAEs, and thus might only be an option for otherwise relatively healthy patients who can tolerate these effects. Importantly, the synergy between anti-PD-1 and anti-CTLA-4 suggests that combinations of either of these antibodies with other checkpoint blockade agents may lead to increased response rates, and perhaps fewer additional irAEs. As discussed previously, preclinical studies targeting the PD-1 pathway in combination with LAG-3, TIM-3, TIGIT, or VISTA (Liu et al. 2015) have shown synergies, giving the impetus for clinical trials with these combinations (Woo et al. 2012; Sakuishi et al. 2010; Johnston et al. 2014).

3.2.2 Targeting T Cell Stimulation

Though most agents to reach the clinic so far have targeted coinhibitory molecules on T cells, there is rationale for targeting costimulatory molecules (using agonistic rather than blocking antibodies) as well. Sending positive signals into T cells may allow them to overcome suppressive signals induced by coinhibitory molecules (Table 1.2). Importantly, this can be done without knowing the dominant coinhibitory pathways driving T cell suppression in a particular tumor. Costimulatory targets include the 4-1BB, OX40, ICOS, GITR, CD40, and CD27 receptors, and many are in clinical trials as single agents (Pardoll 2012; Sharma and Allison 2015; Richman and Vonderheide 2014). Preclinical studies combining costimulatory receptor agonists with checkpoint inhibitors (particularly CTLA-4 or PD-1) have shown enhanced T cell responses to many tumors (Chen et al. 2015; Curran et al. 2011; Marabelle et al. 2013; Redmond et al. 2014). Design and enrollment of clinical trials that test these same combinations in patients are underway.

T cell responses also can be enhanced with cytokines, which have been used in cancer immunotherapy for decades, albeit with generally modest effects. Pro-inflammatory cytokines (e.g., IL-2, IL-15, IL-21) not only can lead to enhanced T cell function, but can also stimulate APCs to present more tumor antigens. Analogously, blockade of immunosuppressive cytokines (e.g., IL-10, TGF) can enhance T cell activation. Thus, clinical efforts to combine these two clinically validated approaches (checkpoint inhibitors and cytokine therapy) are underway (Yu et al. 2010; West et al. 2013; Vanpouille-Box et al. 2015; Brooks et al. 2008).

3.2.3 T Cell Transfer and Vaccines

In cases where checkpoint blockade fails because the underlying T cell response to the tumor is minimal or absent, therapies that can quickly induce or increase this response are needed. One approach is by adoptive transfer of tumor-specific T cells, either harvested from the tumor itself or naïve cells genetically modified to recognize the tumor using TCRs or chimeric antigen receptors (CARs) (Rosenberg and Restifo 2015). This approach has had striking success in blood cancers, and is being actively studied in solid tumors. A major barrier that these cells face upon entry into a solid tumor is the suppressive tumor microenvironment, which may be overcome by combination with checkpoint blockade. In fact, since these approaches involve manipulating T cells in vitro, multiple groups have taken the additional step to further engineer the cells to lack expression of coinhibitory molecules or even modify their cytoplasmic tails so they provide stimulatory rather than inhibitory signals upon ligation, as well as remove the need for antibody administration (Frigault et al. 2015).

Another way to increase T cell responses to a tumor is by therapeutic vaccination. The fundamental goal of tumor vaccines is to activate DCs and induce them to present tumor antigens, in turn stimulating a T cell response against tumors. Several approaches have been tested: administering DCs loaded with tumor antigens, coupling tumor antigens to adjuvant, or injecting irradiated tumor cells modified to promote DC recruitment (GVAX) (Palucka and Banchereau 2013). Preclinical studies showing synergy between GVAX (or derivatives of GVAX) and checkpoint inhibitors have given impetus for clinical trials studying these same combinations (Curran et al. 2010; Duraiswamy et al. 2013; Le et al. 2015b).

3.2.4 Targeting Immune Cells Other than T Cells

The tumor microenvironment is complex, with multiple immunosuppressive cell types that are, by definition, outcompeting any antitumor immune cells (Hanahan and Coussens 2012; Gajewski et al. 2013). There are multiple therapeutic strategies that aim to either diminish immunosuppressive cell types or enhance the antitumor immune cells. Immunosuppressive cells in the tumor microenvironment include Tregs and myeloid-derived suppressor cells (MDSCs), and stromal cells such as cancer-associated fibroblasts (CAFs). Macrophages in the tumor microenvironment can have either antitumor or pro-tumor roles, and the role of B cells in the tumor microenvironment is still unclear. Therapies that deplete or manipulate immunosuppressive cells are emerging. Preclinical work has shown that depletion of MDSCs or CAFs synergizes with checkpoint blockade, as does stimulation of macrophages in the tumor microenvironment (Feig et al. 2013; Highfill et al. 2014; Zhu et al. 2014). CD40 agonistic antibodies, which both enhance T cell stimulation by APCs and enhance macrophage activation, have shown synergy with checkpoint blockade in preclinical models and are being studied in clinical trials (Zippelius et al. 2015).

3.3 Combining Checkpoint Blockade with Non-immunotherapies

It has become increasingly clear that therapies initially thought to target tumor cells specifically also can profoundly affect immune responses (Table 1.3). This understanding provides rationale for combining these therapies with checkpoint blockade in certain settings. In addition, since checkpoint blockade can take weeks to months to have a clinical effect, in some situations it is necessary to start with another therapy that can debulk the tumor, or at least slow tumor growth.

3.3.1 Therapies Targeting Tumor-Specific Mutations

Agents that target specific genetic defects in tumor cells can have profound effects on tumor growth in high percentages of patients with targeted mutations, although the responses are generally not durable. Initially designed to inhibit tumor cells intrinsically, these agents can have tumor cell-extrinsic effects as well, which can elicit a stronger immune response against treated tumors. Perhaps the most well-studied example is agents that target the BRAFV600E mutation, the oncogenic driver commonly found in melanoma and other cancers (Sumimoto et al. 2006). In metastatic melanoma BRAF inhibitor therapy initially leads to an increase in expression of melanocyte differentiation antigens and decreased immunosuppressive cytokine production, coupled with an initial increase in $CD8^+$ T cell infiltration into the tumor (Boni et al. 2010; Cooper et al. 2013a). However, as with other targeted therapies, the response to BRAF inhibitors is often transient. BRAF inhibitor resistance is associated with decreased T cell infiltration and increased PD-L1 expression (Frederick et al. 2013). These effects on the immune response, along with the high response rate but low durability (the inverse of what is seen with checkpoint inhibitors) provide rationale for combining targeted therapies with checkpoint inhibitors (Cooper et al. 2013b). However, clinical studies that combine some BRAF inhibitors with anti-CTLA-4 antibodies have shown increased toxicity, especially when combined with MEK inhibitors (Harding et al. 2012). Preclinical studies have shown synergy between BRAF inhibitors and anti-PD-1 antibodies, and this is now being evaluated clinically (Cooper et al. 2014).

3.3.2 Epigenetic Modifiers and Antiangiogenic Agents

Cancer is now appreciated to be both a genetic and epigenetic disease, and epigenetic changes in tumor cells can be reversed with the goal of returning tumor cells to a normal state (e.g., turn back on a tumor suppressor). Multiple drugs have been developed to target epigenetic modifications in tumor cells, such as methylation and histone modifications. Epigenetic modifiers may increase the expression of tumor antigens that have been repressed, thus allowing either preexisting T cells or new T cells to respond (Heninger et al. 2015). Epigenetic modifiers also can inhibit suppressive Tregs and MDSCs, thereby promoting an antitumor immune response (Bridle et al. 2013; Kim et al. 2014; Shen et al. 2012). The combination of epigenetic modifiers with checkpoint blockade improves T cell function during chronic viral infection in mice, suggesting that this approach may promote antitumor immunity (Zhang et al. 2014). Indeed, anecdotal reports of patients responding to checkpoint inhibitors after receiving epigenetic modifiers have led to the design of clinical trials exploring these combinations more systematically.

Similarly to epigenetic modifiers, antiangiogenic agents can support antitumor immune responses. As tumors grow, they induce the formation of a highly abnormal blood vessel supply. The original motivation for antiangiogenic agents was to prevent the formation of these blood vessels, thereby preventing the supply of nutrients to the tumor. At low doses, antiangiogenic agents can "normalize" this vasculature, which allows for better delivery of agents into the tumor and the infiltration of immune cells (Shrimali et al. 2010; Yang et al. 2009). However, tumor-derived VEGF, a potent angiogenic molecule, can upregulate checkpoint molecules on T cells and induce T cell dysfunction, providing rationale for combining agents that target VEGF with checkpoint blockade (Voron et al. 2015). Moreover, studies of tumor samples from patients treated with ipilimumab suggest that ipilimumab modulates blood vessel formation as part of its therapeutic mechanism (Yuan et al. 2014). Thus, clinical trials are underway to study combined ipilimumab and antiangiogenic therapy (Hodi et al. 2014a).

3.3.3 Radiation Therapy

Radiation therapy accomplishes two tasks that may synergize with checkpoint blockade. First, it debulks and remodels the tumor, potentially allowing the T cell response more time to develop. Second, it leads to immunogenic cell death, potentially increasing tumor-antigen presentation. Multiple mechanisms have been proposed for this immunogenic cell death, including the release of HMGB1 to stimulate DCs via TLR4 or the sensing of tumor cell DNA by the STING-cGAS pathway (Burnette et al. 2011; Deng et al. 2014; Jing et al. 2015; Soukup and Wang 2015; Woo et al. 2014). Radiotherapy seems to result in increased activation of new antitumor T cells. A recent study showed that radiation therapy synergized with blockade of both CTLA-4 and PD-L1; the authors suggested that radiation therapy led to an increased breadth of T cell responses to the tumor, accompanied by the relief of T cell exhaustion from PD-1 blockade and Treg depletion from CTLA-4 blockade (Twyman-Saint Victor et al. 2015).

3.3.4 Chemotherapy

Perhaps most surprising are the strong beneficial effects that conventional chemotherapeutics can have on the antitumor immune response. These drugs are thought to directly kill cancer cells by affecting DNA replication, thereby preventing tumor cell proliferation. However, multiple other modes of action have been elucidated, mostly centered on the stimulation of strong antitumor immune responses (Table 1.3). Similarly to radiation therapy, multiple chemotherapeutic agents induce immunogenic cell death of tumor cells, acting as an endogenous vaccine to stimulate DCs to activate antitumor T cells (Apetoh et al. 2007; Fucikova et al. 2011; Ghiringhelli et al. 2009; Ghiringhelli et al. 2004; Ghiringhelli et al. 2007; Kepp et al. 2014; Lutsiak et al. 2005; Ma et al. 2013; Schiavoni et al. 2011; Sistigu et al. 2014; Tesniere et al. 2010). Furthermore, some chemotherapeutic agents selectively deplete suppressive cells in the tumor microenvironment, such as MDSCs and Tregs (Messina et al. 2012; Ghiringhelli et al. 2004; Ghiringhelli et al. 2007; Schiavoni et al. 2011; Suzuki et al. 2005; Vincent et al. 2010). Interestingly, although chemotherapeutic agents can induce lymphodepletion, this may actually promote antitumor immunity, as suppressed T cells may regain their effector function during the ensuing homeostatic proliferation (i.e., outgrowth to fill the lymphocyte niche). These observations provide motivation for combining chemotherapeutic agents with checkpoint blockade, although clearly the dosing and timing of these therapies (and specific agents) are very critical for realizing their synergistic potential. Several clinical trials of these combinations are underway, with more planned in the near future.

4 Advancing Combination Checkpoint Therapies

4.1 Necessary Next Steps for Advancing Combination Checkpoint Therapies

Many combination checkpoint therapies are making their way to the clinic. Due to the large number of FDA-approved cancer therapies and the vast number currently in clinical trials, it is imperative that the choice of combination therapies to test in patients be rational. A failure to do so may lead to numerous disappointing trial results and exhaust resources and patient populations necessary for finding effective combinations. Towards this goal, we suggest an approach for testing combinations that is based on data from currently ongoing immunotherapy studies and grounded in a sound molecular understanding of the pathways to be targeted: (1) identify the patients most likely to benefit from combination therapy, (2) characterize the mechanisms by which tumors resist immunotherapy, and (3) determine strategies to target these resistance pathways effectively.

Optimal combination therapies will require analyses of the tumor microenvironment of each patient. The emerging principle that checkpoint blockade likely has efficacy only where there is already an ongoing (albeit failing) anti-immune response pre-therapy suggests that this is a primary aspect of the tumor that should be studied. Analytic approaches are needed to distinguish between a lack of an immune response and an active suppression of an immune response. The former type of patients would likely benefit from therapies that promote an immune response (e.g., vaccination, induction of immunogenic cell death), whereas the latter would benefit from therapies that remove suppression (e.g., combination checkpoint blockade, depletion of suppressive cells). These analytic strategies may also benefit patients who develop resistance to checkpoint blockade.

4.2 Understanding Mechanisms of Efficacy of Checkpoint Blockade

A major impediment to the principled combination of checkpoint blockade antibodies with other therapies is an incomplete understanding of their mechanisms of action. Rapid progress is being made in this area. In the clinical setting, tumor biopsies and resections obtained before and after treatment from the same patient are more valuable than equivalent samples obtained from different patients (Cooper et al. 2014). Collaborative efforts (between clinicians and scientists) have the potential to maximize the information obtained from these samples. In the preclinical setting, care must be taken in selection of animal models for studying therapeutic mechanisms of action. Many mouse tumor models do not respond to checkpoint blockade monotherapy (Grosso and Jure-Kunkel 2013). It is important to understand the differences between models that respond and those that do not, and utilize the appropriate models to study mechanism of response and resistance to checkpoint blockade.

For CTLA-4 and PD-1 checkpoint blockade, several fundamental questions remain. The relative effects of anti-CTLA-4 and anti-PD-1 on effector versus Treg cells versus other PD-1 expressing cells (NK cells, myeloid cells) are incompletely understood, and this knowledge may suggest approaches for combination therapy. For example, whereas blockade of PD-1 enhances the function of effector T cells, genetic loss of PD-1 in mouse models actually increases the suppressive capacity of at least a subset of Tregs (Sage et al. 2013), which could in turn inhibit antitumor immunity. Similarly, dissecting the role of PD-L1 and PD-L2 on specific cell types (e.g., immune cells versus tumor cells versus stromal) may lead to mechanistic insights as well as biomarkers that predict response. Future studies also should address the relative effects of checkpoint blockade in the periphery (lymph node, blood) versus the tumor microenvironment, as this information not only will inform the search for biomarkers, but also suggest combination therapeutics. Finally, a molecular understanding of the changes that occur in T cells following checkpoint blockade will greatly refine the combination therapies being explored to enhance T cell function.

Multiple checkpoint blockade antibodies are now available to clinicians but to optimize their therapeutic impact, a better understanding of the similarities and differences between coinhibitory pathways, as well as mechanisms of synergy between coinhibitory pathways is needed. Studying biopsy samples for the relative expression of coinhibitory molecules on T cells and their ligands in the tumor microenvironment will likely help inform the choice of which agent(s) to use, although how to make this choice is still an open question. Insights may come from determining whether synergies between coinhibitory pathways (e.g., PD-1 plus CTLA-4 vs. PD-1 plus LAG-3 vs. PD-1 plus TIM-3) affect similar or different molecular pathways.

While the majority of studies have focused on mechanisms of therapeutic efficacy, relatively little is known about mechanisms of durability and thus questions remain about the necessary length of therapy. Ipilimumab is given in only four doses over 12 weeks, but anti-PD-1 agents are given either every 2 weeks or every 3 weeks indefinitely. Despite the finite length of therapy, the response to ipilimumab seems to be durable, as responders from the original clinical trial remain in remission or with stable disease for many years (Schadendorf et al. 2015). However, because blockade of CTLA-4 and PD-1 likely work by different mechanisms, the durability seen with CTLA-4 blockade does not imply that blockade of PD-1 will have a similar durability. Further work is needed to understand how CTLA-4 and PD-1 blockade affect the generation, function and maintenance of memory T cell subsets. Updates on patients from early clinical trials will begin to answer the question of durability.

4.3 Understanding Mechanisms of Resistance to Checkpoint Blockade

The identification of resistance mechanisms to checkpoint blockade and the development of strategies to circumvent resistance are important steps toward increasing the proportion of patients that respond to therapy. Studies in mouse tumors models in which checkpoint blockade induces tumor regression in certain settings but not others (e.g., larger tumor burden) should provide insights into general principles of therapeutic nonresponsiveness. The potential of such work is illustrated by a recent study showing that elevated beta-catenin signaling in melanoma tumors suppresses spontaneous T cell infiltration into tumors, which is likely a prerequisite for a strong response to checkpoint blockade monotherapy (Spranger et al. 2015). Temporal studies of patient samples (tumor biopsies from patients with recurrence and blood samples from all patients) obtained at multiple time points during checkpoint blockade (during response versus resistance) will be valuable for investigating resistance mechanisms.

Moreover, analyses of immune alterations within human tumor cells and the tumor microenvironment have the potential to identify resistance mechanisms. For example, recently published data from The Cancer Genome Atlas (TCGA) project suggest that tumors may harbor mutations that increase the likelihood of resistance to immunotherapy. Tumors with an increased infiltration of cytolytic effector cells ($CD8^+$ T cells, NK cells) are also more likely to harbor mutations in MHC-I complex subunits, which may impair antigen presentation or in molecules of the extrinsic cell death pathway, which may limit effectiveness of cytolytic effector cells (Rooney et al. 2015). Mutations such as these may be driving the incomplete responses observed in patients and would thus represent a tumor in which another therapy should be pursued.

Additionally, immunophenotyping of patient tumors that fail to respond completely could reveal the increased presence of suppressive cell populations that are preventing the successful reinvigoration of T cells. For example, class-I HDAC inhibitors deplete myeloid-derived suppressor cell (MDSC) populations disproportionately both in vitro and in vivo and synergize with checkpoint blockade, thus representing a strategy for specifically depleting suppressive populations in the tumor microenvironment (Kim et al. 2014).

4.4 Principled Combination of Checkpoint Blockade with Other Immunotherapies

Since immune cell types in addition to T cells can modulate the tumor microenvironment, there is great potential for strategies that combine manipulation of these immune cell types with checkpoint blockade. Here we will discuss principled combination of dendritic cells (DCs), natural killer (NK) cells, and myeloid cell modulation with checkpoint blockade.

Studies of DCs have focused mainly on their use in vaccines, as well as approaches to manipulate endogenous DC populations. The goal of both approaches is a more potent $CD8^+$ T cell response to the tumor, as discussed above. Recent advances in rapid prediction and synthesis of tumor-specific peptide sequences following sequencing of a patient's tumor should enable development of more effective tumor vaccines (Rajasagi et al. 2014). Further work is needed to develop strategies to enhance recruitment and maturation of DCs following peptide vaccination, as well as to improve tumor peptide formulations to promote epitope spreading, the process by which an ongoing immune response to a particular antigen results in "spreading" of the targeted immune response to other antigens. One recent advance involved the preconditioning of a vaccine site with tetanus toxoid in order to enhance DC migration to the lymph node upon vaccination (Mitchell et al. 2015). This approach improved survival of patients with glioblastoma multiforme in a clinical trial. Approaches such as these should be considered in tumors with relatively few infiltrating T cells to induce an immune response that can be supported by combination with checkpoint blockade therapy.

Natural killer (NK) cells are another immune population under intense investigation since NK cells can directly kill tumor cells and mediate the effects of antibody-dependent cellular cytotoxicity. NK cells are particularly important in tumors that downregulate MHCI in an attempt to avoid $CD8^+$ T cell responses, as NK cells attack cells with low MHCI expression. Although NK cells express many of the same coinhibitory receptors as T cells, little is known about the contribution of NK cells to the tumor immunity induced by checkpoint blockade. Intriguingly, a recent study demonstrated that Cbl-b was responsible for regulating NK cell mediated antitumor immunity and that knockdown of Cbl-b induced impressive spontaneous rejection of tumors (Paolino et al. 2014). Further work is need to determine how to modulate NK cell proliferation and effector function alone or in combination with antibodies designed to enhance ADCC or with T cell immunotherapies.

Myeloid cells are the most common immune cell subset in many tumors and often associated with an immunosuppressive M2 macrophage phenotype or myeloid derived suppressor cell phenotype (Lemke and Rothlin 2008; Ruffell et al. 2012). Myeloid derived suppressor cells are a $Gr\text{-}1^+$ immature macrophage or dendritic cell subset characterized by their expression of ARG1 and iNos (Youn and Gabrilovich 2010). Myeloid cells in the tumor microenvironment can exert suppressive effects through the expression of PD-L1 as well as the production of immunosuppressive molecules such IL-10, TGFβ, and nitric oxide (Youn and Gabrilovich 2010). There are a number of strategies under investigation to overcome immunosuppressive effects of myeloid cells including repolarizing them to an M1 phenotype (as is seen in the setting of CSF1R blockade) (Zhu et al. 2014), or blocking their recruitment to the tumor (e.g., by disrupting the CXCR2: CXCL8 axis) (Highfill et al. 2014). In addition, macrophages have an underappreciated role in interfacing with endothelial cells, angiogenesis, and the maintenance of tumor cell vasculature. Tie2^{+} macrophages promote the production of new endothelial cells, which aids in the process of angiogenesis. Perturbation of these interactions decreases tumor cell vasculature and the ability of tumor cells to thrive in a hypoxic environment. Macrophages also can scavenge dead/stressed tumor cells in a non-immunogenic fashion, and strategies to increase the immunogenicity of the tumor through the accumulation of tumor-derived HMGB1 and ATP, two well known immunostimulatory signals in the tumor microenvironment, are under investigation. Lastly, the modulation of the local humoral response may provide a distinct means to promote tumor cell killing by skewing B cells to produce antibodies that participate in complement fixation, ADCC, or FcR-mediated phagocytosis. These approaches are likely to synergize with PD-1 blockade given the distinct mechanisms of action.

4.5 *Principled Combination of Checkpoint Blockade with Non-immunotherapies*

The effects of non-immunotherapeutic approaches on the immune response must be closely examined in order to determine how to optimally combine them with checkpoint blockade. Chemotherapy, targeted therapies, and radiotherapy are often not as effective at inducing tumor regression in the absence of functional immunity (Cooper et al. 2014; Zitvogel et al. 2008). It is clear that innate and adaptive immunity play a critical role in mediating the effects of various non-immunologic cancer therapies (Table 1.3). Traditional therapeutics that elicit immunogenic cell death and increase priming of adaptive immunity, such as chemotherapy with anthracyclines or radiotherapy may synergize with checkpoint blockade. Surgical resection can relieve systemic immunosuppression and perhaps restore T cell function (Danna et al. 2004; Salvadori et al. 2000). A better understanding of the effect of surgical resection of accessible lesions on the immune response to other lesions is needed.

4.6 *Using Biomarkers to Predict Response and Stratify Patients*

Current data indicate that when a patient responds to checkpoint blockade therapy, the response is most often durable (McDermott et al. 2014). However, across different cancer types, sizeable fractions of patients do not respond (Table 1.2). Thus, it is imperative to develop biomarkers that help stratify patients and predict whether a given patient is likely respond to monotherapy, should receive some type of combination therapy, or receive other therapies entirely. To date, three types of biomarkers have been studied intensively, particularly in the context of PD-1 blockade: a high degree of immune infiltrate in the tumor—specifically $CD8^+$ T cells, a high mutational burden/predicted neoepitopes, and expression of PD-L1 by tumor cells or tumor immune cell infiltrates (Snyder et al. 2014; Tumeh et al. 2014; Le et al. 2015a; Herbst et al. 2014; Rizvi et al. 2015a).

Work of Jerome Galon demonstrated the benefit of the immunoscore on patient survival (Anitei et al. 2014). The immunoscore is being investigated for its predictive value for a patient's response to checkpoint blockade. Moreover, with the development of multicolor multiplexed IHC, it is now possible to evaluate $CD8^+$ T cell numbers, as well as their functional status and location within the tumor simultaneously. This approach may lead to identification of biomarkers that will predict whether checkpoint blockade monotherapy will be sufficient to induce an objective response. Ectopic lymphoid follicles are highly correlated with an increase in overall survival in melanoma, breast, and colorectal cancer patients (Messina et al. 2012; Bindea et al. 2013; Gu-Trantien et al. 2013; Huang et al. 2015). The association of these structures with an objective response to checkpoint blockade remains to be investigated.

A higher mutational burden within tumor cells correlates with a better response to checkpoint blockade (Snyder et al. 2014; Le et al. 2015a; Rizvi et al. 2015a). This was initially observed by comparing response rates and mutational burden across different types of cancers, but also is seen in patients with the same type of cancer (e.g., non-small cell lung cancer, colorectal cancer), but with different mutational burdens (Le et al. 2015a; Rizvi et al. 2015a). Together, these data further the hypothesis that tumors that elicit a strong $CD8^+$ T cell response to tumor antigens (e.g., neoantigens) respond better to checkpoint blockade monotherapy than tumors without many mutations and therefore without many tumor antigens. If this is indeed the case, then analysis of the mutational burden of tumor cells, as well as the T cell repertoire in the tumor prior to therapy, may be useful for identifying patients more likely to respond to checkpoint blockade and patients who likely need another intervention prior to checkpoint therapy.

High expression of PD-L1 on tumor cells increases the likelihood of a response to PD-1 pathway blockade, but durable responses are seen in patients with little or no PD-L1 expression. It remains unclear whether optimization of PD-L1 immunohistochemistry will enable better predictive value of PD-L1 expression. Further work is needed to investigate intratumoral heterogeneity of PD-L1 expression, as well as relative expression of PD-L1 in primary and metastatic tumors.

New biomarkers may result from other approaches under investigation. Quantification and characterization of circulating tumor cells in the blood might allow for less invasive analysis of tumor cells, along with real-time monitoring or response to therapy. Similarly, more sensitive tumor DNA detection techniques allow for the real time monitoring of tumor burden in plasma (Anderson 2014). These methods may provide a means to probe the tumor microenvironment via a blood-based assay and enable rapid determination of the efficacy of checkpoint blockade in patients.

4.7 Potential Next-Generation Therapeutic and Diagnostic Strategies

The major goal of combining checkpoint blockade with other therapies is to increase the fraction of patients that have a durable response while minimizing irAEs. The increased rate of irAEs seen with the combination of nivolumab (anti-PD-1) with ipilimumab (anti-CTLA-4) may limit this combination to only otherwise healthy patients, despite the increased durable response rate seen with this therapy. New strategies that target multiple immunosuppressive pathways in parallel and that target these pathways in specific cells, as well as new strategies to study the antitumor immune response are under development and may overcome these limitations.

One potential method for reducing irAEs that result from systemic activation of the immune response is to use targeted antibodies, such as bispecific antibodies or antibodies with modified affinity, both with the goal of targeting specific immune cell populations. Bispecific antibodies have two targets rather than one (as with traditional antibodies). Bispecific antibodies have been used to bring T cells and tumor cells together, but they could be designed to bring T cells and dendritic cells together, draw NK cells to the tumor, and to more specifically target a cell (e.g., a CD8β/PD-1 bispecific antibody that blocks PD-1 specifically on $CD8^+$ T cells to increase their effector function). Another avenue for more specific antibody targeting of immune cells in the tumor involves development of antibodies with a modified affinity such that they only bind cells expressing very high levels of a target molecule.

Many efforts are underway to target multiple coinhibitory pathways (e.g., PD-1, CTLA-4, TIM-3, and LAG-3 in pairwise combinations) in preclinical mouse models and clinical trials. A better understanding of the molecular pathways triggered by coinhibitory receptors is needed to determine shared and unique signaling nodes. This knowledge may reveal new therapeutic targets and strategies. Small molecule inhibitors that target a shared node might potentially replace administration of multiple checkpoint antibodies; this approach may efficiently invigorate dysfunctional $CD8^+$ T cells and potentially decrease the side effects associated with multiple checkpoint inhibition, in addition to being easier to administer and likely less expensive. Furthermore, in engineered T cells (e.g., CAR T cells or adoptive cell transfer) these nodes could be targeted genetically (e.g., using the CRISPR/Cas9 or TALEN systems). In addition, $CD8^+$ T cells could be manipulated to recruit other immune cell populations to the tumor, break down the stromal architecture of the tumor, disrupt tumor vasculature, or potentially support formation of memory $CD8^+$ T cells.

Another way to limit systemic activation of immune cells is to take advantage of advances in drug delivery: both delivery to specific sites and to specific cells. Polymer scaffolds engineered to recruit effector cells and prime them with proper cytokines are being tested in animal models. Such scaffolds could potentially also incorporate checkpoint antibodies. In addition, intratumoral injection approaches may provide a means to stimulate an immune response locally. The potential for this approach is illustrated by studies showing that intratumoral injection of anti-CTLA-4, anti-OX40 plus CpG led to a curative immune response and required 1/100 of the dosage of antibody in mouse tumor models. Directed delivery of checkpoint antibodies to specific cells by targeted nanoparticles or bispecific antibodies may provide even greater specificity by targeting effector cells.

Finally, improvements in cellular and tissue analysis may enable finer methods for evaluating the tumor microenvironment and developing more meaningful immunoscores to more accurately predict if a patient will respond to checkpoint blockade. CyTOF technology coupled with barcoding approaches provides a novel means to identify the spatial location of cells within the tumor and to reconstruct tissue architecture computationally overlaid with quantitation of up to 50 proteins. This approach should make possible functional characterization of immune cell infiltrates in the tumor while maintaining spatial relationships in the tumor. Laser capture microscopy followed by single cell RNAseq provides a complementary approach to investigate the entire transcriptome while preserving tissue structure. These two techniques are powerful tools for investigating clonal heterogeneity of both the immune cells and tumor cells during tumor evolution and determining why tumors regress or progress. This knowledge should aid development of better biomarkers for predicting which patients will respond to checkpoint therapy, monitoring responses to checkpoint blockade and determining if additional interventions are needed to promote tumor eradication.

5 Future Directions

The story of the path of checkpoint blockade antibodies from the lab into the clinic is both exciting and inspirational, requiring the collaboration of physicians, scientists and patients. Checkpoint blockade is now established as a mainstay of medical oncology, but further work is needed to increase the efficacy of checkpoint blockade, and explore the infinite space of potential combination therapies towards the goal of increasing the number of cancer patients who can benefit from checkpoint blockade. New approaches for delivery of checkpoint blockade agents in a targeted manner may help minimize adverse events associated with stimulating the immune system. Multidisciplinary studies of patient biopsies are needed to achieve a mechanistic understanding of checkpoint blockade efficacy and resistance. A better understanding of the effects of non-immunotherapies on the immune response to tumors is needed to design rational combinations. This knowledge will lead to better animal models for studying the vast array of potential combinations, and more personalized combination therapies for patients.

References

Ahmadzadeh, M., et al.: Tumor antigen-specific CD8 T cells infiltrating the tumor express high levels of PD-1 and are functionally impaired. Blood **114**, 1537–1544 (2009). doi:10.1182/blood-2008-12-195792

Alegre, M.L., et al.: Regulation of surface and intracellular expression of CTLA4 on mouse T cells. J. Immunol. **157**, 4762–4770 (1996)

Anderson, A.C.: Tim-3: an emerging target in the cancer immunotherapy landscape. Cancer Immun. Res **2**, 393–398 (2014). doi:10.1158/2326-6066.CIR-14-0039

Anitei, M.G., et al.: Prognostic and predictive values of the immunoscore in patients with rectal cancer. Clin. Cancer Res. **20**, 1891–1899 (2014). doi:10.1158/1078-0432.CCR-13-2830

Ansell, S.M., et al.: PD-1 blockade with nivolumab in relapsed or refractory Hodgkin's lymphoma. N. Engl. J. Med. **372**, 311–319 (2015). doi:10.1056/NEJMoa1411087

Apetoh, L., et al.: Toll-like receptor 4-dependent contribution of the immune system to anticancer chemotherapy and radiotherapy. Nat. Med. **13**, 1050–1059 (2007). doi:10.1038/nm1622

Azuma, T., et al.: B7-H1 is a ubiquitous antiapoptotic receptor on cancer cells. Blood **111**, 3635–3643 (2008). doi:10.1182/blood-2007-11-123141

Balachandran, V.P., et al.: Imatinib potentiates antitumor T cell responses in gastrointestinal stromal tumor through the inhibition of Ido. Nat. Med. **17**, 1094–1100 (2011). doi:10.1038/nm.2438

Barber, D.L., et al.: Restoring function in exhausted CD8 T cells during chronic viral infection. Nature **439**, 682–687 (2006). doi:10.1038/nature04444

Bindea, G., et al.: Spatiotemporal dynamics of intratumoral immune cells reveal the immune landscape in human cancer. Immunity **39**, 782–795 (2013). doi:10.1016/j.immuni.2013.10.003

Boni, A., et al.: Selective BRAFV600E inhibition enhances T-cell recognition of melanoma without affecting lymphocyte function. Cancer Res. **70**, 5213–5219 (2010). doi:10.1158/0008-5472.CAN-10-0118

Brahmer, J.R., et al.: Phase I study of single-agent anti-programmed death-1 (MDX-1106) in refractory solid tumors: safety, clinical activity, pharmacodynamics, and immunologic correlates. J. Clin. Oncol. **28**, 3167–3175 (2010). doi:10.1200/JCO.2009.26.7609

Brahmer, J., et al.: Safety and activity of anti–PD-L1 antibody in patients with advanced cancer. N. Engl. J. Med. **366**, 2455–2465 (2012). doi:10.1056/NEJMoa1200694

Brahmer, J., et al.: Nivolumab versus Docetaxel in Advanced Squamous-Cell Non-Small-Cell Lung Cancer. N. Engl. J. Med. **373**, 123–135 (2015). doi:10.1056/NEJMoa1504627

Bridle, B.W., et al.: HDAC inhibition suppresses primary immune responses, enhances secondary immune responses, and abrogates autoimmunity during tumor immunotherapy. Mol. Ther. **21**, 887–894 (2013). doi:10.1038/mt.2012.265

Brignone, C., Escudier, B., Grygar, C., Marcu, M., Triebel, F.: A phase I pharmacokinetic and biological correlative study of IMP321, a novel MHC class II agonist, in patients with advanced renal cell carcinoma. Clin. Cancer Res. **15**, 6225–6231 (2009). doi:10.1158/1078-0432.CCR-09-0068

Brignone, C., et al.: First-line chemoimmunotherapy in metastatic breast carcinoma: combination of paclitaxel and IMP321 (LAG-3Ig) enhances immune responses and antitumor activity. J. Transl. Med. **8**, 71 (2010). doi:10.1186/1479-5876-8-71

Brooks, D.G., et al.: IL-10 and PD-L1 operate through distinct pathways to suppress T-cell activity during persistent viral infection. Proc. Natl. Acad. Sci. U. S. A. **105**, 20428–20433 (2008). doi:10.1073/pnas.0811139106

Brunet, J.F., et al.: A new member of the immunoglobulin superfamily--CTLA-4. Nature **328**, 267–270 (1987). doi:10.1038/328267a0

Bulliard, Y., et al.: Activating Fc γ receptors contribute to the antitumor activities of immunoregulatory receptor-targeting antibodies. J. Exp. Med. **210**, 1685–1693 (2013). doi:10.1084/jem.20130573

Burnette, B.C., et al.: The efficacy of radiotherapy relies upon induction of type i interferon-dependent innate and adaptive immunity. Cancer Res. **71**, 2488–2496 (2011). doi:10.1158/0008-5472.CAN-10-2820

Camacho, L.H., et al.: Phase I/II trial of tremelimumab in patients with metastatic melanoma. J. Clin. Oncol. **27**, 1075–1081 (2009). doi:10.1200/JCO.2008.19.2435

Chen, W., Jin, W., Wahl, S.M.: Engagement of cytotoxic T lymphocyte-associated antigen 4 (CTLA-4) induces transforming growth factor beta (TGF-beta) production by murine CD4(+) T cells. J. Exp. Med. **188**, 1849–1857 (1998)

Chen, S., et al.: Combination of 4-1BB agonist and PD-1 antagonist promotes antitumor effector/memory CD8 T cells in a poorly immunogenic tumor model. Cancer Immun. Res. **3**, 149–160 (2015). doi:10.1158/2326-6066.CIR-14-0118

Chiba, S., et al.: Tumor-infiltrating DCs suppress nucleic acid-mediated innate immune responses through interactions between the receptor TIM-3 and the alarmin HMGB1. Nat. Immunol. **13**, 832–842 (2012). doi:10.1038/ni.2376

Compagno, D., Laderach, D.J., Gentilini, L., Jaworski, F.M., Rabinovich, G.A.: Delineating the "galectin signature" of the tumor microenvironment. Oncoimmunology **2**, e23565 (2013). doi:10.4161/onci.23565

Cooper, Z., et al.: BRAF inhibition is associated with increased clonality in tumor-infiltrating lymphocytes. Oncoimmunology **2**, e26615 (2013a). doi:10.4161/onci.26615

Cooper, Z., Frederick, D., Ahmed, Z., Wargo, J.: Combining checkpoint inhibitors and BRAF-targeted agents against metastatic melanoma. Oncoimmunology **2**, e24320 (2013b). doi:10.4161/onci.24320

Cooper, Z., et al.: Response to BRAF inhibition in melanoma is enhanced when combined with immune checkpoint blockade. Cancer Immun. Res. **2**, 643–654 (2014). doi:10.1158/2326-6066.CIR-13-0215

Correale, P., et al.: Cetuximab +/– chemotherapy enhances dendritic cell-mediated phagocytosis of colon cancer cells and ignites a highly efficient colon cancer antigen-specific cytotoxic T-cell response *in vitro*. Int. J. Cancer **130**, 1577–1589 (2012). doi:10.1002/ijc.26181

Curran, M., Montalvo, W., Yagita, H., Allison, J.: PD-1 and CTLA-4 combination blockade expands infiltrating T cells and reduces regulatory T and myeloid cells within B16 melanoma tumors. Proc. Natl. Acad. Sci. U. S. A. **107**, 4275–4280 (2010). doi:10.1073/pnas.0915174107

Curran, M., Kim, M., Montalvo, W., Al-Shamkhani, A., Allison, J.: Combination CTLA-4 blockade and 4-1BB activation enhances tumor rejection by increasing T-cell infiltration, proliferation, and cytokine production. PLoS One **6**, 19499 (2011). doi:10.1371/journal.pone.0019499

Danna, E.A., et al.: Surgical removal of primary tumor reverses tumor-induced immunosuppression despite the presence of metastatic disease. Cancer Res. **64**, 2205–2211 (2004)

Dechant, M., et al.: Complement-dependent tumor cell lysis triggered by combinations of epidermal growth factor receptor antibodies. Cancer Res. **68**, 4998–5003 (2008). doi:10.1158/0008-5472.CAN-07-6226

DeKruyff, R.H., et al.: T cell/transmembrane, Ig, and mucin-3 allelic variants differentially recognize phosphatidylserine and mediate phagocytosis of apoptotic cells. J. Immunol. **184**, 1918–1930 (2010). doi:10.4049/jimmunol.0903059

Deng, L., et al.: STING-dependent cytosolic DNA sensing promotes radiation-induced Type I interferon-dependent antitumor immunity in immunogenic tumors. Immunity **41**, 843–852 (2014). doi:10.1016/j.immuni.2014.10.019

Di Giacomo, A.M., et al.: Ipilimumab and fotemustine in patients with advanced melanoma (NIBIT-M1): an open-label, single-arm phase 2 trial. Lancet Oncol. **13**, 879–886 (2012). doi:10.1016/s1470-2045(12)70324-8

Disis, M.L., et al.: Concurrent trastuzumab and HER2/neu-specific vaccination in patients with metastatic breast cancer. J. Clin. Oncol. **27**, 4685–4692 (2009). doi:10.1200/JCO.2008.20.6789

Dougan, M., Dranoff, G.: Immune therapy for cancer. Annu. Rev. Immunol. **27**, 83–117 (2009). doi:10.1146/annurev.immunol.021908.132544

Dummer, R., et al.: A randomized controlled comparison of pembrolizumab and chemotherapy in patients with ipilimumab-refractory melanoma. J. Transl. Med. **13**, O5 (2015). doi:10.1186/1479-5876-13-s1-o5

Duraiswamy, J., Kaluza, K.M., Freeman, G.J., Coukos, G.: Dual blockade of PD-1 and CTLA-4 combined with tumor vaccine effectively restores T-cell rejection function in tumors. Cancer Res. **73**, 3591–3603 (2013). doi:10.1158/0008-5472.CAN-12-4100

Feig, C., et al.: Targeting CXCL12 from FAP-expressing carcinoma-associated fibroblasts synergizes with anti-PD-L1 immunotherapy in pancreatic cancer. Proc. Natl. Acad. Sci. U. S. A. **110**, 20212–20217 (2013). doi:10.1073/pnas.1320318110
Flies, D.B., Sandler, B.J., Sznol, M., Chen, L.: Blockade of the B7-H1/PD-1 pathway for cancer immunotherapy. Yale J. Biol. Med. **84**, 409–421 (2011)
Fourcade, J., et al.: Upregulation of Tim-3 and PD-1 expression is associated with tumor antigen-specific CD8+ T cell dysfunction in melanoma patients. J. Exp. Med. **207**, 2175–2186 (2010). doi:10.1084/jem.20100637
Fox, B., et al.: Defining the critical hurdles in cancer immunotherapy. J. Transl. Med. **9**, 214 (2011). doi:10.1186/1479-5876-9-214
Francisco, L.M., et al.: PD-L1 regulates the development, maintenance, and function of induced regulatory T cells. J. Exp. Med. **206**, 3015–3029 (2009). doi:10.1084/jem.20090847
Francisco, L., Sage, P., Sharpe, A.: The PD-1 pathway in tolerance and autoimmunity. Immunol. Rev. **236**, 219–242 (2010). doi:10.1111/j.1600-065X.2010.00923.x
Frederick, D.T., et al.: BRAF inhibition is associated with enhanced melanoma antigen expression and a more favorable tumor microenvironment in patients with metastatic melanoma. Clin. Cancer Res. **19**, 1225–1231 (2013). doi:10.1158/1078-0432.CCR-12-1630
Freeman, G.J., et al.: CTLA-4 and CD28 mRNA are coexpressed in most T cells after activation. Expression of CTLA-4 and CD28 mRNA does not correlate with the pattern of lymphokine production. J. Immun. **149**, 3795–3801 (1992)
Freeman, G.J., et al.: Cloning of B7-2: a CTLA-4 counter-receptor that costimulates human T cell proliferation. Science **262**, 909–911 (1993a)
Freeman, G.J., et al.: Uncovering of functional alternative CTLA-4 counter-receptor in B7-deficient mice. Science **262**, 907–909 (1993b)
Frigault, M.J., et al.: Identification of chimeric antigen receptors that mediate constitutive or inducible proliferation of T cells. Cancer Immun. Res. **3**, 356–367 (2015). doi:10.1158/2326-6066.CIR-14-0186
Fucikova, J., et al.: Human tumor cells killed by anthracyclines induce a tumor-specific immune response. Cancer Res. **71**, 4821–4833 (2011). doi:10.1158/0008-5472.CAN-11-0950
Gajewski, T., et al.: Cancer immunotherapy strategies based on overcoming barriers within the tumor microenvironment. Curr. Opin. Immunol. **25**, 268–276 (2013). doi:10.1016/j.coi.2013.02.009
Garon, E.B., et al.: Pembrolizumab for the treatment of non-small-cell lung cancer. N. Engl. J. Med. **372**, 2018–2028 (2015). doi:10.1056/NEJMoa1501824
Gautron, A.-S.S., Dominguez-Villar, M., de Marcken, M., Hafler, D.A.: Enhanced suppressor function of TIM-3+ FoxP3+ regulatory T cells. Eur. J. Immunol. **44**, 2703–2711 (2014). doi:10.1002/eji.201344392
Ghiringhelli, F., et al.: CD4+CD25+ regulatory T cells suppress tumor immunity but are sensitive to cyclophosphamide which allows immunotherapy of established tumors to be curative. Eur. J. Immunol. **34**, 336–344 (2004). doi:10.1002/eji.200324181
Ghiringhelli, F., et al.: Metronomic cyclophosphamide regimen selectively depletes CD4+CD25+ regulatory T cells and restores T and NK effector functions in end stage cancer patients. Cancer Immunol. Immunother. **56**, 641–648 (2007). doi:10.1007/s00262-006-0225-8
Ghiringhelli, F., et al.: Activation of the NLRP3 inflammasome in dendritic cells induces IL-1beta-dependent adaptive immunity against tumors. Nat. Med. **15**, 1170–1178 (2009). doi:10.1038/nm.2028
Gibbons, R.M., et al.: B7-H1 limits the entry of effector CD8(+) T cells to the memory pool by upregulating Bim. Oncoimmunology **1**, 1061–1073 (2012). doi:10.4161/onci.20850
Goldberg, M.V., Drake, C.G.: LAG-3 in cancer immunotherapy. Curr. Top. Microbiol. Immunol. **344**, 269–278 (2011). doi:10.1007/82_2010_114
Grohmann, U., et al.: CTLA-4-Ig regulates tryptophan catabolism *in vivo*. Nat. Immunol. **3**, 1097–1101 (2002). doi:10.1038/ni846
Gros, A., et al.: PD-1 identifies the patient-specific CD8(+) tumor-reactive repertoire infiltrating human tumors. J. Clin. Invest. **124**, 2246–2259 (2014). doi:10.1172/JCI73639
Grosso, J., Jure-Kunkel, M.: CTLA-4 blockade in tumor models: an overview of preclinical and translational research. Cancer Immun. **13**, 5 (2013)

Gu-Trantien, C., et al.: CD4+ follicular helper T cell infiltration predicts breast cancer survival. J. Clin. Invest. **123**, 2873–2892 (2013). doi:10.1172/JCI67428

Hamid, O., et al.: Safety and tumor responses with lambrolizumab (anti-PD-1) in melanoma. N. Engl. J. Med. **369**, 134–144 (2013). doi:10.1056/NEJMoa1305133

Hanahan, D., Coussens, L.M.: Accessories to the crime: functions of cells recruited to the tumor microenvironment. Cancer Cell **21**, 309–322 (2012). doi:10.1016/j.ccr.2012.02.022

Harding, J., Pulitzer, M., Chapman, P.: Vemurafenib sensitivity skin reaction after ipilimumab. N. Engl. J. Med. **366**, 866–868 (2012). doi:10.1056/NEJMc1114329

Heninger, E., Krueger, T.E., Lang, J.M.: Augmenting antitumor immune responses with epigenetic modifying agents. Front. Immun. **6**, 29 (2015). doi:10.3389/fimmu.2015.00029

Herbst, R.S., et al.: Predictive correlates of response to the anti-PD-L1 antibody MPDL3280A in cancer patients. Nature **515**, 563–567 (2014). doi:10.1038/nature14011

Highfill, S.L., et al.: Disruption of CXCR2-mediated MDSC tumor trafficking enhances anti-PD1 efficacy. Sci. Transl. Med. **6**, 237ra267 (2014). doi:10.1126/scitranslmed.3007974

Hodi, F., et al.: Improved survival with ipilimumab in patients with metastatic melanoma. N. Engl. J. Med. **363**, 711–723 (2010). doi:10.1056/NEJMoa1003466

Hodi, F.S., et al.: Bevacizumab plus ipilimumab in patients with metastatic melanoma. Cancer Immun. Res. **2**, 632–642 (2014a). doi:10.1158/2326-6066.CIR-14-0053

Hodi, F.S., et al.: Ipilimumab plus sargramostim vs ipilimumab alone for treatment of metastatic melanoma: a randomized clinical trial. JAMA **312**, 1744–1753 (2014b). doi:10.1001/jama.2014.13943

Hsu, Y.F., et al.: Complement activation mediates cetuximab inhibition of non-small cell lung cancer tumor growth *in vivo*. Mol. Cancer **9**, 139 (2010). doi:10.1186/1476-4598-9-139

Huang, Y.-H.H., et al.: CEACAM1 regulates TIM-3-mediated tolerance and exhaustion. Nature **517**, 386–390 (2015). doi:10.1038/nature13848

Hurwitz, A.A., Yu, T.F., Leach, D.R., Allison, J.P.: CTLA-4 blockade synergizes with tumor-derived granulocyte-macrophage colony-stimulating factor for treatment of an experimental mammary carcinoma. Proc. Natl. Acad. Sci. U. S. A. **95**, 10067–10071 (1998)

Jing, W., et al.: Combined immune checkpoint protein blockade and low dose whole body irradiation as immunotherapy for myeloma. J Immunother. Cancer **3**, 2 (2015). doi:10.1186/s40425-014-0043-z

Johnston, R.J., et al.: The immunoreceptor TIGIT regulates antitumor and antiviral CD8(+) T cell effector function. Cancer Cell **26**, 923–937 (2014). doi:10.1016/j.ccell.2014.10.018

Karwacz, K., et al.: PD-L1 co-stimulation contributes to ligand-induced T cell receptor down-modulation on CD8+T cells. EMBO Mol. Med. **3**, 581–592 (2011). doi:10.1002/emmm.201100165

Keir, M.E., Francisco, L.M., Sharpe, A.H.: PD-1 and its ligands in T-cell immunity. Curr. Opin. Immunol. **19**, 309–314 (2007). doi:10.1016/j.coi.2007.04.012

Keir, M.E., Butte, M.J., Freeman, G.J., Sharpe, A.H.: PD-1 and its ligands in tolerance and immunity. Annu. Rev. Immunol. **26**, 677–704 (2008). doi:10.1146/annurev.immunol.26.021607.090331

Kepp, O., et al.: Consensus guidelines for the detection of immunogenic cell death. Oncoimmunology **3**, e955691 (2014). doi:10.4161/21624011.2014.955691

Kim, K., et al.: Eradication of metastatic mouse cancers resistant to immune checkpoint blockade by suppression of myeloid-derived cells. Proc. Natl. Acad. Sci. U. S. A. **111**, 11774–11779 (2014). doi:10.1073/pnas.1410626111

Kirkwood, J.M., et al.: Phase II trial of tremelimumab (CP-675,206) in patients with advanced refractory or relapsed melanoma. Clin. Cancer Res. **16**, 1042–1048 (2010). doi:10.1158/1078-0432.CCR-09-2033

Ko, J.S., et al.: Sunitinib mediates reversal of myeloid-derived suppressor cell accumulation in renal cell carcinoma patients. Clin. Cancer Res. **15**, 2148–2157 (2009). doi:10.1158/1078-0432.CCR-08-1332

Kuehn, H.S., et al.: Immune dysregulation in human subjects with heterozygous germline mutations in CTLA4. Science **345**, 1623–1627 (2014). doi:10.1126/science.1255904

Kujawski, M., et al.: Targeting STAT3 in adoptively transferred T cells promotes their *in vivo* expansion and antitumor effects. Cancer Res. **70**, 9599–9610 (2010). doi:10.1158/0008-5472.CAN-10-1293

Kvistborg, P., et al.: Anti-CTLA-4 therapy broadens the melanoma-reactive CD8+ T cell response. Sci. Transl. Med. **6**, 254ra128 (2014). doi:10.1126/scitranslmed.3008918

Larkin, J., et al.: Combined nivolumab and ipilimumab or monotherapy in untreated melanoma. N. Engl. J. Med. (2015). doi:10.1056/NEJMoa1504030

Larmonier, N., et al.: Imatinib mesylate inhibits CD4+ CD25+ regulatory T cell activity and enhances active immunotherapy against BCR-ABL- tumors. J. Immunol. **181**, 6955–6963 (2008)

Le, D.T., et al.: PD-1 blockade in tumors with mismatch-repair deficiency. N. Engl. J. Med. **372**, 2509–2520 (2015a). doi:10.1056/NEJMoa1500596

Le, D.T., et al.: Safety and survival with GVAX pancreas prime and Listeria Monocytogenes-expressing mesothelin (CRS-207) boost vaccines for metastatic pancreatic cancer. J. Clin. Oncol. **33**, 1325–1333 (2015b). doi:10.1200/JCO.2014.57.4244

Leach, D.R., Krummel, M.F., Allison, J.P.: Enhancement of antitumor immunity by CTLA-4 blockade. Science **271**, 1734–1736 (1996). doi:10.1126/science.271.5256.1734

Lemke, G., Rothlin, C.V.: Immunobiology of the TAM receptors. Nat. Rev. Immunol. **8**, 327–336 (2008). doi:10.1038/nri2303

Liu, J., et al.: Immune-checkpoint proteins VISTA and PD-1 nonredundantly regulate murine T-cell responses. Proc. Natl. Acad. Sci. U. S. A. **112**, 6682–6687 (2015). doi:10.1073/pnas.1420370112

Lozano, E., Dominguez-Villar, M., Kuchroo, V., Hafler, D.A.: The TIGIT/CD226 axis regulates human T cell function. J. Immun. **188**, 3869–3875 (2012). doi:10.4049/jimmunol.1103627

Lutsiak, M.E., et al.: Inhibition of CD4(+)25+ T regulatory cell function implicated in enhanced immune response by low-dose cyclophosphamide. Blood **105**, 2862–2868 (2005). doi:10.1182/blood-2004-06-2410

Ma, Y., et al.: Anticancer chemotherapy-induced intratumoral recruitment and differentiation of antigen-presenting cells. Immunity **38**, 729–741 (2013). doi:10.1016/j.immuni.2013.03.003

Madan, R.A., et al.: Ipilimumab and a poxviral vaccine targeting prostate-specific antigen in metastatic castration-resistant prostate cancer: a phase 1 dose-escalation trial. Lancet Oncol. **13**, 501–508 (2012). doi:10.1016/s1470-2045(12)70006-2

Mangsbo, S.M., Sandin, L.C., Anger, K.: Enhanced tumor eradication by combining CTLA-4 or PD-1 blockade with CpG therapy. J. Immunother. **33**, 225–235 (2010). doi:10.1097/CJI.0b013e3181c01fcb

Marabelle, A., et al.: Depleting tumor-specific Tregs at a single site eradicates disseminated tumors. J. Clin. Invest. **123**, 2447–2463 (2013). doi:10.1172/JCI64859

Marechal, R., et al.: Putative contribution of CD56 positive cells in cetuximab treatment efficacy in first-line metastatic colorectal cancer patients. BMC Cancer **10**, 340 (2010). doi:10.1186/1471-2407-10-340

Marengère, L.E., et al.: Regulation of T cell receptor signaling by tyrosine phosphatase SYP association with CTLA-4. Science **272**, 1170–1173 (1996)

Margolin, K., et al.: Ipilimumab in patients with melanoma and brain metastases: an open-label, phase 2 trial. Lancet Oncol. **13**, 459–465 (2012). doi:10.1016/S1470-2045(12)70090-6

Matsuzaki, J., et al.: Tumor-infiltrating NY-ESO-1-specific CD8+ T cells are negatively regulated by LAG-3 and PD-1 in human ovarian cancer. Proc. Natl. Acad. Sci. U. S. A. **107**, 7875–7880 (2010). doi:10.1073/pnas.1003345107

McDermott, D., et al.: Durable benefit and the potential for long-term survival with immunotherapy in advanced melanoma. Cancer Treat. Rev. **40**, 1056–1064 (2014). doi:10.1016/j.ctrv.2014.06.012

Menard, C., et al.: Natural killer cell IFN-gamma levels predict long-term survival with imatinib mesylate therapy in gastrointestinal stromal tumor-bearing patients. Cancer Res. **69**, 3563–3569 (2009). doi:10.1158/0008-5472.CAN-08-3807

Messina, J.L., et al.: 12-Chemokine gene signature identifies lymph node-like structures in melanoma: potential for patient selection for immunotherapy? Sci. Rep. **2**, 765 (2012). doi:10.1038/srep00765

Mitchell, D.A., et al.: Tetanus toxoid and CCL3 improve dendritic cell vaccines in mice and glioblastoma patients. Nature **519**, 366–369 (2015). doi:10.1038/nature14320

Nakayama, M., et al.: Tim-3 mediates phagocytosis of apoptotic cells and cross-presentation. Blood **113**, 3821–3830 (2009). doi:10.1182/blood-2008-10-185884

Okazaki, T., et al.: PD-1 and LAG-3 inhibitory co-receptors act synergistically to prevent autoimmunity in mice. J. Exp. Med. **208**, 395–407 (2011). doi:10.1084/jem.20100466

Ostrand-Rosenberg, S., Horn, L.A., Haile, S.T.: The programmed death-1 immune-suppressive pathway: barrier to antitumor immunity. J. Immunol. **193**, 3835–3841 (2014). doi:10.4049/jimmunol.1401572

Ozao-Choy, J., et al.: The novel role of tyrosine kinase inhibitor in the reversal of immune suppression and modulation of tumor microenvironment for immune-based cancer therapies. Cancer Res. **69**, 2514–2522 (2009). doi:10.1158/0008-5472.CAN-08-4709

Palucka, K., Banchereau, J.: Dendritic-cell-based therapeutic cancer vaccines. Immunity **39**, 38–48 (2013). doi:10.1016/j.immuni.2013.07.004

Paolino, M., et al.: The E3 ligase Cbl-b and TAM receptors regulate cancer metastasis via natural killer cells. Nature **507**, 508–512 (2014). doi:10.1038/nature12998

Pardoll, D.: The blockade of immune checkpoints in cancer immunotherapy. Nat. Rev. Cancer **12**, 252–264 (2012). doi:10.1038/nrc3239

Park, S., et al.: The therapeutic effect of anti-HER2/neu antibody depends on both innate and adaptive immunity. Cancer Cell **18**, 160–170 (2010). doi:10.1016/j.ccr.2010.06.014

Parry, R.V., et al.: CTLA-4 and PD-1 receptors inhibit T-cell activation by distinct mechanisms. Mol. Cell. Biol. **25**, 9543–9553 (2005). doi:10.1128/MCB.25.21.9543-9553.2005

Peggs, K.S., Quezada, S.A., Chambers, C.A., Korman, A.J., Allison, J.P.: Blockade of CTLA-4 on both effector and regulatory T cell compartments contributes to the antitumor activity of anti-CTLA-4 antibodies. J. Exp. Med. **206**, 1717–1725 (2009). doi:10.1084/jem.20082492

Petrovas, C., et al.: PD-1 is a regulator of virus-specific CD8+ T cell survival in HIV infection. J. Exp. Med. **203**, 2281–2292 (2006). doi:10.1084/jem.20061496

Postow, M.A., et al.: Nivolumab and ipilimumab versus ipilimumab in untreated melanoma. N. Engl. J. Med. **372**, 2006–2017 (2015). doi:10.1056/NEJMoa1414428

Powles, T., et al.: MPDL3280A (anti-PD-L1) treatment leads to clinical activity in metastatic bladder cancer. Nature **515**, 558–562 (2014). doi:10.1038/nature13904

Quigley, M., et al.: Transcriptional analysis of HIV-specific CD8+ T cells shows that PD-1 inhibits T cell function by upregulating BATF. Nat. Med. **16**, 1147–1151 (2010). doi:10.1038/nm.2232

Qureshi, O.S., et al.: Trans-endocytosis of CD80 and CD86: a molecular basis for the cell-extrinsic function of CTLA-4. Science **332**, 600–603 (2011). doi:10.1126/science.1202947

Rajasagi, M., et al.: Systematic identification of personal tumor-specific neoantigens in chronic lymphocytic leukemia. Blood **124**, 453–462 (2014). doi:10.1182/blood-2014-04-567933

Redmond, W.L., Linch, S.N., Kasiewicz, M.J.: Combined targeting of costimulatory (OX40) and coinhibitory (CTLA-4) pathways elicits potent effector T cells capable of driving robust antitumor immunity. Cancer Immun. Res. **2**, 142–153 (2014). doi:10.1158/2326-6066.CIR-13-0031-T

Ribas, A., et al.: Phase III randomized clinical trial comparing tremelimumab with standard-of-care chemotherapy in patients with advanced melanoma. J. Clin. Oncol. **31**, 616–622 (2013). doi:10.1200/JCO.2012.44.6112

Richman, L.P., Vonderheide, R.H.: Role of crosslinking for agonistic CD40 monoclonal antibodies as immune therapy of cancer. Cancer Immun. Res. **2**, 19–26 (2014). doi:10.1158/2326-6066.CIR-13-0152

Rizvi, N.A., et al.: Cancer immunology. Mutational landscape determines sensitivity to PD-1 blockade in non-small cell lung cancer. Science **348**, 124–128 (2015a). doi:10.1126/science.aaa1348

Rizvi, N.A., et al.: Activity and safety of nivolumab, an anti-PD-1 immune checkpoint inhibitor, for patients with advanced, refractory squamous non-small-cell lung cancer (CheckMate 063): a phase 2, single-arm trial. Lancet Oncol. **16**, 257–265 (2015b). doi:10.1016/s1470-2045(15)70054-9

Robert, C., et al.: Ipilimumab plus dacarbazine for previously untreated metastatic melanoma. N. Engl. J. Med. **364**, 2517–2526 (2011). doi:10.1056/NEJMoa1104621

Robert, C., et al.: Anti-programmed-death-receptor-1 treatment with pembrolizumab in ipilimumab-refractory advanced melanoma: a randomised dose-comparison cohort of a phase 1 trial. Lancet **384**, 1109–1117 (2014). doi:10.1016/S0140-6736(14)60958-2

Robert, C., et al.: Nivolumab in previously untreated melanoma without BRAF mutation. N. Engl. J. Med. **372**, 320–330 (2015a). doi:10.1056/NEJMoa1412082

Robert, C., et al.: Pembrolizumab versus ipilimumab in advanced melanoma. N. Engl. J. Med. **372**, 2521–2532 (2015b). doi:10.1056/NEJMoa1503093

Rooney, M.S., Shukla, S.A., Wu, C.J., Getz, G., Hacohen, N.: Molecular and genetic properties of tumors associated with local immune cytolytic activity. Cell **160**, 48–61 (2015). doi:10.1016/j.cell.2014.12.033

Rosenberg, S.A., Restifo, N.P.: Adoptive cell transfer as personalized immunotherapy for human cancer. Science **348**, 62–68 (2015). doi:10.1126/science.aaa4967

Ruffell, B., Affara, N.I., Coussens, L.M.: Differential macrophage programming in the tumor microenvironment. Trends Immunol. **33**, 119–126 (2012). doi:10.1016/j.it.2011.12.001

Sage, P.T., Francisco, L.M., Carman, C.V., Sharpe, A.H.: The receptor PD-1 controls follicular regulatory T cells in the lymph nodes and blood. Nat. Immunol. **14**, 152–161 (2013). doi:10.1038/ni.2496

Sakuishi, K., et al.: Targeting Tim-3 and PD-1 pathways to reverse T cell exhaustion and restore anti-tumor immunity. J. Exp. Med. **207**, 2187–2194 (2010). doi:10.1084/jem.20100643

Salvadori, S., Martinelli, G., Zier, K.: Resection of solid tumors reverses T cell defects and restores protective immunity. J. Immunol. **164**, 2214–2220 (2000). doi:10.4049/jimmunol.164.4.2214

Schadendorf, D., et al.: Pooled analysis of long-term survival data from phase II and phase III trials of ipilimumab in unresectable or metastatic melanoma. J. Clin. Oncol. **33**, 1889–1894 (2015). doi:10.1200/JCO.2014.56.2736

Schiavoni, G., et al.: Cyclophosphamide synergizes with type I interferons through systemic dendritic cell reactivation and induction of immunogenic tumor apoptosis. Cancer Res. **71**, 768–778 (2011). doi:10.1158/0008-5472.CAN-10-2788

Schietinger, A., Greenberg, P.D.: Tolerance and exhaustion: defining mechanisms of T cell dysfunction. Trends Immunol. **35**, 51–60 (2014). doi:10.1016/j.it.2013.10.001

Schubert, D., et al.: Autosomal dominant immune dysregulation syndrome in humans with *CTLA4* mutations. Nat. Med. **20**, 1410–1426 (2014). doi:10.1038/nm.3746

Selby, M.J., et al.: Anti-CTLA-4 antibodies of IgG2a isotype enhance antitumor activity through reduction of intratumoral regulatory T cells. Cancer Immun. Res. **1**, 32–42 (2013). doi:10.1158/2326-6066.CIR-13-0013

Sharma, P., Allison, J.P.: The future of immune checkpoint therapy. Science **348**, 56–61 (2015). doi:10.1126/science.aaa8172

Shen, L., et al.: Class I histone deacetylase inhibitor entinostat suppresses regulatory T cells and enhances immunotherapies in renal and prostate cancer models. PLoS One **7**, e30815 (2012). doi:10.1371/journal.pone.0030815

Sheppard, K.A., et al.: PD-1 inhibits T-cell receptor induced phosphorylation of the ZAP70/CD3zeta signalosome and downstream signaling to PKCtheta. FEBS Lett. **574**, 37–41 (2004). doi:10.1016/j.febslet.2004.07.083

Shin, D.S., Ribas, A.: The evolution of checkpoint blockade as a cancer therapy: what's here, what's next? Curr. Opin. Immunol. **33**, 23–35 (2015). doi:10.1016/j.coi.2015.01.006

Shrimali, R.K., et al.: Antiangiogenic agents can increase lymphocyte infiltration into tumor and enhance the effectiveness of adoptive immunotherapy of cancer. Cancer Res. **70**, 6171–6180 (2010). doi:10.1158/0008-5472.CAN-10-0153

Simpson, T., et al.: Fc-dependent depletion of tumor-infiltrating regulatory T cells co-defines the efficacy of anti-CTLA-4 therapy against melanoma. J. Exp. Med. **210**, 1695–1697 (2013). doi:10.1084/jem.20130579

Sistigu, A., et al.: Cancer cell-autonomous contribution of type I interferon signaling to the efficacy of chemotherapy. Nat. Med. **20**, 1301–1309 (2014). doi:10.1038/nm.3708

Snyder, A., et al.: Genetic basis for clinical response to CTLA-4 blockade in melanoma. N. Engl. J. Med. **371**, 2189–2199 (2014). doi:10.1056/NEJMoa1406498

Soukup, K., Wang, X.: Radiation meets immunotherapy - a perfect match in the era of combination therapy? Int. J. Radiat. Biol. **91**, 299–305 (2015). doi:10.3109/09553002.2014.995383

Spranger, S., et al.: Up-regulation of PD-L1, IDO, and T(regs) in the melanoma tumor microenvironment is driven by CD8(+) T cells. Sci. Transl. Med. **5**, 200ra116 (2013). doi:10.1126/scitranslmed.3006504

Spranger, S., et al.: Mechanism of tumor rejection with doublets of CTLA-4, PD-1/PD-L1, or IDO blockade involves restored IL-2 production and proliferation of CD8(+) T cells directly within the tumor microenvironment. J. Immunother. Cancer **2**, 3 (2014). doi:10.1186/2051-1426-2-3

Spranger, S., Bao, R., Gajewski, T.F.: Melanoma-intrinsic beta-catenin signalling prevents anti-tumour immunity. Nature **523**, 231–235 (2015). doi:10.1038/nature14404

Stagg, J., et al.: Anti-ErbB-2 mAb therapy requires type I and II interferons and synergizes with anti-PD-1 or anti-CD137 mAb therapy. Proc. Natl. Acad. Sci. U. S. A. **108**, 7142–7147 (2011). doi:10.1073/pnas.1016569108

Sumimoto, H., Imabayashi, F., Iwata, T., Kawakami, Y.: The BRAF-MAPK signaling pathway is essential for cancer-immune evasion in human melanoma cells. J. Exp. Med. **203**, 1651–1656 (2006). doi:10.1084/jem.20051848

Suzuki, E., Kapoor, V., Jassar, A.S., Kaiser, L.R., Albelda, S.M.: Gemcitabine selectively eliminates splenic Gr-1+/CD11b+myeloid suppressor cells in tumor-bearing animals and enhances antitumor immune activity. Clin. Cancer Res. **11**, 6713–6721 (2005). doi:10.1158/1078-0432.CCR-05-0883

Tarhini, A.A., et al.: Safety and efficacy of combination immunotherapy with interferon alfa-2b and tremelimumab in patients with stage IV melanoma. J. Clin. Oncol. **30**, 322–328 (2012). doi:10.1200/JCO.2011.37.5394

Taube, J.M., et al.: Colocalization of inflammatory response with B7-h1 expression in human melanocytic lesions supports an adaptive resistance mechanism of immune escape. Sci. Transl. Med. **4**, 127ra137 (2012). doi:10.1126/scitranslmed.3003689

Teply, B.A., Lipson, E.J.: Identification and management of toxicities from immune checkpoint-blocking drugs. Oncology **28**(Suppl 3), 30–38 (2014)

Tesniere, A., et al.: Immunogenic death of colon cancer cells treated with oxaliplatin. Oncogene **29**, 482–491 (2010). doi:10.1038/onc.2009.356

Tivol, E.A., et al.: Loss of CTLA-4 leads to massive lymphoproliferation and fatal multiorgan tissue destruction, revealing a critical negative regulatory role of CTLA-4. Immunity **3**, 541–547 (1995)

Topalian, S.L., Sharpe, A.H.: Balance and imbalance in the immune system: life on the edge. Immunity **41**, 682–684 (2014). doi:10.1016/j.immuni.2014.11.005

Topalian, S., et al.: Safety, activity, and immune correlates of anti–PD-1 antibody in cancer. N. Engl. J. Med. **366**, 2443–2454 (2012). doi:10.1056/NEJMoa1200690

Topalian, S., et al.: Survival, durable tumor remission, and long-term safety in patients with advanced melanoma receiving nivolumab. J. Clin. Oncol. **32**, 1020–1030 (2014). doi:10.1200/JCO.2013.53.0105

Topalian, S.L., Drake, C.G., Pardoll, D.M.: Immune checkpoint blockade: a common denominator approach to cancer therapy. Cancer Cell **27**, 450–461 (2015). doi:10.1016/j.ccell.2015.03.001

Tumeh, P.C., et al.: PD-1 blockade induces responses by inhibiting adaptive immune resistance. Nature **515**, 568–571 (2014). doi:10.1038/nature13954

Twyman-Saint Victor, C., et al.: Radiation and dual checkpoint blockade activate non-redundant immune mechanisms in cancer. Nature **520**, 373–377 (2015). doi:10.1038/nature14292

van der Merwe, P.A., Bodian, D.L., Daenke, S., Linsley, P., Davis, S.J.: CD80 (B7-1) binds both CD28 and CTLA-4 with a low affinity and very fast kinetics. J. Exp. Med. **185**, 393–403 (1997)

van Elsas, A., Hurwitz, A.A., Allison, J.P.: Combination immunotherapy of B16 melanoma using anti-cytotoxic T lymphocyte-associated antigen 4 (CTLA-4) and granulocyte/macrophage colony-stimulating factor (GM-CSF)-producing vaccines induces rejection of subcutaneous and metastatic tumors accompanied by autoimmune depigmentation. J. Exp. Med. **190**, 355–366 (1999)

Vanneman, M., Dranoff, G.: Combining immunotherapy and targeted therapies in cancer treatment. Nat. Rev. Cancer **12**, 237–251 (2012). doi:10.1038/nrc3237

Vanpouille-Box, C., et al.: TGFβ is a master regulator of radiation therapy-induced antitumor immunity. Cancer Res. **75**, 2232–2242 (2015). doi:10.1158/0008-5472.CAN-14-3511

Vincent, J., et al.: 5-Fluorouracil selectively kills tumor-associated myeloid-derived suppressor cells resulting in enhanced T cell-dependent antitumor immunity. Cancer Res. **70**, 3052–3061 (2010). doi:10.1158/0008-5472.CAN-09-3690

Voron, T., et al.: VEGF-A modulates expression of inhibitory checkpoints on CD8+ T cells in tumors. J. Exp. Med. **212**, 139–148 (2015). doi:10.1084/jem.20140559

Waterhouse, P., et al.: Lymphoproliferative disorders with early lethality in mice deficient in Ctla-4. Science **270**, 985–988 (1995)

West, E.E., et al.: PD-L1 blockade synergizes with IL-2 therapy in reinvigorating exhausted T cells. J. Clin. Invest. **123**, 2604–2615 (2013). doi:10.1172/JCI67008

Westin, J.R., et al.: Safety and activity of PD1 blockade by pidilizumab in combination with rituximab in patients with relapsed follicular lymphoma: a single group, open-label, phase 2 trial. Lancet Oncol. **15**, 69–77 (2014). doi:10.1016/s1470-2045(13)70551-5

Wherry, E.J.: T cell exhaustion. Nat. Immunol. **131**, 492–499 (2011). doi:10.1038/ni.2035

Wing, K., et al.: CTLA-4 control over Foxp3+ regulatory T cell function. Science **322**, 271–275 (2008). doi:10.1126/science.1160062

Wolchok, J.D., et al.: Nivolumab plus ipilimumab in advanced melanoma. N. Engl. J. Med. **369**, 122–133 (2013). doi:10.1056/NEJMoa1302369

Woo, S.R., et al.: Immune inhibitory molecules LAG-3 and PD-1 synergistically regulate T-cell function to promote tumoral immune escape. Cancer Res. **72**, 917–927 (2012). doi:10.1158/0008-5472.CAN-11-1620

Woo, S.R., et al.: STING-dependent cytosolic DNA sensing mediates innate immune recognition of immunogenic tumors. Immunity **41**, 830–842 (2014). doi:10.1016/j.immuni.2014.10.017

Yang, D.H., et al.: The dysfunction and abnormal signaling pathway of dendritic cells loaded by tumor antigen can be overcome by neutralizing VEGF in multiple myeloma. Leuk. Res. **33**, 665–670 (2009). doi:10.1016/j.leukres.2008.09.006

Youn, J.I., Gabrilovich, D.I.: The biology of myeloid-derived suppressor cells: the blessing and the curse of morphological and functional heterogeneity. Eur. J. Immunol. **40**, 2969–2975 (2010). doi:10.1002/eji.201040895

Yu, P., Steel, J.C., Zhang, M., Morris, J.C., Waldmann, T.A.: Simultaneous blockade of multiple immune system inhibitory checkpoints enhances antitumor activity mediated by interleukin-15 in a murine metastatic colon carcinoma model. Clin. Cancer Res. **16**, 6019–6028 (2010). doi:10.1158/1078-0432.CCR-10-1966

Yuan, J., et al.: Pretreatment serum VEGF is associated with clinical response and overall survival in advanced melanoma patients treated with ipilimumab. Cancer Immun. Res. **2**, 127–132 (2014). doi:10.1158/2326-6066.CIR-13-0163

Zhang, F., et al.: Epigenetic manipulation restores functions of defective CD8(+) T cells from chronic viral infection. Mol. Ther. **22**, 1698–1706 (2014). doi:10.1038/mt.2014.91

Zhu, C., et al.: The Tim-3 ligand galectin-9 negatively regulates T helper type 1 immunity. Nat. Immunol. **6**, 1245–1252 (2005). doi:10.1038/ni1271

Zhu, Y., et al.: CSF1/CSF1R blockade reprograms tumor-infiltrating macrophages and improves response to T-cell checkpoint immunotherapy in pancreatic cancer models. Cancer Res. **74**, 5057–5069 (2014). doi:10.1158/0008-5472.CAN-13-3723

Zimmer, L., et al.: Phase II DeCOG-study of ipilimumab in pretreated and treatment-naive patients with metastatic uveal melanoma. PLoS One **10**, e0118564 (2015). doi:10.1371/journal.pone.0118564

Zippelius, A., Schreiner, J., Herzig, P., Muller, P.: Induced PD-L1 expression mediates acquired resistance to agonistic anti-CD40 treatment. Cancer Immunol Res **3**, 236–244 (2015). doi:10.1158/2326-6066.CIR-14-0226

Zitvogel, L., et al.: The anticancer immune response: indispensable for therapeutic success? J. Clin. Invest. **118**, 1991–2001 (2008). doi:10.1172/JCI35180

Chapter 2
Novel Immunomodulatory Pathways in the Immunoglobulin Superfamily

Paul D. Rennert

Abbreviations

APC	Antigen presenting cells
CEACAM1	Carcinoembryonic antigen-related cell adhesion molecule 1
DC	Dendritic cells
ICOS	Inducible T-cell costimulator
IgSF	Immunoglobulin superfamily
ITIM	Immunoreceptor tyrosine-based inhibition motif
LAG-3	Lymphocyte activation gene-3
MDSC	Myeloid-derived suppressor cells
MHC	Major histocompatibility complex
PS	Phosphatidylserine
PVR	Poliovirus receptor
TCR	T cell receptor
TIGIT	T cell immunoglobulin and ITIM domain
TIL	Tumor-infiltrating lymphocytes
TIM	T cell immunoglobulin mucin
VISTA	V-domain immunoglobulin (Ig)-containing suppressor of T-cell activation

P.D. Rennert (✉)
Sugarcone Biotech LLC, Holliston, MA 01746, USA

Aleta Biotherapeutics, Natick, MA 01760, USA
e-mail: rennertp@sugarconebiotech.com

P.D. Rennert (ed.), *Novel Immunotherapeutic Approaches to the Treatment of Cancer*, DOI 10.1007/978-3-319-29827-6_2

1 Introduction

The immunoglobulin superfamily (IgSF) is a large and highly diverse assemblage of related proteins that regulate many different biological processes. The name of the family is based on early studies demonstrating sequence similarity between the antibody (immunoglobulin) variable and constant domains, showing an ancestral link, and the subsequent identification of proteins with similar sequences, suggesting broad diversification and evolution (Williams and Barclay 1988). Antibodies, the T cell receptors (TCR), and the major histocompatibility complex (MHC), among others, are made up of multiple Ig domain chains that assemble to form the final protein, facilitating antigen presentation/recognition (Fig. 2.1a). The individual Ig domains within this family contain a conserved intra-chain disulfide bond that serves to stabilize the domain. These individual structural domains consist of two “sheets” that consist of beta-strands, as illustrated for a generic Ig-domain (Fig. 2.1b). Many IgSF proteins consist of single chains that string together one or more Ig-domains, each with its own intrinsic features. IgSF proteins can have from one to many such domains, and these are characterized as variable (V) domains, as in Fig. 2.1b, or constant (C) domains based on sequence and structural similarity to the domains characterized in antibodies (Fig. 2.1a). Beyond the conserved core motifs, the family has diverged drastically, and many unique and unusual structural features have evolved.

Within the IgSF there are many different proteins that contribute to the regulation of the immune response to cancer. These include the canonical regulatory

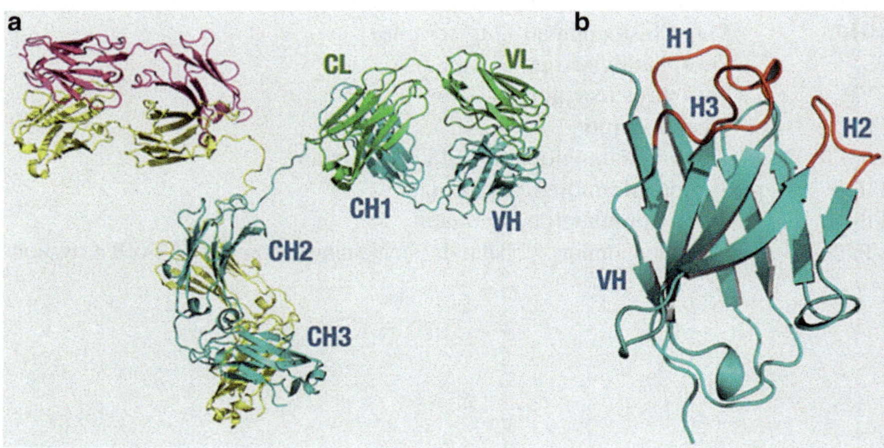

Fig 2.1 The IgSF shares conserved structural motifs. (**a**) The IgSF was identified based on homology to antibodies, cell surface and secreted immunoglobulins that have multiple Ig-domains. The illustration shows an IgG antibody having distinct Variable and Constant domains. (**b**) Each Ig-domain contains at least one disulfide bond that serves to stabilize the protein. A single IgV-like domain is shown: the beta stands form sheets that are connected by loops of varying lengths. In antibodies the loops are referred to as CDRs, and these are essential for the recognition of antigen. Image credit: http://www.blopig.com/blog/

Table 2.1 IgSF proteins named in this review

Common name	Synonyms	CD designation	IgSF subclass
B7-1	B7/BB1	CD80	B7
B7-2	ETC-1	CD86	B7
CD28	MGC138290, Tp44	CD28	CD28
CTLA4	GSE, GRD4, IDDM12, CELIAC3	CD152	CD28
PD-1	PCDP1, SLEB2	CD-279	PD-1
PD-L1	B7-H1	CD-274	PD-L1
PD-L2	B7-DC	CD-273	PD-L1
CEACAM1	NCA-160	CD66a	CEA
CEACAM5	CEA	CD66e	CEA
ICOS	AILIM	CD278	CD28
ICOS-L	B7-H2, B7RP-1, GL50	CD275	Butyrophilin
LAG-3	None	CD223	CD4
TIGIT	VSIG9; VSTM3; WUCAM	None assigned	Nectin/PVR
TIM-3	HAVCR2, TIMD3	CD366	TIM
Galectin-9	Ecalectin, tumor antigen HOM-HD-21	None assigned	Galectin
VISTA	PD-L3, B7H5, C10orf54, Dies1, PD1H, Gi24 precursor, SISP1	None assigned	Singleton?

proteins within the B7/CD28 pathway that control T cell activation and those within the PD-L1/PD-1 pathway that control T cell effector function and persistence. Therapeutics that antagonize these pathways—ipilimumab (anti-CTLA4 antibody; Yervoy™), nivolumab (anti-PD-1 antibody, Opdivo™), and pembrolizumab (anti-PD-1 antibody, Keytruda™) are now the foundational drugs for the immunotherapy of cancer (Mahoney et al. 2015).

The IgSF has been extensively studied in an attempt to identify additional immune regulatory proteins and pathways. Such investigations have revealed critical control pathways on lymphocytes (T, B, and NK cells), on myeloid lineage cells (monocytes, macrophages, and dendritic cells (DC)), on mesenchymal cells (epithelial, endothelial, and stromal) and on many types of tumor cells. This review covers six late preclinical development and clinical stage IgSF proteins being targeted with therapeutics for the treatment of cancer, highlighting key preclinical data. The proteins discussed represent a small sample of the diverse subfamilies within the IgSF. Many of the proteins mentioned have had multiple names assigned to them; Table 2.1 summarizes the nomenclature of many of the proteins mentioned in this review.

2 CEACAM1

CEACAM1 (Carcinoembryonic antigen-related cell adhesion molecule 1; CD66a, Table 2.1) was first characterized as a cell–cell adhesion molecule detected on leukocytes, epithelial cells, and endothelial cells, and is a member of the CEA family

Table 2.2 Development stage of IgSF proteins discussed in this review

Common name	Companies	Therapeutic designation	Development stage	Clinical trials
CEACAM1	Merck	CM24	Phase 1	NCT02346955
	Agenus	None	Preclinical	n/a
ICOS	Jounce	None	Preclinical	n/a
LAG-3	Bristol-Myers Squibb	BMS986016	Phase 1	NCT01968109
	Prima Biomed	IMP321	Phase 2	None active
	Novartis	LAG525	Phase 1	NCT02460224
TIGIT	Roche/Genentech	None	Preclinical	n/a
TIM-3	Novartis	None	IND	n/a
VISTA	ImmuNext/Jannsen	None	Preclinical	n/a

(Table 2.2). The encoded protein has been shown to mediate cell adhesion primarily via homophilic CEACAM1–CEACAM1 interactions. Heterophilic protein binding has also been described, including interactions with other CEACAM family members, notably CEACAM5 (CD66e). The complexity of CEACAM1 mediated biology is underscored by the multifaceted regulation of protein expression, notably by differential splicing of CEACAM1 mRNA. This regulation yields 11 distinct CEACAM1 isoforms in humans that have different extracellular domain configurations that can signal via distinct pathways intracellularly (Chen et al. 2009). All CEACAM1 isoforms possess the most N-terminal IgV-domain that includes the protein homodimerization site (Fig. 2.2). The so-called "long" form, CEACAM1L, signals through ITIM domains and has clear inhibitory activity in T cells (Nagaishi et al. 2006), wherein CEACAM1 associates with the TCR complex. Homophilic binding that engages CEACAM1L in trans (i.e., between different cells) results in tyrosine phosphorylation of the intracellular ITIM (immunoreceptor tyrosine-based inhibition motif) domains. Phospho-ITIM motifs recruit the inhibitory phosphatase SHP1 to the TCR/CD3 complex, leading to CD3 and ZAP-70 dephosphorylation, thus terminating TCR-signaling (Chen et al. 2008). The activity of membrane-bound CEACAM1 isoforms is also regulated at the level of protein dimerization, whereby the dimeric form is in an inactive state and the monomeric form is active. A recent study demonstrated that CEACAM1 and TIM-3 (T cell immunoglobulin mucin-3) are expressed together and TIM-3 appears able to regulate the cell surface expression of CEACAM1. This may be yet another mechanism for the regulation of CEACAM1 expression. Finally, the protein is heavily glycosylated, adding yet another layer of biophysical complexity.

This complexity at the mRNA and protein level may in part explain conflicting data regarding the role of CEACAM1 in cancer immunity. Early studies suggested both tumor-suppressive and tumor-supportive roles for CEACAM1 in different cancer indications. While differences in tumor biology may explain the disparate findings, this may also be due to the use of different reagents (proteins and anti-CEACAM1 antibodies) and the in vitro nature of many of the studies. Indeed it has recently become clear that CEACAM1 is actively immunosuppressive in many cancers, with

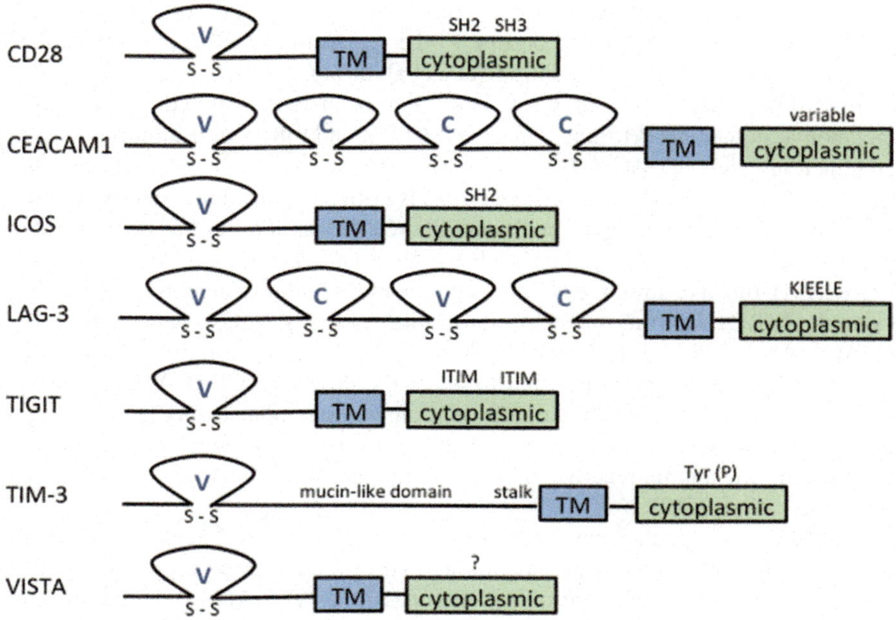

Fig. 2.2 Diversity within the IgSF. Ig-domains can number from one to many across IgSF proteins, and both variable (V) and constant (C) domains can be used. In addition, many IgSF proteins have incorporated distinct functionalities, illustrated by the presence of a mucin-like domain in the TIM proteins and distinct cytoplasmic domains across the family members shown. *TM* transmembrane, *Tyr (P)* tyrosine phosphorylation

robust expression of the protein both on tumor-infiltrating lymphocytes (TIL) and the tumor cells themselves. The remarkable degree of expression on both tumor cells and TIL was elegantly shown by the cCAM BioTherapeutics group (see AACR 2015 Abstract #6211: http://www.abstractsonline.com/).

Beyond the details of CEACAM1 expression has emerged very compelling data that support therapeutic targeting of this protein. Accumulating clinical evidence shows that increased CEACAM1 expression is correlated with poor clinical prognosis in diverse cancers (Xi et al. 2008). The precise nature of the CEACAM1 isoforms expressed in distinct tumor types is poorly understood, but several mechanisms seem to be at work, perhaps in concert, to support tumor survival and dissemination. CEACAM1 is associated with invasiveness of tumors through effects on the cell cytoskeletal machinery and resulting cellular morphology. CEACAM1 on tumor-associated endothelium has been shown to promote angiogenesis via VEGF secretion. Finally, CEACAM1 expressed on tumor cells can bind to CEACAM1 and perhaps other proteins on T cells, disabling the antitumor immune response. CEACAM1 modulation of NK cell activity has also been investigated, particularly in the context of antitumor responses. It was demonstrated that CEACAM1 expression on activated NK cells inhibited NKG2D-mediated NK activity, including signaling and the induction of cytotoxic activity (Hosomi et al. 2013). This activity appears to be due to the regulation of NKG2D cell surface expression by CEACAM1 signaling (Chen et al. 2011).

In addition, expression of CEACAM1 has been demonstrated in metastatic melanoma, non-small cell lung cancer (NSCLC), and other solid tumors, often in conjunction with CEACAM1+ TIL. This expression pattern suggests that CEACAM1–CEACAM1 interaction *in trans* is utilized by the tumor cells to disable TIL function. Preclinical work with anti-CEACAM1 antibodies has demonstrated that blocking CEACAM1 binding leads to enhanced cytotoxic TIL activity against CEACAM1-positive tumor cell lines and in mouse tumor models in vivo. For example, MRG1 is a mouse IgG1 monoclonal antibody (IgG1) that binds to the CEACAM1-specific N-terminal Ig-domain with high affinity ($K_D = 2nM$). N-terminal directed antibodies bind to all of the described CEACAM1 isoforms. MRG1 inhibits CEACAM1 homophilic binding without inducing ADCC or agonistic signaling, and was demonstrated to enhance the cytotoxic activity of adoptively transferred, melanoma-reactive TIL in a human melanoma xenograft model (Ortenberg et al. 2012).

cCAM Biotherapeutics has further developed the antibody CM-24 for the treatment of multiple oncological indications. The preclinical development of this antibody suggests the promise of this therapeutic target. CM24 is a high-affinity humanized anti-CEACAM1 IgG4 monoclonal antibody (see AACR 2015 Abstract #262: http://www.abstractsonline.com/). CM24 blocks intercellular CEACAM1 homotypic interactions, i.e., between tumor cells and T cells or NK cells. Molecularly, CM24 reversed TIL inhibition by restoring ZAP70 phosphorylation and associated TCR/CD3 complex signaling. As a consequence, CM24 enhanced the cytotoxic activity of CD8+ TIL and NK cells, increasing secretion of granzyme B and IFNγ and improving tumor cell killing. cCAM also presented in vitro data suggesting synergistic activity with anti-PD-1 antagonism. The in vitro data was mirrored by results from in vivo tumor xenograft models showing the CM24 had antitumor activity (Ortenberg et al. 2012). cCAM began enrolling patients into a Phase 1 trial in the spring of 2015 (NCT02346955). This is an open-label, multidose escalation study primarily focused on establishing a safe dose. Objective responses to therapy will be measured as well, as a secondary endpoint. The company was acquired by Merck in June of 2015.

An antibody phage display library developed at the University of Urbino (Italy) was used to develop a high-affinity scFV panel against CEACAM1 (Moricoli et al. 2014). A scFv is a single chain antibody fragment consisting of the Vh and Vl chains, linked together, and is suitable for creating full antibodies by standard genetic engineering. Some of these assets were licensed into the private company DIATHEVA and then acquired by the US biotechnology company Agenus Inc in July of 2015.

The licensing activity around CEACAM1 illustrates the importance with which this pathway is viewed. True validation will only come from the clinical studies, and we will not see readouts from those until 2017 at the earliest. There is significant interest in other family members, particularly CEACAMs 5, 6, and 8. An anti-human CEACAM scFv (MA39) isolated from a phage-display library was demonstrated to bind an epitope shared by CEACAMs 1, 5, and 6, a very interesting specificity (Pavoni et al. 2006). Also of note, an anti-CEACAM5 antibody-drug conjugate (IMMU-130) is in Phase 2 clinical trials in colorectal cancer. IMMU-130 caused dose-limiting neutropenia in Phase 1 clinical trials, although was otherwise well-tolerated. Alternative dosing regimens are being tested in Phase 2 (see ASCO 2014 Abstract #3106: http://meetinglibrary.asco.org/content/128066-144). It will be of keen interest to monitor this family for additional drug development activity.

3 ICOS

The concept of T cell costimulation in immunity began with the observation that triggering TCR signaling with one activation signal, such as a purified soluble peptide/MHC complex, or an anti-CD2 antibody, or an anti-CD3 antibody, was insufficient to drive T cell differentiation, proliferation, effector function, and survival. A "second signal" was needed, and it was clear that antigen-presenting cells (APC) such as DC, monocytes/macrophages and B cells, could present such a signal (Jenkins et al. 1988). In the very early days of costimulation biology, molecular DNA library screening was used to clone CD28, the canonical T cell costimulatory receptor (Aruffo and Seed 1987). Over the next few years the CD28 ligands were discovered: B7-1 (CD80) and B7-2 (CD86) (reviewed in Sharpe and Freeman 2002). CD28 is a very unique receptor with only two closely relatives: CTLA4, with which it competes for binding to the B7-1 and B7-2 ligands, and a second protein called ICOS (Inducible T-cell costimulator) (Gonzalo et al. 2001). ICOS is rather divergent from CD28, with limited amino acid sequence similarity, although sharing key structural features such as a single IgV-like domain and cytoplasmic domain homology (Fig. 2.2). The ligand for ICOS was initially called B7H2 (B7 Homology 2, Table 2.1) to indicate relatedness to B7-1 and B7-2; however, the degree of homology is very weak. ICOS-L is more closely related to the butyrophilins (Table 2.1). I note in passing that there is a tendency to label IgSF proteins with even more spurious homology as relatives of B7-1/B7-2 (or more recently PD-1 and PD-L1) in an attempt to capture reflected glory from these critically important immune checkpoint proteins. As we learn more about the homology within the IgSF such claims have become weaker, as demonstrated by several recent elegant protein systematics papers (Yap et al. 2014; Rubinstein et al. 2013).

Regardless, ICOS and its ligand, ICOS-L (CD278 and CD275, respectively, Table 2.1) are critically important in their own right. ICOS is expressed on activated T cells and mediates T cell activation in response to binding by ICOS-L expressed on B cells and APC (Sharpe 2009). Diverse functions have been ascribed to ICOS, the most important of which may be to propagate and sustain T follicular T cells that drive germinal center reactions and the development of antibody secreting B cells. A well-defined additional role in the development of the Th17 T cell lineage has been described. Compelling genetic data has accumulated about this pathway. ICOS or ICOS-L gene-deficient ("knockout") mice, and patients with inactivating ICOS mutations, suffer severe defects in the development of B cell dependent antibody responses to pathogen challenge. ICOS knockout mice and mice treated with antagonist anti-ICOS antibodies are resistant to the development of autoimmune diseases in multiple mouse models (Simpson et al. 2010). The human ICOS deficiency causes a common variable immunodeficiency and patients have reduced CD4+ T cell subtypes, lack protective antibodies and have a markedly reduced pool of memory B cells (Yong et al. 2009; Warnatz et al. 2006; Salzer et al. 2004). Conversely, hyperactivity of the pathway may be associated with autoimmune disease, including lupus, primary biliary cirrhosis, and perhaps type 1 diabetes. Because the CD28, CTLA4 and ICOS genes are closely linked on human chromosome 2q33, it is difficult to assign autoimmune susceptibility to genetic alterations in ICOS (Coyle et al. 2000).

Activation of ICOS might prove beneficial in the setting of immunotherapy targeting cancer. Recent work has demonstrated that high ICOS expression on circulating T cells correlate with a productive clinical response to CTLA4 blockade, suggesting that influencing this pathway, which is downstream of the primary T cell activation mediated by CD28, may be an appropriate means of boosting the response rate in patients receiving anti-CTLA4, i.e., ipilimumab (Ng Tang et al. 2013). Mechanistically, ICOS expression is upregulated when T cells are activated through the TCR and costimulated via CD28 signaling, as is the case in the context of anti-CTLA-4 therapeutics. In an important preclinical study, ICOS activation was synergistic with CTLA4 blockade in melanoma and pancreatic cancer models (Fan et al. 2014). It was also demonstrated that in patients treated with ipilimumab, the $ICOS^+$ T cell population contained the highest proportion of tumor-antigen-specific and IFN-γ secreting CD4+ T cells (Liakou et al. 2008). These studies, and several others, suggest that ICOS is a marker of functional TIL within tumors. This is driving significant drug-development interest in understanding how best to stimulate and expand ICOS+ TIL (Capece et al. 2012).

Activation of the pathway will require an agonist agent, either a soluble ICOS-L molecule or an agonist antibody to ICOS itself. Few agonist antibodies targeting ICOS have been developed. The approach has certainly been cautious, as prior experience targeting the related CD28 protein with an activating antibody caused disastrous acute inflammation and multiorgan failure (Suntharalingam et al. 2006). Jounce Therapeutics recently disclosed an ICOS agonist program in IND-enabling studies and other agonist agents can be found in patent databases, with Bristol-Myers Squibb a notable contributor. However, therapeutics have not reached the clinic yet and we cannot know if these agents will be safe and efficacious until they are used to treat patients. One area of concern is the potential for "cytokine storm" toxicity, as was triggered by the Tegenero anti-CD28 agonist antibody TGN1412. More worrisome in the long term may be an association of ICOS activity with autoimmunity. As has been seen with anti-CTLA4 and anti-PD-1 pathway antagonists, autoimmune toxicity is a very real threat to patients. In particular, combining an ICOS agonist with other immune checkpoint therapeutics like the anti-CTLA4 antibody ipilimumab will have to be done with keen awareness of the potential for significant adverse autoimmunity.

4 LAG-3

LAG-3 (Lymphocyte activation gene-3, CD223) is a homologue of CD4, a protein expressed on T cells (CD4+ T cells) and several other cell types. LAG-3 and CD4 have a very similar protein structure consisting of four Ig-domains (Fig. 2.2). The most N-terminal domain in each protein contains the ligand-binding site. CD4 is an essential co-receptor within the TCR cell surface membrane complex and functions by amplifying the TCR signal via recruitment of Lck, a tyrosine kinase that is essential for transducing the TCR signaling cascade. Both CD4 and the TCR bind the MHC class II (MHCII) protein complex found on APC. MHCII is an IgSF protein that functions by presenting foreign peptides to the TCR thereby triggering an immune response: CD4+ T cells will only respond to peptides that are bound within the MHCII complex. CD4 binds MHCII at a region distinct from the TCR binding domains, thus, both proteins can bind simultaneously, ensuring that the Lck tyrosine kinase is brought proximal to the TCR intracellular domain. LAG-3 is also a ligand for MHCII and binds with a higher affinity than CD4. Binding of LAG-3 to MHCII disrupts CD4 binding and thereby negatively regulates TCR signaling (Turnis et al. 2012). An indication that LAG-3 was important in immune regulation came when expression of the protein was identified on regulatory T cells (Tregs) that inhibit activated T cell effector function (Huang et al. 2004). LAG-3 is expressed along with PD-1 and TIM-3 on chronically "exhausted" CD8+ T cells that can no longer respond productively to antigen stimulation. Exhausted CD8+ TIL are considered to be an indication of a suppressed antitumor immune response. Importantly, LAG-3 is also expressed on tumor cells of many types, suggesting that the tumor is using this protein to shield it from productive antitumor immunity. Since both TIL and tumor cells can express LAG-3 within a tumor, teasing apart the relative roles of protein expression in these two compartments is complex and perhaps unnecessary.

Mechanistic data is limited but consistent with the hypothesis that LAG-3 negatively regulates immune responses. For example, transfection of naive CD4+ T cells with LAG-3 was sufficient to drive those cells into a Treg phenotype with immunosuppressive function (Huang et al. 2004). In this and several additional studies it was shown that Tregs require signaling through LAG-3 (Workman and Vignali 2005). Of interest, the manner in which LAG-3 signals to regulate cellular responses remains unknown, except that the signaling requires an amino acid motif, KIEELE, that appears to be unique to this protein. LAG-3 also negatively regulates CD8+ T cell activity, albeit via a poorly understood mechanism (Sierro et al. 2011; Grosso et al. 2007).

Notably, blockade of LAG-3 and PD-1 using antagonist antibodies synergistically reactivated exhausted CD8+ T cells in a model of chronic immune challenge via viral infection (Blackburn et al. 2009). Such models are thought to mimic the exhausted T cell state that tumors induce in TIL to inactivate them. In another study, mice rendered gene-deficient for both LAG-3 and PD-1 were shown to reject even poorly immunogenic tumors. The distinct roles played by LAG-3 and PD-1 in regulating immune responses are clearly seen in the doubly gene-deficient mice, which develop aggressive autoimmune disease as they age. However, combination blockade using biologic therapies appears to be both effective and tolerable in preclinical mouse tumor models (Woo et al. 2012). LAG-3$^+$/PD-1$^+$ TIL isolated from ovarian cancer patients were shown to have a defective immune response to tumor antigen stimulation (Matsuzaki et al. 2010). T cell responses could be restored in the presence of antagonists of LAG-3 and PD-1, to a degree that was significantly higher than anti-PD-1 antibody treatment alone. However, LAG-3 blockade alone was insufficient to restore antitumor T cell activity. From the perspective of translational medicine and biomarker development, these data suggest that dual antagonism of LAG-3 and PD-1 may be indicated in tumors where PD-1 and LAG-3 are coexpressed on TIL, or in tumors where PD-L1 and LAG-3 are expressed on tumor cells. One can envision additional expression patterns that might suggest synergy leading to increased patient response rates and the degree of response to therapy in response to combination therapy.

Several LAG-3 antagonists are in clinical development (Table 2.2). The first therapeutic developed to target LAG-3 activity was a LAG-3-Fc fusion protein created by Immuntep, called IMP321. IMP321 showed biological activity and modest clinical responses in several advanced solid tumor types (Sierro et al. 2011). The IMP321 program was acquired by Prima Biomed, however there has been no further clinical development presented to date. Bristol-Myers Squibb has developed an anti-LAG-3 antibody (BMS986016) that is in a Phase 1 clinical trial in advanced solid tumors as a monotherapy and in combination with the anti-PD-1 antibody nivolumab (Table 2.2). Novartis acquired anti-LAG-3 assets through the acquisition of CoStim Inc., and anti-LAG-3 antibody LAG525 will be analyzed as monotherapy and in combination with a new anti-PD-1 antibody, named PDR001, also from Novartis (Table 2.2). The trial had not yet enrolled patients in July 2015. In preclinical development is a LAG-3/PD-1 bispecific antibody created by Tesaro and partnered with AnaptysBio. Other programs with less visibility are likely underway.

Like the CD28/CTLA4 and ICOS pathways, LAG-3 activity is intimately tied to TCR engagement and signaling. This places LAG-3 "upstream" in the hierarchy of immune checkpoint inhibitors that control T cell activation and proliferation. With additional roles in NK cell and APC function, it is anticipated that LAG-3 will be a significant new immune checkpoint pathway. Early clinical results are expected in late 2016 or early 2017.

5 TIGIT

TIGIT (T cell immunoglobulin and ITIM domain) is an IgSF protein with diverse and very interesting functional activities. Like PD-1, LAG-3, and TIM-3, TIGIT can be expressed on exhausted CD8+ T cells. However, much of the function of this protein appears to be due to its modulation of both T cell and NK cell function (Lozano et al. 2012; Stanietsky et al. 2009). TIGIT interacts with members of the Polovirus Receptor (PVR) family within the IgSF that also includes DNAM-1 (CD226), CD96, and CD112 (PVRL2), CD155 (PVR), other nectins, and related proteins (Rubinstein et al. 2013). Many of the proteins within the PVR family are characterized by diverse ligand–receptor interactions. TIGIT can interact with CD155, CD112, and the related nectin family member CD113/PVRL3. Mechanistically, TIGIT function appears dependent on engagement of CD155 expressed on immature or resting DC. This interaction blocks DC maturation that is normally triggered by DNAM-1 binding to CD155. That is, the binding events are competitive. TIGIT binds CD155 with a higher affinity than DNAM-1 and will outcompete DNAM-1 when present in equimolar concentrations or even less. This means, as is usual for negative regulatory signals, TIGIT-mediated immunosuppression of DC maturation will override activation (Pauken and Wherry 2014; Lozano et al. 2012).

The interaction is complex. Two TIGIT/CD155 dimers form a hetero-tetramer having a TIGIT/TIGIT cis-homodimer at the center. Each TIGIT molecule binds to one CD155 molecule (Stengel et al. 2012). This cis–trans interaction requires cell–cell contact and adhesion. These data suggest that antagonism of either TIGIT homodimerization or TIGIT–CD155 interaction could be an effective means of blocking TIGIT-mediated negative signaling. The importance of TIGIT-mediated DC suppression is illustrated by the TIGIT gene knockout mouse, which exacerbates mouse autoimmune models (de Andrade et al. 2014; Levin et al. 2011). TIGIT activity has been shown to disable tumor antigen-specific TIL function and also to identify potent Treg T cells (Chauvin et al. 2015; Joller et al. 2014). Genentech researchers demonstrated that co-blockade of TIGIT and PD-L1 resulted in tumor rejection by restoring the function of exhausted CD8+ TIL (Johnston et al. 2014). However, the in vivo studies used very high amounts of ADCC-competent anti-TIGIT antibody, which certainly complicates interpretation (Mahoney et al. 2015). This raises the question of whether lower doses, when properly controlled for IgG isotype, were ineffective. Regardless, and in support of the Genentech antibody experiments, TIGIT knockout mice showed reduced tumor growth in a syngeneic melanoma model (Sema Kurtulus et al. 2014). Further, an anti-TIGIT antibody was synergistic with an anti-TIM-3 antibody in controlling tumor growth (Sema Kurtulus et al. 2014). The early data accumulating around TIGIT and interacting proteins suggest that targeting TIGIT may be especially beneficial in tumor environments where both T cells and NK cells are demonstrated to be present and DC maturation may be stimulated, as in tumors in which tertiary lymphoid organization is observed.

6 TIM-3

TIM-3 is a cell surface protein expressed on T cells and is a receptor within the subfamily of TIM (T cell-immunoglobulin-mucin domain) proteins (Table 2.2) (McIntire et al. 2001). The TIM family was initially identified in a study of the genetic basis for the differential asthmatic activity seen in divergent in-bred mouse strains (McIntire et al. 2001). As with LAG-3, much of the early data on the role of TIM-3 came from studies of T cells “exhausted” by chronic viral exposure. TIM-3 is highly expressed on exhausted CD8+ T cells, and blockade of TIM-3 can reverse this exhausted state, allowing T cells to again respond to viral antigen challenge. CD8+ T cells that express both TIM-3 and PD-1 were more refractory to viral antigen than cells expressing just PD-1, suggesting a biological rationale for combination therapy (Jin et al. 2010). Human TIM-3 is also expressed by NK cells, NKT cells, and APCs including DC and macrophages. Thus antibodies targeting TIM-3 may impact immune responses in many different ways depending on the specific isotype of the antibody (Mahoney et al. 2015).

It is less clear mechanistically how this pathway is regulated. Much of the difficulty encountered in studying TIM-3 (and other TIM proteins, notably TIM-1) is due to the "sticky" nature of these proteins. Indeed, under standard assay conditions engineered soluble TIM-1-Fc and TIM-3-Fc proteins were shown to bind promiscuously to diverse cell types (Wilker et al. 2007). As a consequence, numerous putative TIM ligands have been proposed, and the role of any specific ligand remains controversial. Indeed, nearly all studies done using TIM fusion proteins in vivo or in vitro must be viewed with caution given their propensity for nonspecific binding.

The best-studied TIM protein ligand is phosphatidylserine (PS). PS has been demonstrated to bind to TIM-1, TIM-3 and TIM-4 proteins (mouse and human) and the co-crystal structures have been determined (Freeman et al. 2010). Biologically, PS is associated with apoptotic (i.e., physiologically regulated) cell death, a process that is thought to be immunologically silent. In chronic viral infection it is perhaps the overwhelming amount of cell death occurring that is sufficient to "exhaust" T cells, in part via TIM-3 engagement. Blocking TIM-3 in the context of an antitumor immune response may be efficacious because the ability of the immune system to recognize dead and dying tumor cells is altered (DeKruyff et al. 2010). Indeed, the role of PS in TIM-family biology is remarkable. TIM-1 has even been coopted by filoviruses (Ebola, Marburg), alpha viruses (Yellow Fever), and other classes as a receptor used by the virus to infect cells (Moller-Tank et al. 2013; Moller-Tank and Maury 2014; Moller-Tank et al. 2014). In this setting viral particles hijack PS, which then binds to TIM-1 (and TIM-4), facilitating cell binding and internalization. Although TIM-1 has been targeted with a toxin-conjugated monoclonal antibody for the treatment of renal cell carcinoma, this is not strictly speaking an immune checkpoint based immunotherapy approach. Recently, TIM-1 was identified as a critical control protein involved in lymphocyte trafficking (Angiari et al. 2014) and such activity may complicate anti-TIM-1 drug development.

Other ligands proposed for TIM-3 include galectin-9, HMGB1, and CEACAM1 (Freeman et al. 2010; Zhu et al. 2005; Huang et al. 2014). Of these, galectin-9 has been the most studied (Sakuishi et al. 2011). We recently proposed that galectin-9, by binding specific sugar residues on multiple glycoproteins (such as the TCR, 4-1BB, and TIM-3), may act as a general enhancer of glycoprotein receptor signaling by increasing crosslinking after a canonical ligand has bound (Madireddi et al. 2014; Mahoney et al. 2015). In this regard, galectin-9 may regulate TIM-3 signaling after PS binds. Finally, as mentioned earlier, CEACAM1 may play a role in regulating the cell surface expression of TIM-3 (Huang et al. 2014). Regardless of the difficulties in discerning biologically relevant protein ligand–TIM-3 interactions, the potency of the TIM-3 pathway in antitumor immunity is apparent.

Preclinical studies using TIM-3 antagonists and the TIM-3 gene-deficient mouse in transplantation, autoimmunity and antigen challenge models established the importance of TIM-3 in immunity (Freeman et al. 2010). As noted above the characterization of TIM-3+/PD-1+/CD8+ TIL as exhausted T cells suggested a role for TIM-3 in antitumor immunity. Studies done using preclinical syngeneic tumor challenge models further built on the expression data. In the murine syngeneic tumor models all TIM-3-positive TIL coexpressed PD-1 (Sakuishi et al. 2010). This suggests that these TIL populations contain exhausted T cells. Supporting this hypothesis, the efficacy of TIM-3 antagonists synergized with PD-1 blockade. TIM-3 antagonism was also enhanced with agonist anti-4-1BB antibody therapy (Guo et al. 2013) again highlighting the synergy between relief from immunosuppression and T cell stimulation.

Such studies raise the critical question of when it is clinically relevant to apply anti-TIM-3 therapy. The preclinical data suggest that coexpression of TIM-3 with PD-1 and/or LAG-3 on TIL may a relevant indication that combination therapy is warranted. TIM-3 expression was correlated with tumor clinical stage and ex vivo T cell immunocompetence in a small cohort of colorectal cancer patients (Xu et al. 2015). In a study of clear cell renal cancer patients TIM-3 expression was detected on lymphocytes, cancer cells and tumor-associated macrophages (TAM), and high TIM-3 expression was positively correlated with shorter progression-free survival (Komohara et al. 2015). Of note an increased number of TAMs was correlated with high TIM-3 expression in patients. These observations, among others in the literature, highlight the complex role that TIM-3 may play in different tumor settings. While no TIM-3 antagonists were in clinical trials by July 2015, a number are in development, and a Novartis trial is expected to begin by the end of 2015 (Table 2.2).

7 VISTA

From the perspective of immune checkpoint combination therapy, VISTA (V-domain immunoglobulin (Ig)-containing suppressor of T-cell activation) appears particularly attractive. VISTA is highly expressed on both myeloid cells and T cells. In the context of the tumor microenvironment, myeloid-derived suppressor cells (MDSC) and Tregs express VISTA at an elevated level. Evolutionarily, VISTA is a surprising protein and perhaps a "singleton," meaning it has no close relatives (Table 2.1). It has minimal homology to other immune checkpoint proteins such as the B7s, CD28 or CTLA4, PD-1 or the PD-Ls. Nor is it particularly closely related to protein families that share homology with B7s, such as the butyrophilins (Rubinstein et al. 2013; Yap et al. 2014). The function of the protein appears somewhat similar to other negative immune regulators. Deletion of the *VISTA* gene in mice resulted in spontaneous T-cell activation, increased neoantigen response, and age-related inflammation. Notably, VISTA gene-deficient mice developed nervous system autoimmunity when bred onto an autoimmune-prone transgenic mouse strain. These results suggest a role for VISTA in controlling T cell responses. Further work using the gene-deficient mouse model measured immune responses against tumor-associated antigens. VISTA gene-deficient mice had enhanced responses to melanoma cells expressing the OVA antigen, however control of tumor growth required peptide vaccination in the presence of Toll-like receptor (TLR) agonists (Wang et al. 2014). While these results were taken as evidence that innate immune (TLR) stimulation was a component of VISTA T cell function, it seems likely in retrospect that TLR/peptide vaccination engaged other VISTA-dependent cells. For example, anti-VISTA antibody blockade increased the infiltration, proliferation, and effector function of TIL in a melanoma model while blocking Treg function, similar to the effect on T cells seen with PD-1 blockade. However, VISTA blockade also decreased the number of MDSC and increased the presence of activated DC within the tumor microenvironment, effects that may be directly due to VISTA function on myeloid lineage cells (Le Mercier et al. 2014). Indeed, in human colon cancer and lung cancer samples, VISTA expression was predominantly found on CD11b+ myeloid cells within the tumor microenvironment. VISTA expressed on APCs was shown to suppress CD4+ T cell and CD8+ T-cell proliferation and cytokine production and induces the induction of Treg T cells (Le Mercier et al. 2014; Wang et al. 2011).

With these results we are beginning to see potentially important clues as to the use of VISTA antagonists in the context of other immune therapeutics that specifically target T cells. In such a setting VISTA antagonism may have a synergistic impact on the T cell response while also affecting the immunosuppressive myeloid lineages in the TME. VISTA drug development has lagged behind some of the other targets described in this review. A collaboration between ImmuNext and Janssen (a division of Johnson & Johnson) was formed to develop anti-VISTA antibodies and VISTA-Fc fusion proteins. Immunext has announced the enrollment and dosing of the first patient with their anti-VISTA antibody.

8 Summary

The IgSF contains diverse proteins that regulate immune responses. A small sample of the available data is presented in this review, but this is not to suggest that the list is complete or even contains the most important proteins and pathways. For example, the large butyrophilin and siglec families within the IgSF are likely to contain important immune modulatory targets. Thus, the list of potential therapeutic targets will only grow longer in the coming years. A critical issue as we examine the IgSF for additional therapeutic targets is the development of guidelines for the rational deployment of diverse therapeutics in different cancer indications. To the extent that combination therapy may engage different arms of the immune response they should show additive or synergistic effect and the mechanism of action of each therapeutic must be well characterized. In addition, understanding the patterns of expression of target ligands and receptors within the tumor, on tumor associated cells, in tumor-draining lymph nodes and in the circulation will be critical to developing rational combinations between IgSF-directed therapeutics and with other immunomodulatory agents. Preclinical and clinical studies now underway will further our understanding of how best to target specific pathways for the treatment of specific tumor indications, tailored perhaps, to individual patients. That is certainly a lofty goal, and we are lucky to be in the field of cancer immunotherapy at this extraordinary and exciting time, when such a goal can realistically be formulated.

References

Angiari, S., Donnarumma, T., Rossi, B., Dusi, S., Pietronigro, E., Zenaro, E., Della Bianca, V., Toffali, L., Piacentino, G., Budui, S., Rennert, P., Xiao, S., Laudanna, C., Casasnovas, J.M., Kuchroo, V.K., Constantin, G.: TIM-1 glycoprotein binds the adhesion receptor P-selectin and mediates T cell trafficking during inflammation and autoimmunity. Immunity **40**, 542–553 (2014)

Aruffo, A., Seed, B.: Molecular cloning of a CD28 cDNA by a high-efficiency COS cell expression system. Proc. Natl. Acad. Sci. U. S. A. **84**, 8573–8577 (1987)

Blackburn, S.D., Shin, H., Haining, W.N., Zou, T., Workman, C.J., Polley, A., Betts, M.R., Freeman, G.J., Vignali, D.A., Wherry, E.J.: Coregulation of CD8+ T cell exhaustion by multiple inhibitory receptors during chronic viral infection. Nat. Immunol. **10**, 29–37 (2009)

Capece, D., Verzella, D., Fischietti, M., Zazzeroni, F., Alesse, E.: Targeting costimulatory molecules to improve antitumor immunity. J. Biomed. Biotechnol. **2012**, 926321 (2012)

Chauvin, J.M., Pagliano, O., Fourcade, J., Sun, Z., Wang, H., Sander, C., Kirkwood, J.M., Chen, T.H., Maurer, M., Korman, A.J., Zarour, H.M.: TIGIT and PD-1 impair tumor antigen-specific CD8(+) T cells in melanoma patients. J. Clin. Invest. **125**, 2046–2058 (2015)

Chen, Z., Chen, L., Qiao, S.W., Nagaishi, T., Blumberg, R.S.: Carcinoembryonic antigen-related cell adhesion molecule 1 inhibits proximal TCR signaling by targeting ZAP-70. J. Immunol. **180**, 6085–6093 (2008)

Chen, Z., Chen, L., Blumberg, R.S.: Editorial: CEACAM1: fine-tuned for fine-tuning. J. Leukoc. Biol. **86**, 195–197 (2009)

Chen, Z., Chen, L., Baker, K., Olszak, T., Zeissig, S., Huang, Y.H., Kuo, T.T., Mandelboim, O., Beauchemin, N., Lanier, L.L., Blumberg, R.S.: CEACAM1 dampens antitumor immunity by down-regulating NKG2D ligand expression on tumor cells. J. Exp. Med. **208**, 2633–2640 (2011)

Coyle, A.J., Lehar, S., Lloyd, C., Tian, J., Delaney, T., Manning, S., Nguyen, T., Burwell, T., Schneider, H., Gonzalo, J.A., Gosselin, M., Owen, L.R., Rudd, C.E., Gutierrez-Ramos, J.C.: The CD28-related molecule ICOS is required for effective T cell-dependent immune responses. Immunity **13**, 95–105 (2000)

DE Andrade, L.F., Smyth, M.J., Martinet, L.: DNAM-1 control of natural killer cells functions through nectin and nectin-like proteins. Immunol. Cell Biol. **92**, 237–244 (2014)

Dekruyff, R.H., Bu, X., Ballesteros, A., Santiago, C., Chim, Y.L., Lee, H.H., Karisola, P., Pichavant, M., Kaplan, G.G., Umetsu, D.T., Freeman, G.J., Casasnovas, J.M.: T cell/transmembrane, Ig, and mucin-3 allelic variants differentially recognize phosphatidylserine and mediate phagocytosis of apoptotic cells. J. Immunol. **184**, 1918–1930 (2010)

Fan, X., Quezada, S.A., Sepulveda, M.A., Sharma, P., Allison, J.P.: Engagement of the ICOS pathway markedly enhances efficacy of CTLA-4 blockade in cancer immunotherapy. J. Exp. Med. **211**, 715–725 (2014)

Freeman, G.J., Casasnovas, J.M., Umetsu, D.T., Dekruyff, R.H.: TIM genes: a family of cell surface phosphatidylserine receptors that regulate innate and adaptive immunity. Immunol. Rev. **235**, 172–189 (2010)

Gonzalo, J.A., Delaney, T., Corcoran, J., Goodearl, A., Gutierrez-Ramos, J.C., Coyle, A.J.: Cutting edge: the related molecules CD28 and inducible costimulator deliver both unique and complementary signals required for optimal T cell activation. J. Immunol. **166**, 1–5 (2001)

Grosso, J.F., Kelleher, C.C., Harris, T.J., Maris, C.H., Hipkiss, E.L., DE Marzo, A., Anders, R., Netto, G., Getnet, D., Bruno, T.C., Goldberg, M.V., Pardoll, D.M., Drake, C.G.: LAG-3 regulates CD8+ T cell accumulation and effector function in murine self- and tumor-tolerance systems. J. Clin. Invest. **117**, 3383–3392 (2007)

Guo, Z., Cheng, D., Xia, Z., Luan, M., Wu, L., Wang, G., Zhang, S.: Combined TIM-3 blockade and CD137 activation affords the long-term protection in a murine model of ovarian cancer. J. Transl. Med. **11**, 215 (2013)

Hosomi, S., Chen, Z., Baker, K., Chen, L., Huang, Y.H., Olszak, T., Zeissig, S., Wang, J.H., Mandelboim, O., Beauchemin, N., Lanier, L.L., Blumberg, R.S.: CEACAM1 on activated NK cells inhibits NKG2D-mediated cytolytic function and signaling. Eur. J. Immunol. **43**, 2473–2483 (2013)

Huang, C.T., Workman, C.J., Flies, D., Pan, X., Marson, A.L., Zhou, G., Hipkiss, E.L., Ravi, S., Kowalski, J., Levitsky, H.I., Powell, J.D., Pardoll, D.M., Drake, C.G., Vignali, D.A.: Role of LAG-3 in regulatory T cells. Immunity **21**, 503–513 (2004)

Huang, Y.H., Zhu, C., Kondo, Y., Anderson, A.C., Gandhi, A., Russell, A., Dougan, S.K., Petersen, B.S., Melum, E., Pertel, T., Clayton, K.L., Raab, M., Chen, Q., Beauchemin, N., Yazaki, P.J., Pyzik, M., Ostrowski, M.A., Glickman, J.N., Rudd, C.E., Ploegh, H.L., Franke, A., Petsko, G.A., Kuchroo, V.K., Blumberg, R.S.: CEACAM1 regulates TIM-3-mediated tolerance and exhaustion. Nature **517**, 386–390 (2014)

Jenkins, M.K., Ashwell, J.D., Schwartz, R.H.: Allogeneic non-T spleen cells restore the responsiveness of normal T cell clones stimulated with antigen and chemically modified antigen-presenting cells. J. Immunol. **140**, 3324–3330 (1988)

Jin, H.T., Anderson, A.C., Tan, W.G., West, E.E., Ha, S.J., Araki, K., Freeman, G.J., Kuchroo, V.K., Ahmed, R.: Cooperation of Tim-3 and PD-1 in CD8 T-cell exhaustion during chronic viral infection. Proc. Natl. Acad. Sci. U. S. A. **107**, 14733–14738 (2010)

Johnston, R.J., Comps-Agrar, L., Hackney, J., Yu, X., Huseni, M., Yang, Y., Park, S., Javinal, V., Chiu, H., Irving, B., Eaton, D.L., Grogan, J.L.: The immunoreceptor TIGIT regulates antitumor and antiviral CD8(+) T cell effector function. Cancer Cell **26**, 923–937 (2014)

Joller, N., Lozano, E., Burkett, P.R., Patel, B., Xiao, S., Zhu, C., Xia, J., Tan, T.G., Sefik, E., Yajnik, V., Sharpe, A.H., Quintana, F.J., Mathis, D., Benoist, C., Hafler, D.A., Kuchroo, V.K.: Treg cells expressing the coinhibitory molecule TIGIT selectively inhibit proinflammatory Th1 and Th17 cell responses. Immunity **40**, 569–581 (2014)

Komohara, Y., Morita, T., Annan, D.A., Horlad, H., Ohnishi, K., Yamada, S., Nakayama, T., Kitada, S., Suzu, S., Kinoshita, I., Dosaka-Akita, H., Akashi, K., Takeya, M., Jinushi, M.: The coordinated actions of TIM-3 on cancer and myeloid cells in the regulation of tumorigenicity and clinical prognosis in clear cell renal cell carcinomas. Cancer Immuno. Res. **3**, 999–1007 (2015)

Le Mercier, I., Chen, W., Lines, J.L., Day, M., Li, J., Sergent, P., Noelle, R.J., Wang, L.: VISTA regulates the development of protective antitumor immunity. Cancer Res. **74**, 1933–44 (2014)

Levin, S.D., Taft, D.W., Brandt, C.S., Bucher, C., Howard, E.D., Chadwick, E.M., Johnston, J., Hammond, A., Bontadelli, K., Ardourel, D., Hebb, L., Wolf, A., Bukowski, T.R., Rixon, M.W., Kuijper, J.L., Ostrander, C.D., West, J.W., Bilsborough, J., Fox, B., Gao, Z., Xu, W., Ramsdell, F., Blazar, B.R., Lewis, K.E.: Vstm3 is a member of the CD28 family and an important modulator of T-cell function. Eur. J. Immunol. **41**, 902–915 (2011)

Liakou, C.I., Kamat, A., Tang, D.N., Chen, H., Sun, J., Troncoso, P., Logothetis, C., Sharma, P.: CTLA-4 blockade increases IFNgamma-producing CD4+ICOShi cells to shift the ratio of effector to regulatory T cells in cancer patients. Proc. Natl. Acad. Sci. U. S. A. **105**, 14987–14992 (2008)

Lozano, E., Dominguez-Villar, M., Kuchroo, V., Hafler, D.A.: The TIGIT/CD226 axis regulates human T cell function. J. Immunol. **188**, 3869–3875 (2012)

Madireddi, S., Eun, S.Y., Lee, S.W., Nemcovicova, I., Mehta, A.K., Zajonc, D.M., Nishi, N., Niki, T., Hirashima, M., Croft, M.: Galectin-9 controls the therapeutic activity of 4-1BB-targeting antibodies. J. Exp. Med. **211**, 1433–1448 (2014)

Mahoney, K.M., Rennert, P.D., Freeman, G.J.: Combination cancer immunotherapy and new immunomodulatory targets. Nat. Rev. Drug Discov. **14**, 561–584 (2015)
Matsuzaki, J., Gnjatic, S., Mhawech-Fauceglia, P., Beck, A., Miller, A., Tsuji, T., Eppolito, C., Qian, F., Lele, S., Shrikant, P., Old, L.J., Odunsi, K.: Tumor-infiltrating NY-ESO-1-specific CD8+ T cells are negatively regulated by LAG-3 and PD-1 in human ovarian cancer. Proc. Natl. Acad. Sci. U. S. A. **107**, 7875–7880 (2010)
Mcintire, J.J., Umetsu, S.E., Akbari, O., Potter, M., Kuchroo, V.K., Barsh, G.S., Freeman, G.J., Umetsu, D.T., Dekruyff, R.H.: Identification of Tapr (an airway hyperreactivity regulatory locus) and the linked Tim gene family. Nat. Immunol. **2**, 1109–1116 (2001)
Moller-Tank, S., Maury, W.: Phosphatidylserine receptors: enhancers of enveloped virus entry and infection. Virology **468–470**, 565–580 (2014)
Moller-Tank, S., Kondratowicz, A.S., Davey, R.A., Rennert, P.D., Maury, W.: Role of the phosphatidylserine receptor TIM-1 in enveloped-virus entry. J. Virol. **87**, 8327–8341 (2013)
Moller-Tank, S., Albritton, L.M., Rennert, P.D., Maury, W.: Characterizing functional domains for TIM-mediated enveloped virus entry. J. Virol. **88**, 6702–6713 (2014)
Moricoli, D., Laguardia, M.E., Carbonella, D.C., Balducci, M.C., Dominici, S., Fiori, V., Serafini, G., Flego, M., Cianfriglia, M., Magnani, M.: Isolation of a new human scFv antibody recognizing a cell surface binding site to CEACAM1. Large yield production, purification and characterization in E. coli expression system. Protein Expr. Purif. **93**, 38–45 (2014)
Nagaishi, T., Pao, L., Lin, S.H., Iijima, H., Kaser, A., Qiao, S.W., Chen, Z., Glickman, J., Najjar, S.M., Nakajima, A., Neel, B.G., Blumberg, R.S.: SHP1 phosphatase-dependent T cell inhibition by CEACAM1 adhesion molecule isoforms. Immunity **25**, 769–781 (2006)
Ng Tang, D., Shen, Y., Sun, J., Wen, S., Wolchok, J.D., Yuan, J., Allison, J.P., Sharma, P.: Increased frequency of ICOS+ CD4 T cells as a pharmacodynamic biomarker for anti-CTLA-4 therapy. Cancer Immuno. Res. **1**, 229–234 (2013)
Ortenberg, R., Sapir, Y., Raz, L., Hershkovitz, L., Ben Arav, A., Sapoznik, S., Barshack, I., Avivi, C., Berkun, Y., Besser, M.J., Ben-Moshe, T., Schachter, J., Markel, G.: Novel immunotherapy for malignant melanoma with a monoclonal antibody that blocks CEACAM1 homophilic interactions. Mol. Cancer Ther. **11**, 1300–1310 (2012)
Pauken, K.E., Wherry, E.J.: TIGIT and CD226: tipping the balance between costimulatory and coinhibitory molecules to augment the cancer immunotherapy toolkit. Cancer Cell **26**, 785–787 (2014)
Pavoni, E., Flego, M., Dupuis, M.L., Barca, S., Petronzelli, F., Anastasi, A.M., D'Alessio, V., Pelliccia, A., Vaccaro, P., Monteriu, G., Ascione, A., DE Santis, R., Felici, F., Cianfriglia, M., Minenkova, O.: Selection, affinity maturation, and characterization of a human scFv antibody against CEA protein. BMC Cancer **6**, 41 (2006)
Rubinstein, R., Ramagopal, U.A., Nathenson, S.G., Almo, S.C., Fiser, A.: Functional classification of immune regulatory proteins. Structure **21**, 766–776 (2013)
Sakuishi, K., Apetoh, L., Sullivan, J.M., Blazar, B.R., Kuchroo, V.K., Anderson, A.C.: Targeting Tim-3 and PD-1 pathways to reverse T cell exhaustion and restore anti-tumor immunity. J. Exp. Med. **207**, 2187–2194 (2010)
Sakuishi, K., Jayaraman, P., Behar, S.M., Anderson, A.C., Kuchroo, V.K.: Emerging Tim-3 functions in antimicrobial and tumor immunity. Trends Immunol. **32**, 345–349 (2011)
Salzer, U., Maul-Pavicic, A., Cunningham-Rundles, C., Urschel, S., Belohradsky, B.H., Litzman, J., Holm, A., Franco, J.L., Plebani, A., Hammarstrom, L., Skrabl, A., Schwinger, W., Grimbacher, B.: ICOS deficiency in patients with common variable immunodeficiency. Clin. Immunol. **113**, 234–240 (2004)
Sema Kurtulus, S., Kaori Sakuishi, K., Huiyuan Zhang, H., Nicole Joller, N., Dewar Tan, D., Mark Smyth, M., Vijay Kuchroo, V., Ana Anderson, A. (2014) Mechanisms of TIGIT-driven immune suppression in cancer. J. Immunother. Cancer **2** (Suppl 3)**,** (abstract O13)
Sharpe, A.H.: Mechanisms of costimulation. Immunol. Rev. **229**, 5–11 (2009)
Sharpe, A.H., Freeman, G.J.: The B7-CD28 superfamily. Nat. Rev. Immunol. **2**, 116–126 (2002)
Sierro, S., Romero, P., Speiser, D.E.: The CD4-like molecule LAG-3, biology and therapeutic applications. Expert Opin. Ther. Targets **15**, 91–101 (2011)

Simpson, T.R., Quezada, S.A., Allison, J.P.: Regulation of CD4 T cell activation and effector function by inducible costimulator (ICOS). Curr. Opin. Immunol. **22**, 326–332 (2010)
Stanietsky, N., Simic, H., Arapovic, J., Toporik, A., Levy, O., Novik, A., Levine, Z., Beiman, M., Dassa, L., Achdout, H., Stern-Ginossar, N., Tsukerman, P., Jonjic, S., Mandelboim, O.: The interaction of TIGIT with PVR and PVRL2 inhibits human NK cell cytotoxicity. Proc. Natl. Acad. Sci. U. S. A. **106**, 17858–17863 (2009)
Stengel, K.F., Harden-Bowles, K., Yu, X., Rouge, L., Yin, J., Comps-Agrar, L., Wiesmann, C., Bazan, J.F., Eaton, D.L., Grogan, J.L.: Structure of TIGIT immunoreceptor bound to poliovirus receptor reveals a cell-cell adhesion and signaling mechanism that requires cis-trans receptor clustering. Proc. Natl. Acad. Sci. U. S. A. **109**, 5399–5404 (2012)
Suntharalingam, G., Perry, M.R., Ward, S., Brett, S.J., Castello-Cortes, A., Brunner, M.D., Panoskaltsis, N.: Cytokine storm in a phase 1 trial of the anti-CD28 monoclonal antibody TGN1412. N. Engl. J. Med. **355**, 1018–1028 (2006)
Turnis, M.E., Korman, A.J., Drake, C.G., Vignali, D.A.: Combinatorial Immunotherapy: PD-1 may not be LAG-ing behind any more. Oncoimmunology **1**, 1172–1174 (2012)
Wang, L., Rubinstein, R., Lines, J.L., Wasiuk, A., Ahonen, C., GUO, Y., Lu, L.F., Gondek, D., Wang, Y., Fava, R.A., Fiser, A., Almo, S., Noelle, R.J.: VISTA, a novel mouse Ig superfamily ligand that negatively regulates T cell responses. J. Exp. Med. **208**, 577–592 (2011)
Wang, L., Le Mercier, I., Putra, J., Chen, W., Liu, J., Schenk, A.D., Nowak, E.C., Suriawinata, A.A., Li, J., Noelle, R.J.: Disruption of the immune-checkpoint VISTA gene imparts a proinflammatory phenotype with predisposition to the development of autoimmunity. Proc. Natl. Acad. Sci. U. S. A. **111**, 14846–14851 (2014)
Warnatz, K., Bossaller, L., Salzer, U., Skrabl-Baumgartner, A., Schwinger, W., VAN DER Burg, M., VAN Dongen, J.J., Orlowska-Volk, M., Knoth, R., Durandy, A., Draeger, R., Schlesier, M., Peter, H.H., Grimbacher, B.: Human ICOS deficiency abrogates the germinal center reaction and provides a monogenic model for common variable immunodeficiency. Blood **107**, 3045–3052 (2006)
Wilker, P.R., Sedy, J.R., Grigura, V., Murphy, T.L., Murphy, K.M.: Evidence for carbohydrate recognition and homotypic and heterotypic binding by the TIM family. Int. Immunol. **19**, 763–773 (2007)
Williams, A.F., Barclay, A.N.: The immunoglobulin superfamily--domains for cell surface recognition. Annu. Rev. Immunol. **6**, 381–405 (1988)
Woo, S.R., Turnis, M.E., Goldberg, M.V., Bankoti, J., Selby, M., Nirschl, C.J., Bettini, M.L., Gravano, D.M., Vogel, P., Liu, C.L., Tangsombatvisit, S., Grosso, J.F., Netto, G., Smeltzer, M.P., Chaux, A., Utz, P.J., Workman, C.J., Pardoll, D.M., Korman, A.J., Drake, C.G., Vignali, D.A.: Immune inhibitory molecules LAG-3 and PD-1 synergistically regulate T-cell function to promote tumoral immune escape. Cancer Res. **72**, 917–927 (2012)
Workman, C.J., Vignali, D.A.: Negative regulation of T cell homeostasis by lymphocyte activation gene-3 (CD223). J. Immunol. **174**, 688–695 (2005)
Xi, L., Feber, A., Gupta, V., Wu, M., Bergemann, A.D., Landreneau, R.J., Litle, V.R., Pennathur, A., Luketich, J.D., Godfrey, T.E.: Whole genome exon arrays identify differential expression of alternatively spliced, cancer-related genes in lung cancer. Nucleic Acids Res. **36**, 6535–6547 (2008)
Xu, B., Yuan, L., Gao, Q., Yuan, P., Zhao, P., Yuan, H., Fan, H., Li, T., Qin, P., Han, L., Fang, W., Suo, Z.: Circulating and tumor-infiltrating Tim-3 in patients with colorectal cancer. Oncotarget **6**, 20592 (2015)
Yap, E.H., Rosche, T., Almo, S., Fiser, A.: Functional clustering of immunoglobulin superfamily proteins with protein-protein interaction information calibrated hidden Markov model sequence profiles. J. Mol. Biol. **426**, 945–961 (2014)
Yong, P.F., Salzer, U., Grimbacher, B.: The role of costimulation in antibody deficiencies: ICOS and common variable immunodeficiency. Immunol. Rev. **229**, 101–113 (2009)
Zhu, C., Anderson, A.C., Schubart, A., Xiong, H., Imitola, J., Khoury, S.J., Zheng, X.X., Strom, T.B., Kuchroo, V.K.: The Tim-3 ligand galectin-9 negatively regulates T helper type 1 immunity. Nat. Immunol. **6**, 1245–1252 (2005)

Chapter 3
Parallel Costimulation of Effector and Regulatory T Cells by OX40, GITR, TNFRSF25, CD27, and CD137: Implications for Cancer Immunotherapy

Taylor H. Schreiber

Abbreviations

ADCC	Antibody-dependent cellular cytotoxicity
APC	Antigen presenting cell
DR3	Death receptor 3
EAE	Experimental autoimmune encephalomyelitis
Ig	Immunoglobulin
TCR	T cell receptor
Teff	Effector T cell
Treg	Regulatory T cells

1 Introduction

Cancer immunotherapy is quickly gaining momentum based on the rapid clinical uptake of checkpoint inhibitory antibodies (anti-CTLA-4, anti-PD-1/L1 blocking antibodies) in many tumor types. Clinical responses to these agents occur in a minority of patients; however, those responses tend to be dramatic and provide long-term survival with low or no evidence of disease for the lucky few. As a result of this success, it is very likely that clinical responses can be extended to a majority of patients with appropriate combination immunotherapy. Thus, prioritization of appropriate combination strategies has become a formidable task for many physicians, patients

T.H. Schreiber (✉)
Heat Biologics, Inc., Durham, North Carolina, USA

Pelican Therapeutics, Inc., Durham, North Carolina, USA

The University of Miami, Coral Gables, FL, USA
e-mail: taylor@pelicantherapeutics.com

P.D. Rennert (ed.), *Novel Immunotherapeutic Approaches to the Treatment of Cancer*, DOI 10.1007/978-3-319-29827-6_3

and biopharmaceutical companies challenged with understanding the complexity of the human immune system and predicting which pathways may synergize with one another to provide a safe and superior therapeutic benefit (Mahoney et al. 2015).

Because immune homeostasis is maintained by a hierarchy of both positive (costimulatory) and negative (inhibitory/checkpoint) signals, one of the high priority combination therapies currently being evaluated includes a checkpoint inhibitory antibody coupled with a T cell costimulatory antibody or fusion protein. Part of the attraction of this strategy results from the observation that because the immune system is poised for nonresponsiveness even in tumor naïve patients, addition of a T cell costimulatory therapy may provide true synergy with checkpoint inhibitors. There seem to be fewer targets for T cell costimulation than for checkpoint inhibition, and the list of costimulatory molecules that are in clinical testing and development is currently limited to OX40 (TNFRSF4, CD134), GITR (TNFRSF18, CD357), CD40 (TNFRSF5), CD137 (TNFRSF9, 4-1BB), CD27 (TNFRSF7), DR3 (TNFRSF25), and ICOS (CD278). There is a significant amount of preclinical literature for most of these targets, but because few of them have been systematically evaluated in head-to-head studies, it remains difficult to evaluate relative distinctions and potency between molecules. This complicates our ability to develop a comprehensive understanding of how the underlying biology of these receptors evolved, and to provide insight into the all-important question of how each receptor serves to differentially tune adaptive immune responses.

For each costimulatory receptor–ligand pair, the literature consists of studies conducted in both murine tumor model systems and autoimmune disease models. This is largely a result of the fact that each receptor can be found on both CD4+ or CD8+ effector T cells (Teff) as well as on CD4+FoxP3+ regulatory T cells (Treg), which led to early hypothesis generation in both oncology and inflammatory disease. Studies have revealed that stimulation of each receptor can lead to functional changes in either Teff or Treg biology that can either enhance or inhibit immunopathology. Intriguingly, sometimes the same target when activated with the same treatment regimen can produce seemingly contradictory results, which underscores the complexity of these interactions when studied in different model systems. Some examples include reports that OX40, GITR, CD27, CD137, and TNFRSF25 agonists can all lead to the simultaneous activation of Teff and Treg, which in some autoimmune disease models and contexts leads to the suppression of immunopathology, and in other models causes tumor regression and autoreactivity.

The underlying complexity of this biology relates to; (1) whether or not each receptor requires prior engagement of the T cell receptor by its cognate antigen, (2) whether there is preferential activation of Treg versus Teff, and (3) whether the mechanism of costimulation leads to proliferation, enhanced cytokine production, loss of effector function or to changes in the differentiation, maturation or survival status of the targeted T cell.

The purpose of this chapter is to provide a review of the literature on OX40, GITR, CD137, TNFRSF25, and CD27 in an effort to highlight how the biology of each receptor may be unique. The predominant focus is on the relative costimulatory activity of each receptor on Treg cells versus Teff cells, and comparisons are made between individual targets for areas where the biology has been broadly studied. In most cases, agonistic antibodies or fusion proteins have been used to study the biology of these receptors, and it should be taken as an overall caveat that the effector functions of each reagent (Fc binding, cross-linking, etc.) may augment interpretations made for each native receptor.

In general, TNF receptors exist in the hierarchy of T cell costimulators beneath the T cell receptor (TCR) and B7/Ig family of molecules. As a result, one line of thought is that stimulation of the TNF superfamily receptors with agonistic therapeutics may lead to less toxicity and a broader therapeutic window than stimulation of the B7 family of costimulatory molecules (CD28 and potentially ICOS). In addition to being generally dependent upon prior TCR engagement for activity, the expression patterns of these TNF receptors on T cells tends to be limited to antigen-experienced (activated) or "memory" T cells, as opposed to antigen-naïve T cells. However, there are exceptions even to these basic ground rules. The sections below provide a summary of the literature for the activities of each of these costimulators on the function of CD4+ and CD8+ effector T cells (Teff) as well as CD4+FoxP3+ regulatory T cells (Treg). The core activities that have been systematically studied for each receptor are also summarized in Table 3.1 (Treg) and Table 3.2 (Teff).

Table 3.1 Regulatory T cell functions of OX40, GITR, TNFRSF25, CD137 and CD27

CD4+FoxP3+ T regulatory cell functions					
	OX40	GITR	TNFRSF25	CD137	CD27
Expression	+	+	+	+	+
Suppressive activity	↓	↓	↓	↓	↔
Proliferation	↕	↕	↑	↑	↑
Depletion	↔	↕	↔	↔	↔
pTreg induction	↓	↔	↓	↓	↔
Conversion to Teff	↔	↔	N.D.	N.D.	N.D.
Survival	↔	↕	↔	N.D.	↑

+ denotes constitutive expression, ↓ denotes decreased activity, ↔ denotes no change in activity, ↑ denotes increased activity, ↕ denotes that both increased and decreased activity are reported in the literature, N.D. denotes a lack of evidence in the literature

Table 3.2 Effector T cell functions of OX40, GITR, TNFRSF25, CD137 and CD27

CD4+ or CD8+ effector T cell functions					
	OX40	GITR	TNFRSF25	CD137	CD27
Expression	Activated	Activated	Activated	Activated	Naive
TCR dependent	Yes	Yes	Yes	No	Yes
Proliferation at priming	CD4>CD8	↕	CD8>CD4	CD8>CD4	↕
Proliferation at boosting	CD4>CD8	N.D.	CD8>CD4	CD8>CD4 AICD?	↔
Cytokine expression	↑	↔	↑	↑	↔
Survival	↑	N.D.	N.D.	↕	↑

↓ denotes decreased activity, ↔ denotes no change in activity, ↑ denotes increased activity, ↕ denotes that both increased and decreased activity are reported in the literature, N.D. denotes a lack of evidence in the literature

2 OX40 (TNFRSF4, CD134)

Out of the targets discussed, there is perhaps the broadest knowledge and clinical enthusiasm for clinical development of OX40 agonists in oncology. There are a series of phase I clinical trials either in progress or completed with a murine anti-human OX40 agonistic antibody (Providence Cancer Center), a human OX40L-Fc fusion protein (Medimmune/Astra-Zeneca) and a human OX40 agonist antibody (Medimmune/Astra-Zeneca and Genentech/Roche). In addition, OX40 agonists have been disclosed by several other pharmaceutical and biotechnology companies and are expected to enter the clinic within the next few years. Clinical progress for OX40 agonists is likely due to the fact that it was one of the first costimulatory receptors to be discovered, and also because the preclinical literature for OX40 is largely convergent on the underlying biology (Calderhead et al. 1993; Mallett et al. 1990; Godfrey et al. 1994).

Similar to the other costimulators being discussed here, OX40 is expressed by both CD4+ and CD8+ conventional T cells as well as by CD4+FoxP3+ regulatory T cells (Treg). Expression of OX40 is generally low in naïve effector T cell Teff, but is rapidly upregulated upon TCR ligation and also highly expressed by Treg cells (Calderhead et al. 1993; Takeda et al. 2004; Vu et al. 2007; Gramaglia et al. 1998). In addition, OX40-ligand (OX40L, CD252, TNFRSF4) expression is tightly regulated and predominantly provided by antigen presenting cells (APCs) following innate inflammatory signals. The kinetics of ligand upregulation are rapid, with maximal expression observed within 2–3 days, followed by equally rapid downregulation by 4–5 days (Gramaglia et al. 1998). This suggests that the physiologic role of OX40/OX40L interaction will be restricted to a specific tissue microenvironment that has detected the possible presence of a pathogen, and wherein OX40L provided by an APC may serve to costimulate the activity of a Teff or Treg expressing OX40 within the same tissue microenvironment over a period of several days (Weinberg et al. 1996). Therefore, it is important to recognize that because transgenic expression or gene knockout of a particular receptor or ligand results in life-long perturbation of an otherwise spatiotemporally restricted signaling axis, and conclusions reached with these models may not fully recapitulate the native biology.

In general, OX40 appears to be a more potent costimulator of CD4+ T cells (both Teff and Treg) than for CD8+ T cells (Schreiber et al. 2012). Most studies agree that OX40 stimulated proliferation of CD4+ Teff requires initial activation through the TCR, either by APC or anti-CD3 antibody stimulation that appears independent of the CD28/B7 axis (Takeda et al. 2004; Gramaglia et al. 1998; Duan et al. 2008; Kroemer et al. 2007; Akiba et al. 1999; Gopisetty et al. 2013). Following costimulation through OX40, CD4+ Teff exhibit enhanced proliferation both in vitro and in vivo, and ligation of OX40 also contributes to enhanced survival and generation of memory CD4 T cells (Takeda et al. 2004; Kroemer et al. 2007; Xiao et al. 2008; Song et al. 2004). In animal models predisposed to the development of autoimmune disease, the enhanced activation of CD4+ T cells contributes to immunopathology, which can be mitigated by antibody blockade or genetic deletion of the axis (Weinberg et al. 1996; Weinberg et al. 1999; Gaspal et al. 2011).

Many of the early studies have also reported effects of the OX40 axis on Treg, consistent with the high expression of OX40 by most Treg. Similar to its effects on CD4+ Teff, OX40 can stimulate proliferation of Treg in the context of TCR ligation (Takeda et al. 2004; Duan et al. 2008; Gopisetty et al. 2013; Curti et al. 2013; Hirschhorn-Cymerman et al. 2009; Xiao et al. 2012). In addition to causing Treg proliferation, OX40 is also reported to inhibit the suppressive activity of Treg and to block the formation of new Treg (peripherally induced Treg, iTreg or pTreg) (Vu et al. 2007; Duan et al. 2008; Kroemer et al. 2007; So and Croft 2007; Voo et al. 2013). The inhibition of Treg suppressive activity by OX40 appears to require persistent engagement of OX40 by OX40L or a receptor agonistic antibody (Vu et al. 2007; Griseri et al. 2010).

Due to the costimulatory activity of OX40 on Teff cells and the inhibition of Treg suppressive activity by OX40, the activity of an OX40 agonistic antibody (clone OX86) was investigated in a series of murine tumor models (Hirschhorn-Cymerman et al. 2009; Bulliard et al. 2014; Kjaergaard et al. 2000; Redmond et al. 2014; Takeda et al. 2010; Weinberg et al. 2000). These reports demonstrate variable activity across the B16 melanoma, 4T1 breast carcinoma, CT26 colon carcinoma, MCA205 sarcoma and TRAMP prostate carcinoma. High-dose (300–400 μg) OX86 treatment led to complete rejection of established CT26 tumors, which correlated with increased intra-tumoral CD8+ T cells (Bulliard et al. 2014). In general, however, treatment of established tumors with OX40 agonists as monotherapy does not lead to dramatic efficacy (B16, 4T1, MCA205 and TRAMP models) (Hirschhorn-Cymerman et al. 2009; Redmond et al. 2014; Takeda et al. 2010). Despite the relative lack of tumor rejection, the immunologic readouts in these models show increased proliferation of both Treg and CD8+ T cells within the tumor microenvironment, and a general shift in the balance of Teff to Treg in favor of Teff cells and greater expression of IFNγ by tumor infiltrating Teff cells.

Taken together, the data demonstrate that OX40 is a pro-inflammatory, costimulatory receptor with preferential expression and activity in CD4+ Teff and Treg cells, but is also capable of stimulating CD8+ T cells, at least during priming (Schreiber et al. 2012; Ruby et al. 2007). Preliminary analysis of human peripheral blood T cell responses from patients treated with a murine anti-human OX40 agonist antibody (9B12) appear to demonstrate similar effects in human T cell to those shown in murine T cells (Curti et al. 2013). The simultaneous proliferation and transient inhibition of Treg suppressive function is shared by other family members and is discussed further below.

3 GITR (TNFRSF18, CD357)

Glucocorticoid induced TNF receptor family-related gene (GITR) is one of the more recently described T cell costimulatory molecules that also modulates both Treg and Teff function. GITR is expressed at low levels by naïve CD4+ and CD8+ T cells as well as B cells and monocytes, and is induced in T cells upon activation

(Shimizu et al. 2002). GITR ligand (GITR-L) is expressed by APCs, predominantly B cells, and seems to be downregulated by activation—the reverse of what has been observed with most TNF ligands (Stephens et al. 2004).

Much of our understanding of GITR comes from studies using an agonistic monoclonal antibody, DTA-1 (IgG2a), which was raised against Tregs as a functional clone able to block Treg mediated suppression of Teff proliferation (Shimizu et al. 2002). This first report by Shimizu et al. suggested that DTA-1 was not able to stimulate Teff proliferation, but was soon followed by an conflicting report by Stephens et al., suggesting that not only does GITR cause CD4+ or CD8+ T cell proliferation, but that the reason GITR blocks Treg suppression is a result of making Teff resistant to suppression by Treg, termed "licensing" (Shimizu et al. 2002; Stephens et al. 2004).

A role for GITR stimulation in enhancing immunopathology was reported from both autoimmune disease and tumor models in early studies of this pathway. For example, in experimental autoimmune encephalomyelitis (EAE), DTA-1 treatment was shown to exacerbate disease pathology by direct stimulation of Teff cells, independent of its effects on Treg (Kohm et al. 2004). Relatively high doses of antibody were required for the effect (500 μg/mouse, ~25 mg/kg), and were also used in a parallel study demonstrating that DTA-1 increased CD4+ and CD8+ T cell accumulation in Meth A sarcomas, leading to tumor rejection in up to 90 % of treated mice (Ko et al. 2005). Interestingly, the timing of DTA-1 administration had a profound effect on tumor rejection. Early treatment (4 days prior to tumor establishment) or late treatment (12 days post tumor establishment) provided very little benefit, while treatment on day 8 of tumor establishment led to a strong response. This is quite different from OX40 and CD137 (as well as anti-PD-1/L1 and anti-CTLA-4), where the effect of agonistic antibody treatment progressively diminishes as tumors become larger. Similar efficacy was also seen in an established CT26 or RENCA tumor model, where up to 80 % tumor rejection was observed with DTA-1 or Fc-mGITRL fusion protein treatment, mediated by CD4+ and CD8+ effector T cells (Zhou et al. 2007; Hu et al. 2008).

All of the studies referenced to this point were in relative agreement that stimulation of GITR led to (1) increased CD4+ and CD8+ effector cell accumulation, (2) dampened the suppressive effects of Treg, (3) had relatively little influence on Teff phenotype and importantly, (4) did not lead to Treg depletion or instability (Snell et al. 2010; van Olffen et al. 2009). In a study using a much higher dose of DTA-1 (1 mg/mouse, ~50 mg/kg), GITR stimulation was reported to enhance tumor rejection by specifically decreasing Treg within tumors, which lead to a shift in the balance of Teff to Treg in favor of Teff (Cohen et al. 2010). This study was followed up by a report demonstrating that Treg from tumor-bearing mice are more susceptible to GITR mediated depletion than Treg from non-tumor bearing mice. This report also raised the possibility that GITR stimulation may lead to downregulation of FoxP3 and conversion of Treg to Teff (Schaer et al. 2013).

Contemporaneous with the reports of GITR mediated Treg depletion, it was reported that GITR can also support the proliferation of Treg, and that B cell expressed GITR-L (where it is endogenously expressed) supports Treg homeostasis and prevents autoimmunity (Liao et al. 2010; Ray et al. 2012). Another report suggested that the multitude of effects that can be observed following GITR ligation are context dependent, and that different responses in Treg and Teff can be seen in lymphopenia, as compared to autoimmunity, as compared to intra-tumorally (Ephrem et al. 2013). This is likely not far from the truth; however, many unresolved questions remain that may influence the application of GITR agonistic agents to cancer patients.

4 DR3 (TNFRSF25)

TNFRSF25 is the most recently identified family member and is the only death-domain containing costimulatory molecule with an expression pattern and function consistent with the others discussed herein. TNFRSF25 was identified on the basis of a putative death domain and has been given a series of names: DR3, Apo-3, LARD, and TRAMP, with DR3 (death receptor 3) as the most commonly used in the literature (Bodmer et al. 1997; Chinnaiyan et al. 1996; Kitson et al. 1996; Marsters et al. 1996; Screaton et al. 1997). Interestingly, TNFRSF25 has the highest homology to TNFR1 out of all family members, which likely implies early evolutionary divergence. In contrast to TNFR1, TNFRSF25 is expressed almost exclusively by lymphocytes (CD4+, CD8+, NK, NKT), and the level of expression is highest in antigen-experienced memory cells and recently activated T cells (Schreiber and Podack 2013). This texpression profile is extremely similar to that of OX40, which is a close neighbor on chromosome 1 together with CD137 and GITR (Bodmer et al. 2002).

TNFRSF25 binds a single ligand, TL1A, which is a toll-like receptor (TLR) and FcγR inducible ligand predominantly expressed by dendritic cells and macrophages (Migone et al. 2002). The transcriptional kinetics of upregulation and downregulation of TL1A very closely mimic those of OX40L. In mice, TL1A is only reported to interact with TNFRSF25; however, in humans it can also bind decoy receptor 3 (DcR3) (Migone et al. 2002). In keeping with other family members, the functional signaling unit of TL1A appears to be a homo-trimer, interacting with a homo-trimerized TNFRSF25 (Jin et al. 2007a; Jin et al. 2007b).

In transformed tumor cell lines, overexpression of TNFRSF25 or ligation by TL1A leads to the recruitment of "complex 2" (TRAF2/FADD), caspase 3 activation, and apoptosis (Chinnaiyan et al. 1996; Ashkenazi and Dixit 1998). In primary cells, however, TNFRSF25 ligation leads to recruitment of "complex 1" (TRAF2/TRADD), NF-κB activation, survival, proliferation, and effector function. The cues which distinguish between activation of "complex 1" versus "complex 2" remain unclear; however, it has been proposed that increased activity of cIAP2 in primary cells guides signaling in favor of "complex 1"(Warzocha and Salles 1998; Wen et al. 2003). Regardless of the mechanism, the principal functions of TNFRSF25 in primary cells do not include activation of the death domain or apoptosis.

Many of the initial studies of TL1A and TNFRSF25 were performed using transgenic or knockout mouse models in autoimmune disease settings (allergic lung inflammation, EAE, arthritis and inflammatory bowel disease). In all cases, expression of either TL1A or TNFRSF25 was associated with increased disease pathology. Pathology was associated with increased effector cytokine suppression and T cell activation, across each of the CD4+ effector lineages (Th1, Th2, Th9, and Th17) as well as CD8+ and NKT cells. Thus, TNFRSF25 appeared to be a particularly broad-acting T cell costimulator that, if anything, was hazardous to express (Schreiber et al. 2011).

Although Tregs were known to express TNFRSF25 the role of this receptor in modulating Treg function was not clarified by early studies using KO and transgenic animal models. Both TL1A-Ig fusion proteins and TNFRSF25 agonist antibodies were generated by Podack and colleagues, and these agents were observed to stimulate rapid, specific and profound proliferation of CD4+FoxP3+ Treg in mice (Schreiber et al. 2010; Khan et al. 2013). Studying Treg biology in response to TNFRSF25 agonists quickly became a tool with which to better understand the overall biology of the axis. In these studies it was determined that TNFRSF25 signaling in T cells is absolutely dependent upon TCR recognition of MHC-bound cognate antigen ((Schreiber et al. 2010) and Schreiber, unpublished data). Following TCR engagement, TNFRSF25 signaling becomes permissive in T cells and functions to increase the sensitivity of T cells to IL-2 via the IL-2R (Migone et al. 2002; Schreiber et al. 2010). This is associated with increased phosphorylation of Akt on S-475 and downstream activation of FoxO3-family transcription factors (Schreiber, unpublished data). Thus, a potential unifying explanation for the diverse effects of TNFRSF25 across Treg, CD8 and CD4 T cell subsets is likely a result of its role as a TCR-dependent IL-2 sensitizer. This effect is not mediated by increased IL-2 receptor subunit expression or enhanced STAT5 phosphorylation, but may be linked to PTEN inhibition ((Schreiber et al. 2010) and unpublished data).

Like CD137 agonist antibodies, TNFRSF25 agonists can also enhance both immunopathology (desirable in oncology) and tolerance (desirable in inflammation and transplant). In contrast to CD137 agonists, however, TNFRSF25 agonists lead to predictable effects based on the timing of administration of the agonist in proximity to the potentially offending antigen. In inflammation and transplant models, TNFRSF25 agonists must be used in the neo-adjuvant setting (as monotherapy at least) in order to bias the effect of TNFRSF25 toward Treg proliferation. The reason for this is that Treg, but not Teff, regularly encounter cognate "self" antigen, and therefore are preferentially sensitive to TNFRSF25 stimulation. Neo-adjuvant administration of TNFRSF25 agonists leads to Treg expansion, which inhibits pathology in inflammation, transplant and graft-versus-host disease models (Schreiber et al. 2010; Khan et al. 2013; Wolf et al. 2012). If, however, TNFRSF25 agonists are administered in a setting of active inflammation (an existing tumor, combined with a vaccine, during active autoimmunity), disease pathology is increased through the activation of Teff cells (Schreiber et al. 2012; Migone et al. 2002; Bamias et al. 2006; Bull et al. 2008; Fang et al. 2008; Meylan et al. 2008; Meylan et al. 2011; Pappu et al. 2008; Slebioda et al. 2011; Taraban et al. 2011).

Despite the presence of the death domain, there is currently no evidence of specific depletion of effector subsets in animals treated with TNFRSF25 agonists, as has been described for CD137.

In addition to modulating Treg proliferation, TNFRSF25 also inhibits the suppressive activity of Treg and blocks the *de novo* induction of Treg from conventional CD4 cells (Schreiber and Podack 2013; Schreiber et al. 2010; Khan et al. 2013; Meylan et al. 2011). These effects are consistent with what has been described for OX40 and GITR, and may result from conserved biology in these family members. The evolutionary logic for TNFRSF25 in driving Teff and Treg proliferation, inhibiting Treg suppressive function and blocking *de novo* Treg induction remains incompletely characterized. However, it has been described as an overall mechanism to focus the clonality of an immune response toward foreign pathogens, while dampening bystander inflammation against self or commensal antigens (Schreiber and Podack 2013).

5 CD137 (TNFRSF9, 4-1BB)

Like OX40 and CD27, CD137 was identified early as a gene associated with activated CD4+ and CD8+ T cells (Kwon and Weissman 1989). Compared to the other targets discussed, there is the greatest amount of published clinical data available for CD137 agonist antibodies, which have been investigated in at least 12 clinical trials in the US and more worldwide (recently reviewed; (Yonezawa et al. 2015; Melero et al. 2013)). Despite the rapid progression of CD137 agonist antibodies into the clinic, significant questions remain in our understanding of CD137 mediated T cell activation. Like the other TNF receptors being discussed, the CD137 field is split between studies in autoimmunity and studies in oncology. What makes the CD137 agonist literature unique, however, is that the same agonistic antibodies can be applied therapeutically to both prevent autoimmunity and enhance antitumor immunity.

CD137 is expressed at barely detectable levels on naïve CD4+ and CD8+ T cells, but is strongly upregulated following activation in CD4+ and CD8+ T cells as well as natural killer cells (Kwon and Weissman 1989; Croft 2003; Vinay and Kwon 1998; Watts 2005). In addition, CD137 is constitutively expressed in Treg cells (Gavin et al. 2002; McHugh et al. 2002). Interestingly, CD137 expression appears to be downstream of IL-2 signaling in T cells, which is clearly distinct from OX40 and TNFRSF25 (Elpek et al. 2007). The early literature showed that CD137 stimulation using either agonist antibodies or 4-1BBL fusion proteins stimulated proliferation of both CD4+ and CD8+ T cells, and that generally, proliferation was greater for CD8+ T cells. In addition to causing proliferation, CD137 stimulation increased effector cytokine production by activated T cells, especially IFNγ, and could be used to stimulate effective antitumor immunity in a large number of preclinical tumor models. Generally speaking, CD137 agonists were effective as monotherapy in what are considered the "immunogenic" tumor models (including MCA205 and GL261), but worked only in combinations in the "non-immunogenic" tumor models (including B16, C3, TC1, ID8, AG104, EMT6, M109) (McMillin et al. 2006; Shi and Siemann 2006; Curran et al. 2011; Vinay and Kwon 2012; Guo et al. 2013; Kohrt et al. 2014; Melero et al. 1997; Melero et al. 2008). Effective combinations included certain vaccines, radiation therapy, certain chemotherapy as well as combinations with other immunomodulatory antibodies (Uno et al. 2006). The need for combination therapy in non-immunogenic tumors is likely related to antigen release as a result of tumor lysis, which leads to activation of a T cell response that can be costimulated through CD137. More recent data using targeted therapies such as cetuximab has demonstrated rapid upregulation of CD137 by human NK cells, which can then be further costimulated by CD137 agonist antibodies to reject established tumors in an NK and CD8 dependent manner (Kohrt et al. 2014).

Treg cells express CD137 constitutively, and CD137 appears to control several important aspects of Treg function (Gavin et al. 2002; McHugh et al. 2002; Elpek et al. 2007; So et al. 2008). Treg proliferation is stimulated by CD137 in vitro in the presence of anti-CD3 or APC and IL-2, and has also been reported in vivo following administration of CD137 agonist antibodies (either 3H3 or LOB 12.3) in both tumor-free and tumor-bearing mice. Treg that are expanded through CD137 remain highly suppressive to Teff cells following removal of CD137 agonists, but suppression is attenuated in the continuous presence of an agonist (Elpek et al. 2007; Zheng et al. 2004). Similar to some reports of GITR agonists, CD137 stimulated Teff cells may also become "licensed" to resist suppression by Treg cells.

Given the activity of CD137 agonist antibodies in facilitating tumor rejection, it is surprising that the same antibodies also have activity in preventing autoimmune disease (Foell et al. 2003; Seo et al. 2004; Sun et al. 2002a; Sun et al. 2002b). While it is true that TNFRSF25 agonists can be applied in both settings, the use of TNFRSF25 agonists in autoimmunity and transplantation is purely in the neo-adjuvant settings, whereas with CD137 agonists the setting can be therapeutic. In studies that proved to be a harbinger of later clinical data, chronic stimulation through CD137 was found to cause significantly different immunological outcomes than short-term stimulation (Niu et al. 2007; Lee et al. 2009). Importantly, long-term treatment with CD137 agonist antibodies was found to cause IFNγ associated depletion of early B cells and also activation induced cell death in both CD4+ T cells and NK cells. This is in contrast to short-term stimulation, which in addition to the activities described above, leads to upregulation of PI3K, Akt and Bcl-x_L (Starck et al. 2005). The contribution of CD137 agonist antibodies to reducing immunopathology in autoimmune disease appears related to depletion of autoreactive T cell clones in certain settings. A careful understanding of how human CD137 agonist clones behave, and the timing of administration, will clearly be important to influencing whether or not CD137 stimulation leads to enhanced or inhibited antitumor immunity.

The effects of CD137 agonists appear highly similar to those of TNFRSF25 on both Teff and Treg cells, and both appear more specific to CD8+ stimulation than GITR, OX40 or CD27. The clearest distinction between CD137 and TNFRSF25 appears to be related to TCR and IL-2 dependence. CD137 is the only co-stimulator being discussed that can cause T cell activation (particularly memory cells) in the absence of TCR stimulation, potentially because CD137 activation can directly augment signaling through the TCR (Niu et al. 2007; Nam et al. 2005). TNFRSF25 is exquisitely dependent upon TCR recognition of cognate antigen in the context of MHC molecules for subsequent IL-2 dependent proliferation of T cells. IL-2 dependent expression of CD137 may, therefore, provide an additional regulatory mechanism to prevent antigen-independent proliferation of autoreactive T cells outside of an inflammatory microenvironment with high concentrations of IL-2. A complete characterization of the memory response to CD137 stimulation is lacking, but the high expression of KLRG-1 and decreased memory response to CD137 stimulation in some reports may also indicate that the risk of off-target activation by CD137 is mitigated by programmed inhibition of memory immunity.

There have been at least seven clinical trials testing the activity of CD137 agonistic antibodies in melanoma, non-small cell lung cancer and other metastatic solid tumor indications (recently reviewed in (Yonezawa et al. 2015; Melero et al. 2013). Some clinical responses were observed; however, trials were terminated in phase II as a result of lethal hepatotoxicity at doses as low as 1 mg/kg. Today, several phase I trials have been reinitiated, largely advancing the work of Kohrt and colleagues to enhance responses to targeted antibodies including rituximab, cetuximab, and elotuzumab.

6 CD27 (TNFRSF7)

CD27 was one of the earliest identified TNF receptors, and was designated as such based on binding of several different antibodies (CLB-CD 27/1, 9F4, OKT 18A, VIT 14, and S152) raised against human lymphocytes (Bigler et al. 1988; van Lier et al. 1987). CD27 can be found on naïve as well as activated CD4+ and CD8+ T cells, NK cells and also B cells (Gravestein et al. 1995; Takeda et al. 2000; Tesselaar et al. 2003). Although early studies indicated that CD27 stimulation provides expansion and survival of T cells (CD8 more than CD4), some discordance persists in the literature in defining the context and functional consequence of CD70 signaling to CD27; and whether this promotes or prevents immunopathology. A warning to this discordance was noted in one of the earlier reviews on the axis, where Borst and colleagues commented; "Targeting CD27-CD70 for therapy is attractive, but should take into account the fact that constitutive CD27 stimulation culminates in lethal immunodeficiency" (Borst et al. 2005).

The early observation that CD27 stimulates T cell proliferation was refined by the observation that although increased numbers of T cells are detected in CD27 stimulated cultures, it is due to increased accumulation and survival of T cells rather than increased proliferation (Hendriks et al. 2003). This finding was further investigated several years later and shown to be due to increased development of CD8+CD127+KLRG1- memory precursor cells, which lead to overall enhancement of CD8 memory responses (Dong et al. 2012). The mechanism is not entirely clear; however, blunted responses to IL-12 during priming appear to be partially involved (Dong et al. 2012). Stimulation of CD27 using agonist antibodies also led to increased persistence, but not proliferation of CD8+ T cells within established murine melanoma and contributed to antitumor immunity (Roberts et al. 2010).

Similar to the other costimulators discussed, the context of CD27 costimulation is critical to the resulting effector T cell response. Transgenic expression of CD70 both by B cells and dendritic cells can lead to the development of systemic autoimmunity and death (Arens et al. 2001; Keller et al. 2008). Interestingly, when CD70 is provided by CD11c+ dendritic cells, it promotes CD8+ priming to typically tolerogenic antigen stimulation, memory formation, and effective tumor immunity (Keller et al. 2008). The proliferation of CD8+ cells is enhanced when CD70 is provided by dendritic cells, but not B cells. Given the phenotypic similarity in these two mouse strains albeit with mechanistic distinction in effector activation, it is possible that B cell derived CD70 promotes autoimmunity through preferential and unique inactivation of Treg cells. This possibility would mirror reports of B cell derived GITRL providing important signals for the maintenance of Treg and prevention of autoimmunity (van Olffen et al. 2009; Ray et al. 2012).

Treg cells also express high levels of CD27, and it has been associated with the most highly suppressive Treg in some tissues (Mack et al. 2009). Within the thymic medulla, CD70 expression is also important for the development of self-reactive "natural" Treg (nTreg or tTreg) (Coquet et al. 2013). Within transplanted tumor fragments, CD27 stimulation has been reported to promote Treg proliferation and contribute to tumor progression (Riether et al. 2012; Claus et al. 2012). In other reports, CD27 stimulation promotes CD8+ T cell persistence in tumors and decreased PD-1 expression, leading to improved tumor control without rejection (Roberts et al. 2010). As a result, both CD27 stimulation and CD27 blockade have been proposed as strategies to enhance antitumor immunity (Riether et al. 2012; Thomas et al. 2014).

A monoclonal antibody targeting CD27 (1F5, CDX-1127) has entered clinical development for the treatment of human cancer. Interestingly, this antibody is agonistic and causes human T cell proliferation when it is bound to the surface of the culture vessel together with an anti-CD3 antibody. However, in human tumor xenografts, the antitumor activity of this antibody is due to antibody-dependent cellular cytotoxicity (ADCC), and not agonistic activity (Vitale et al. 2012). Other reports confirm that the agonistic activity of this antibody is only observed when the antibody is cross-linked or plate-bound, and preclinical data in human CD27 transgenic mice demonstrate dependence upon Fc receptor binding (FcγRI and IV) for antitumor activity, which is not yet directly linked to agonistic activity (Thomas et al. 2014; He et al. 2013). As a result, the clinical data generated with CDX-1127 is needed to inform whether clinical benefit (if observed) is related to effector cell activation, ADCC mediated Treg or tumor cell depletion, or both.

7 Conclusions

Adaptive immune responses are clearly complex, and are regulated by a nonlinear but generally hierarchical series of Ig and TNF superfamily molecules downstream of the T cell receptor. Integration of the signaling pathways downstream of these membrane receptors modulates T cell sensitivity to particular cytokines, which in turn governs cell cycle regulation, survival, and effector function within individual subsets of T cells. In reviewing the activities of OX40, GITR, TNFRSF25, CD137, and CD27, it is clear that many characteristics are overlapping, and distinctions are subtle and context dependent.

Beginning with the expression patterns of each receptor, the data suggest that the primary roles of GITR and CD27 may be unique from OX40, TNFRSF25, and CD137. CD27, expressed at relatively high levels by naïve CD4+ and CD8+ T cells, is unique in its effects to facilitate T cell survival and memory without being directly pro-proliferative. The role for CD70 expression in the thymus is likely to facilitate the survival of thymic-derived Treg cells recognizing self-antigen. In general, the effects of CD27 appear to be more pronounced on effector CD8 cells than effector CD4 cells. The expression of GITR-L is unique in that it is mostly localized to B cells, and that it is downregulated upon B cell activation. This expression pattern, combined with the constitutive expression of GITR by highly suppressive Treg, suggests that B cell derived GITR-L is important for the homeostatic maintenance of Treg cells. There are clearly complexities to the GITR axis, however, and a multitude of reported functions including the depletion or conversion of Treg to Teff cells. Interestingly, these sorts of effects have only been reported with GITR agonist antibody doses that exceed any dose range currently being tested for OX40, CD137, or CD27 agonist antibodies in clinical studies by between 5 and 100-fold (an equivalent of approximately 50 mg/kg).

OX40, TNFRSF25, and CD137 are all quite similar in that they are expressed at very low levels by naïve T cells, their ligands are virtually absent on non-activated APCs, and both the receptors and ligands are rapidly upregulated by both populations following innate stimulation. These receptors are also constitutively expressed by Treg, and can influence the proliferation, dampen suppressive activity and block induction of new Treg cells. Although TNFRSF25 seems to deliver a stronger proliferative signal to Treg than either OX40 or CD137, this may be due to the underlying mechanism of increasing IL-2 sensitivity in Treg, which constitutively express high amounts of CD25 as well. A distinction between OX40 and both TNFRSF25 and CD137 appears to be the preferential stimulation of memory CD4+ Teff cells; which is not necessarily apparent in studies that analyze only the primary immune response to an antigen. A clear distinction in the functional outcome of TNFRSF25 and CD137 signaling has yet to be systematically characterized. Both receptors seem to preferentially activate CD8+ T cells over CD4+ T cells, and both receptors are related to IL-2 signaling in T cells. In the case of TNFRSF25, it seems to function as an IL-2 sensitizer, whereas CD137 expression is dependent upon IL-2 and leads to the potentiation of TCR signaling. This suggests differential signaling pathways downstream of CD137 and TNFRSF25, and the mechanism by which TNFRSF25 leads to increased T cell sensitivity to IL-2 may be related to increased phospho-PTEN (T Schreiber, unpublished data). In general, however, it appears that short-term stimulation of CD137 provides a proliferative burst to CD8+ T cells whereas stimulation of TNFRSF25 seems to provide a more sustained proliferative signal that is correlated with increased memory CD8+ T cell responses.

It is important to recognize that OX40, CD137, GITR, TNFRSF25, and CD27 all have antitumor activity, which is generally limited to immunogenic tumor models. The preclinical tumor models in which agonistic antibodies to these receptors have been investigated all inform *only* to the activity of these receptors in the context of a primary immune response with short-term exposure to an agonistic antibody. This is because orthotopic tumor models are lethal within relatively short periods of time, wherein there is very limited time for maturation of T cells into bona fide "memory" cells. It is not possible, on the basis of a literature review, to draw conclusions as to the relative potency of each of these receptors in facilitating an antitumor immune response. This is because each tumor model is unique, even models with the same name (e.g., B16) may be testing cell lines that have been propagated in culture so long that the underlying immunogenicity/tumorigenicity of the tumors are distinct. Additionally, the doses of antibody used vary widely and have not been standardized and the timing of treatment relative to tumor dose and inoculation can be quite varied. What can be safely concluded, however, is that the activity of agonist antibodies for any of these costimulators is unlikely to be impressive when administered as monotherapy.

The observation of therapeutic tumor immunity following treatment with costimulatory receptor agonists, concurrent with expansion of both Teff and Treg, has perplexed many in the field. The nonredundant role for Treg in preventing autoimmunity and the observation that Treg depletion (using anti-CD25 antibodies or FoxP3-DTR mouse strains) leads to improved tumor control in many mouse models has supported the overall hypothesis that Treg are generally antagonistic to tumor immunity. This hypothesis does not take into account a significant amount of recent evidence demonstrating that durable immunity actually requires concurrent proliferation of both Treg and Teff cells. These recent studies have shown that during the contraction phase of an immune response, Treg are actually required for the formation of effective memory CD8+ T cells. The mechanism for this interaction seems to involve IL-10 and TGF-β, which are necessary for CD8+ memory formation by "insulating" memory precursor cells from the inflammatory milieu in a resolving immune response (de Goer de Herve et al. 2012; Graham et al. 2014; Laidlaw et al. 2015; Pace et al. 2012). These data suggest that concurrent Teff and Treg activation by some TNF receptors may in fact be vital to a durable CD8+ T cell response, an effect that is not accurately modeled by short-term orthotopic mouse tumor models.

Because monotherapy with T cell costimulatory agents is unlikely to lead to significant efficacy in humans, the focus on combination regimens should be on the basis of the underlying mechanism, not any particular tumor survival curve from a preclinical study. The current clinical trials with CD137 agonists given in combination with targeted agents are a good example. In this case, mechanistic preclinical data strongly indicate that targeted agents lead to increased expression of CD137 on NK cells, which could be targeted with CD137 agonists to enhance ADCC of target-antibody coated tumor cells. This is a significantly different direction than was taken with the initial CD137 agonist trials, which more directly investigated the effects of pure agonism of CD8+ T cells, and led to significant toxicity. Many monotherapy phase I trials are now underway with GITR and OX40 agonists, which may be valuable in defining toxicity and certain aspects of the pharmacokinetics and pharmacodynamics of the agents being tested. To maximize the clinical potential of this promising class of agents, however, investigators should strongly consider innovative combination trial designs, even in phase I, and work closely with regulatory agencies to ensure that those designs can be as informative as possible in validating the mechanistic insights provided from preclinical studies.

References

Akiba, H., Oshima, H., Takeda, K., Atsuta, M., Nakano, H., Nakajima, A., et al.: CD28-independent costimulation of T cells by OX40 ligand and CD70 on activated B cells. J. Immunol. **162**, 7058–7066 (1999)

Arens, R., Tesselaar, K., Baars, P.A., van Schijndel, G.M., Hendriks, J., Pals, S.T., et al.: Constitutive CD27/CD70 interaction induces expansion of effector-type T cells and results in IFNgamma-mediated B cell depletion. Immunity **15**, 801–812 (2001)

Ashkenazi, A., Dixit, V.M.: Death receptors: signaling and modulation. Science **281**, 1305–1308 (1998)

Bamias, G., Mishina, M., Nyce, M., Ross, W.G., Kollias, G., Rivera-Nieves, J., et al.: Role of TL1A and its receptor DR3 in two models of chronic murine ileitis. Proc. Natl. Acad. Sci. U. S. A. **103**, 8441–8446 (2006)

Bigler, R.D., Bushkin, Y., Chiorazzi, N.: S152 (CD27). A modulating disulfide-linked T cell activation antigen. J. Immunol. **141**, 21–28 (1988)

Bodmer, J.L., Burns, K., Schneider, P., Hofmann, K., Steiner, V., Thome, M., et al.: TRAMP, a novel apoptosis-mediating receptor with sequence homology to tumor necrosis factor receptor 1 and Fas(Apo-1/CD95). Immunity **6**, 79–88 (1997)

Bodmer, J.L., Schneider, P., Tschopp, J.: The molecular architecture of the TNF superfamily. Trends Biochem. Sci. **27**, 19–26 (2002)

Borst, J., Hendriks, J., Xiao, Y.: CD27 and CD70 in T cell and B cell activation. Curr. Opin. Immunol. **17**, 275–281 (2005)

Bull, M.J., Williams, A.S., Mecklenburgh, Z., Calder, C.J., Twohig, J.P., Elford, C., et al.: The death receptor 3-TNF-like protein 1A pathway drives adverse bone pathology in inflammatory arthritis. J. Exp. Med. **205**, 2457–2464 (2008)

Bulliard, Y., Jolicoeur, R., Zhang, J., Dranoff, G., Wilson, N.S., Brogdon, J.L.: OX40 engagement depletes intratumoral Tregs via activating FcgammaRs, leading to antitumor efficacy. Immunol. Cell Biol. **92**, 475–480 (2014)

Calderhead, D.M., Buhlmann, J.E., van den Eertwegh, A.J., Claassen, E., Noelle, R.J., Fell, H.P.: Cloning of mouse Ox40: a T cell activation marker that may mediate T-B cell interactions. J. Immunol. **151**, 5261–5271 (1993)

Chinnaiyan, A.M., O'Rourke, K., Yu, G.L., Lyons, R.H., Garg, M., Duan, D.R., et al.: Signal transduction by DR3, a death domain-containing receptor related to TNFR-1 and CD95. Science **274**, 990–992 (1996)

Claus, C., Riether, C., Schurch, C., Matter, M.S., Hilmenyuk, T., Ochsenbein, A.F.: CD27 signaling increases the frequency of regulatory T cells and promotes tumor growth. Cancer Res. **72**, 3664–3676 (2012)

Cohen, A.D., Schaer, D.A., Liu, C., Li, Y., Hirschhorn-Cymmerman, D., Kim, S.C., et al.: Agonist anti-GITR monoclonal antibody induces melanoma tumor immunity in mice by altering regulatory T cell stability and intra-tumor accumulation. PLoS One **5**, e10436 (2010)

Coquet, J.M., Ribot, J.C., Babala, N., Middendorp, S., van der Horst, G., Xiao, Y., et al.: Epithelial and dendritic cells in the thymic medulla promote CD4+Foxp3+ regulatory T cell development via the CD27-CD70 pathway. J. Exp. Med. **210**, 715–728 (2013)

Croft, M.: Co-stimulatory members of the TNFR family: keys to effective T-cell immunity? Nat. Rev. Immunol. **3**, 609–620 (2003)

Curran, M.A., Kim, M., Montalvo, W., Al-Shamkhani, A., Allison, J.P.: Combination CTLA-4 blockade and 4-1BB activation enhances tumor rejection by increasing T-cell infiltration, proliferation, and cytokine production. PLoS One **6**, e19499 (2011)

Curti, B.D., Kovacsovics-Bankowski, M., Morris, N., Walker, E., Chisholm, L., Floyd, K., et al.: OX40 is a potent immune-stimulating target in late-stage cancer patients. Cancer Res. **73**, 7189–7198 (2013)

de Goer de Herve, M.G., Jaafoura, S., Vallee, M., Taoufik, Y.: FoxP3(+) regulatory CD4 T cells control the generation of functional CD8 memory. Nat. Commun. **3**, 986 (2012)

Dong, H., Franklin, N.A., Roberts, D.J., Yagita, H., Glennie, M.J., Bullock, T.N.: CD27 stimulation promotes the frequency of IL-7 receptor-expressing memory precursors and prevents IL-12-mediated loss of CD8(+) T cell memory in the absence of CD4(+) T cell help. J. Immunol. **188**, 3829–3838 (2012)

Duan, W., So, T., Croft, M.: Antagonism of airway tolerance by endotoxin/lipopolysaccharide through promoting OX40L and suppressing antigen-specific Foxp3+ T regulatory cells. J. Immunol. **181**, 8650–8659 (2008)

Elpek, K.G., Yolcu, E.S., Franke, D.D., Lacelle, C., Schabowsky, R.H., Shirwan, H.: Ex vivo expansion of CD4+CD25+FoxP3+ T regulatory cells based on synergy between IL-2 and 4-1BB signaling. J. Immunol. **179**, 7295–7304 (2007)

Ephrem, A., Epstein, A.L., Stephens, G.L., Thornton, A.M., Glass, D., Shevach, E.M.: Modulation of Treg cells/T effector function by GITR signaling is context-dependent. Eur. J. Immunol. **43**, 2421–2429 (2013)

Fang, L., Adkins, B., Deyev, V., Podack, E.R.: Essential role of TNF receptor superfamily 25 (TNFRSF25) in the development of allergic lung inflammation. J. Exp. Med. **205**, 1037–1048 (2008)

Foell, J., Strahotin, S., O'Neil, S.P., McCausland, M.M., Suwyn, C., Haber, M., et al.: CD137 costimulatory T cell receptor engagement reverses acute disease in lupus-prone NZB x NZW F1 mice. J. Clin. Invest. **111**, 1505–1518 (2003)

Gaspal, F., Withers, D., Saini, M., Bekiaris, V., McConnell, F.M., White, A., et al.: Abrogation of CD30 and OX40 signals prevents autoimmune disease in FoxP3-deficient mice. J. Exp. Med. **208**, 1579–1584 (2011)

Gavin, M.A., Clarke, S.R., Negrou, E., Gallegos, A., Rudensky, A.: Homeostasis and anergy of CD4(+)CD25(+) suppressor T cells in vivo. Nat. Immunol. **3**, 33–41 (2002)

Godfrey, W.R., Fagnoni, F.F., Harara, M.A., Buck, D., Engleman, E.G.: Identification of a human OX-40 ligand, a costimulator of CD4+ T cells with homology to tumor necrosis factor. J. Exp. Med. **180**, 757–762 (1994)

Gopisetty, A., Bhattacharya, P., Haddad, C., Bruno Jr., J.C., Vasu, C., Miele, L., et al.: OX40L/Jagged1 cosignaling by GM-CSF-induced bone marrow-derived dendritic cells is required for the expansion of functional regulatory T cells. J. Immunol. **190**, 5516–5525 (2013)

Graham, J.B., Da Costa, A., Lund, J.M.: Regulatory T cells shape the resident memory T cell response to virus infection in the tissues. J. Immunol. **192**, 683–690 (2014)

Gramaglia, I., Weinberg, A.D., Lemon, M., Croft, M.: Ox-40 ligand: a potent costimulatory molecule for sustaining primary CD4 T cell responses. J. Immunol. **161**, 6510–6517 (1998)

Gravestein, L.A., Nieland, J.D., Kruisbeek, A.M., Borst, J.: Novel mAbs reveal potent co-stimulatory activity of murine CD27. Int. Immunol. **7**, 551–557 (1995)

Griseri, T., Asquith, M., Thompson, C., Powrie, F.: OX40 is required for regulatory T cell-mediated control of colitis. J. Exp. Med. **207**, 699–709 (2010)

Guo, Z., Cheng, D., Xia, Z., Luan, M., Wu, L., Wang, G., et al.: Combined TIM-3 blockade and CD137 activation affords the long-term protection in a murine model of ovarian cancer. J. Transl. Med. **11**, 215 (2013)

He, L.Z., Prostak, N., Thomas, L.J., Vitale, L., Weidlick, J., Crocker, A., et al.: Agonist anti-human CD27 monoclonal antibody induces T cell activation and tumor immunity in human CD27-transgenic mice. J. Immunol. **191**, 4174–4183 (2013)

Hendriks, J., Xiao, Y., Borst, J.: CD27 promotes survival of activated T cells and complements CD28 in generation and establishment of the effector T cell pool. J. Exp. Med. **198**, 1369–1380 (2003)

Hirschhorn-Cymerman, D., Rizzuto, G.A., Merghoub, T., Cohen, A.D., Avogadri, F., Lesokhin, A.M., et al.: OX40 engagement and chemotherapy combination provides potent antitumor immunity with concomitant regulatory T cell apoptosis. J. Exp. Med. **206**, 1103–1116 (2009)

Hu, P., Arias, R.S., Sadun, R.E., Nien, Y.C., Zhang, N., Sabzevari, H., et al.: Construction and preclinical characterization of Fc-mGITRL for the immunotherapy of cancer. Clin. Cancer Res. **14**, 579–588 (2008)

Jin, T., Kim, S., Guo, F., Howard, A., Zhang, Y.Z.: Purification and crystallization of recombinant human TNF-like ligand TL1A. Cytokine **40**, 115–122 (2007a)

Jin, T., Guo, F., Kim, S., Howard, A., Zhang, Y.Z.: X-ray crystal structure of TNF ligand family member TL1A at 2.1A. Biochem. Biophys. Res. Commun. **364**, 1–6 (2007b)

Keller, A.M., Schildknecht, A., Xiao, Y., van den Broek, M., Borst, J.: Expression of costimulatory ligand CD70 on steady-state dendritic cells breaks CD8+ T cell tolerance and permits effective immunity. Immunity **29**, 934–946 (2008)

Khan, S.Q., Tsai, M.S., Schreiber, T.H., Wolf, D., Deyev, V.V., Podack, E.R.: Cloning, expression, and functional characterization of TL1A-Ig. J. Immunol. **190**, 1540–1550 (2013)

Kitson, J., Raven, T., Jiang, Y.P., Goeddel, D.V., Giles, K.M., Pun, K.T., et al.: A death-domain-containing receptor that mediates apoptosis. Nature **384**, 372–375 (1996)

Kjaergaard, J., Tanaka, J., Kim, J.A., Rothchild, K., Weinberg, A., Shu, S.: Therapeutic efficacy of OX-40 receptor antibody depends on tumor immunogenicity and anatomic site of tumor growth. Cancer Res. **60**, 5514–5521 (2000)

Ko, K., Yamazaki, S., Nakamura, K., Nishioka, T., Hirota, K., Yamaguchi, T., et al.: Treatment of advanced tumors with agonistic anti-GITR mAb and its effects on tumor-infiltrating Foxp3 + CD25 + CD4+ regulatory T cells. J. Exp. Med. **202**, 885–891 (2005)

Kohm, A.P., Williams, J.S., Miller, S.D.: Cutting edge: ligation of the glucocorticoid-induced TNF receptor enhances autoreactive CD4+ T cell activation and experimental autoimmune encephalomyelitis. J. Immunol. **172**, 4686–4690 (2004)

Kohrt, H.E., Colevas, A.D., Houot, R., Weiskopf, K., Goldstein, M.J., Lund, P., et al.: Targeting CD137 enhances the efficacy of cetuximab. J. Clin. Invest. **124**, 2668–2682 (2014)

Kroemer, A., Xiao, X., Vu, M.D., Gao, W., Minamimura, K., Chen, M., et al.: OX40 controls functionally different T cell subsets and their resistance to depletion therapy. J. Immunol. **179**, 5584–5591 (2007)

Kwon, B.S., Weissman, S.M.: cDNA sequences of two inducible T-cell genes. Proc. Natl. Acad. Sci. U. S. A. **86**, 1963–1967 (1989)

Laidlaw, B.J., Cui, W., Amezquita, R.A., Gray, S.M., Guan, T., Lu, Y., et al.: Production of IL-10 by CD4(+) regulatory T cells during the resolution of infection promotes the maturation of memory CD8(+) T cells. Nat. Immunol. **16**, 871–879 (2015)

Lee, S.W., Salek-Ardakani, S., Mittler, R.S., Croft, M.: Hypercostimulation through 4-1BB distorts homeostasis of immune cells. J. Immunol. **182**, 6753–6762 (2009)

Liao, G., Nayak, S., Regueiro, J.R., Berger, S.B., Detre, C., Romero, X., et al.: GITR engagement preferentially enhances proliferation of functionally competent CD4 + CD25 + FoxP3+ regulatory T cells. Int. Immunol. **22**, 259–270 (2010)

Mack, D.G., Lanham, A.M., Palmer, B.E., Maier, L.A., Fontenot, A.P.: CD27 expression on CD4+ T cells differentiates effector from regulatory T cell subsets in the lung. J. Immunol. **182**, 7317–7324 (2009)

Mahoney, K.M., Rennert, P.D., Freeman, G.J.: Combination cancer immunotherapy and new immunomodulatory targets. Nat. Rev. Drug Discov. **14**, 561–584 (2015)

Mallett, S., Fossum, S., Barclay, A.N.: Characterization of the MRC OX40 antigen of activated CD4 positive T lymphocytes--a molecule related to nerve growth factor receptor. EMBO J. **9**, 1063–1068 (1990)

Marsters, S.A., Sheridan, J.P., Donahue, C.J., Pitti, R.M., Gray, C.L., Goddard, A.D., et al.: Apo-3, a new member of the tumor necrosis factor receptor family, contains a death domain and activates apoptosis and NF-kappa B. Curr. Biol.. **6**, 1669–1676 (1996)

McHugh, R.S., Whitters, M.J., Piccirillo, C.A., Young, D.A., Shevach, E.M., Collins, M., et al.: CD4(+)CD25(+) immunoregulatory T cells: gene expression analysis reveals a functional role for the glucocorticoid-induced TNF receptor. Immunity **16**, 311–323 (2002)

McMillin, D.W., Hewes, B., Gangadharan, B., Archer, D.R., Mittler, R.S., Spencer, H.T.: Complete regression of large solid tumors using engineered drug-resistant hematopoietic cells and anti-CD137 immunotherapy. Hum. Gene Ther. **17**, 798–806 (2006)

Melero, I., Shuford, W.W., Newby, S.A., Aruffo, A., Ledbetter, J.A., Hellstrom, K.E., et al.: Monoclonal antibodies against the 4-1BB T-cell activation molecule eradicate established tumors. Nat. Med. **3**, 682–685 (1997)

Melero, I., Murillo, O., Dubrot, J., Hervas-Stubbs, S., Perez-Gracia, J.L.: Multi-layered action mechanisms of CD137 (4-1BB)-targeted immunotherapies. Trends Pharmacol. Sci. **29**, 383–390 (2008)

Melero, I., Hirschhorn-Cymerman, D., Morales-Kastresana, A., Sanmamed, M.F., Wolchok, J.D.: Agonist antibodies to TNFR molecules that costimulate T and NK cells. Clin. Cancer Res. **19**, 1044–1053 (2013)

Meylan, F., Davidson, T.S., Kahle, E., Kinder, M., Acharya, K., Jankovic, D., et al.: The TNF-family receptor DR3 is essential for diverse T cell-mediated inflammatory diseases. Immunity **29**, 79–89 (2008)

Meylan, F., Song, Y.J., Fuss, I., Villarreal, S., Kahle, E., Malm, I.J., et al.: The TNF-family cytokine TL1A drives IL-13-dependent small intestinal inflammation. Mucosal immunol. **4**, 172–185 (2011)

Migone, T.S., Zhang, J., Luo, X., Zhuang, L., Chen, C., Hu, B., et al.: TL1A is a TNF-like ligand for DR3 and TR6/DcR3 and functions as a T cell costimulator. Immunity **16**, 479–492 (2002)

Nam, K.O., Kang, W.J., Kwon, B.S., Kim, S.J., Lee, H.W.: The therapeutic potential of 4-1BB (CD137) in cancer. Curr. Cancer Drug Targets **5**, 357–363 (2005)

Niu, L., Strahotin, S., Hewes, B., Zhang, B., Zhang, Y., Archer, D., et al.: Cytokine-mediated disruption of lymphocyte trafficking, hemopoiesis, and induction of lymphopenia, anemia, and thrombocytopenia in anti-CD137-treated mice. J. Immunol. **178**, 4194–4213 (2007)

Pace, L., Tempez, A., Arnold-Schrauf, C., Lemaitre, F., Bousso, P., Fetler, L., et al.: Regulatory T cells increase the avidity of primary CD8+ T cell responses and promote memory. Science **338**, 532–536 (2012)

Pappu, B.P., Borodovsky, A., Zheng, T.S., Yang, X., Wu, P., Dong, X., et al.: TL1A-DR3 interaction regulates Th17 cell function and Th17-mediated autoimmune disease. J. Exp. Med. **205**, 1049–1062 (2008)

Ray, A., Basu, S., Williams, C.B., Salzman, N.H., Dittel, B.N.: A novel IL-10-independent regulatory role for B cells in suppressing autoimmunity by maintenance of regulatory T cells via GITR ligand. J. Immunol. **188**, 3188–3198 (2012)

Redmond, W.L., Linch, S.N., Kasiewicz, M.J.: Combined targeting of costimulatory (OX40) and coinhibitory (CTLA-4) pathways elicits potent effector T cells capable of driving robust antitumor immunity. Cancer Immun. Res. **2**, 142–153 (2014)

Riether, C., Schurch, C., Ochsenbein, A.F.: Modulating CD27 signaling to treat cancer. Oncoimmunology **1**, 1604–1606 (2012)

Roberts, D.J., Franklin, N.A., Kingeter, L.M., Yagita, H., Tutt, A.L., Glennie, M.J., et al.: Control of established melanoma by CD27 stimulation is associated with enhanced effector function and persistence, and reduced PD-1 expression of tumor infiltrating CD8(+) T cells. J. Immunother. **33**, 769–779 (2010)

Ruby, C.E., Redmond, W.L., Haley, D., Weinberg, A.D.: Anti-OX40 stimulation in vivo enhances CD8+ memory T cell survival and significantly increases recall responses. Eur. J. Immunol. **37**, 157–166 (2007)

Schaer, D.A., Budhu, S., Liu, C., Bryson, C., Malandro, N., Cohen, A., et al.: GITR pathway activation abrogates tumor immune suppression through loss of regulatory T cell lineage stability. Cancer Immun. Res. **1**, 320–331 (2013)

Schreiber, T.H., Podack, E.R.: Immunobiology of TNFSF15 and TNFRSF25. Immunol. Res. **57**, 3–11 (2013)

Schreiber, T.H., Wolf, D., Tsai, M.S., Chirinos, J., Deyev, V.V., Gonzalez, L., et al.: Therapeutic Treg expansion in mice by TNFRSF25 prevents allergic lung inflammation. J. Clin. Invest. **120**, 3629–3640 (2010)

Schreiber, T.H., Wolf, D., Podack, E.R.: The role of TNFRSF25:TNFSF15 in disease... health? Adv. Exp. Med. Biol. **691**, 289–298 (2011)

Schreiber, T.H., Wolf, D., Bodero, M., Gonzalez, L., Podack, E.R.: T cell costimulation by TNFR superfamily (TNFRSF)4 and TNFRSF25 in the context of vaccination. J. Immunol. **189**, 3311–3318 (2012)

Screaton, G.R., Xu, X.N., Olsen, A.L., Cowper, A.E., Tan, R., McMichael, A.J., et al.: LARD: a new lymphoid-specific death domain containing receptor regulated by alternative pre-mRNA splicing. Proc. Natl. Acad. Sci. U. S. A. **94**, 4615–4619 (1997)

Seo, S.K., Choi, J.H., Kim, Y.H., Kang, W.J., Park, H.Y., Suh, J.H., et al.: 4-1BB-mediated immunotherapy of rheumatoid arthritis. Nat. Med. **10**, 1088–1094 (2004)

Shi, W., Siemann, D.W.: Augmented antitumor effects of radiation therapy by 4-1BB antibody (BMS-469492) treatment. Anticancer Res. **26**, 3445–3453 (2006)

Shimizu, J., Yamazaki, S., Takahashi, T., Ishida, Y., Sakaguchi, S.: Stimulation of CD25(+) CD4(+) regulatory T cells through GITR breaks immunological self-tolerance. Nat. Immunol. **3**, 135–142 (2002)

Slebioda, T.J., Rowley, T.F., Ferdinand, J.R., Willoughby, J.E., Buchan, S.L., Taraban, V.Y., et al.: Triggering of TNFRSF25 promotes CD8(+) T-cell responses and anti-tumor immunity. Eur. J. Immunol. **41**, 2606–2611 (2011)

Snell, L.M., McPherson, A.J., Lin, G.H., Sakaguchi, S., Pandolfi, P.P., Riccardi, C., et al.: CD8 T cell-intrinsic GITR is required for T cell clonal expansion and mouse survival following severe influenza infection. J. Immunol. **185**, 7223–7234 (2010)

So, T., Croft, M.: Cutting edge: OX40 inhibits TGF-beta- and antigen-driven conversion of naive CD4 T cells into CD25+Foxp3+ T cells. J. Immunol. **179**, 1427–1430 (2007)

So, T., Lee, S.W., Croft, M.: Immune regulation and control of regulatory T cells by OX40 and 4-1BB. Cytokine Growth Factor Rev. **19**, 253–262 (2008)

Song, J., Salek-Ardakani, S., Rogers, P.R., Cheng, M., Van Parijs, L., Croft, M.: The costimulation-regulated duration of PKB activation controls T cell longevity. Nat. Immunol. **5**, 150–158 (2004)

Starck, L., Scholz, C., Dorken, B., Daniel, P.T.: Costimulation by CD137/4-1BB inhibits T cell apoptosis and induces Bcl-xL and c-FLIP(short) via phosphatidylinositol 3-kinase and AKT/protein kinase B. Eur. J. Immunol. **35**, 1257–1266 (2005)

Stephens, G.L., McHugh, R.S., Whitters, M.J., Young, D.A., Luxenberg, D., Carreno, B.M., et al.: Engagement of glucocorticoid-induced TNFR family-related receptor on effector T cells by its ligand mediates resistance to suppression by CD4+CD25+ T cells. J. Immunol. **173**, 5008–5020 (2004)

Sun, Y., Chen, H.M., Subudhi, S.K., Chen, J., Koka, R., Chen, L., et al.: Costimulatory molecule-targeted antibody therapy of a spontaneous autoimmune disease. Nat. Med. **8**, 1405–1413 (2002a)

Sun, Y., Lin, X., Chen, H.M., Wu, Q., Subudhi, S.K., Chen, L., et al.: Administration of agonistic anti-4-1BB monoclonal antibody leads to the amelioration of experimental autoimmune encephalomyelitis. J. Immunol. **168**, 1457–1465 (2002b)

Takeda, K., Oshima, H., Hayakawa, Y., Akiba, H., Atsuta, M., Kobata, T., et al.: CD27-mediated activation of murine NK cells. J. Immunol. **164**, 1741–1745 (2000)

Takeda, I., Ine, S., Killeen, N., Ndhlovu, L.C., Murata, K., Satomi, S., et al.: Distinct roles for the OX40-OX40 ligand interaction in regulatory and nonregulatory T cells. J. Immunol. **172**, 3580–3589 (2004)

Takeda, K., Kojima, Y., Uno, T., Hayakawa, Y., Teng, M.W., Yoshizawa, H., et al.: Combination therapy of established tumors by antibodies targeting immune activating and suppressing molecules. J. Immunol. **184**, 5493–5501 (2010)

Taraban, V.Y., Slebioda, T.J., Willoughby, J.E., Buchan, S.L., James, S., Sheth, B., et al.: Sustained TL1A expression modulates effector and regulatory T-cell responses and drives intestinal goblet cell hyperplasia. Mucosal immunol. **4**, 186–196 (2011)

Tesselaar, K., Xiao, Y., Arens, R., van Schijndel, G.M., Schuurhuis, D.H., Mebius, R.E., et al.: Expression of the murine CD27 ligand CD70 in vitro and in vivo. J. Immunol. **170**, 33–40 (2003)

Thomas, L.J., He, L.Z., Marsh, H., Keler, T.: Targeting human CD27 with an agonist antibody stimulates T-cell activation and antitumor immunity. Oncoimmunology **3**, e27255 (2014)

Uno, T., Takeda, K., Kojima, Y., Yoshizawa, H., Akiba, H., Mittler, R.S., et al.: Eradication of established tumors in mice by a combination antibody-based therapy. Nat. Med. **12**, 693–698 (2006)

van Lier, R.A., Borst, J., Vroom, T.M., Klein, H., Van Mourik, P., Zeijlemaker, W.P., et al.: Tissue distribution and biochemical and functional properties of Tp55 (CD27), a novel T cell differentiation antigen. J. Immunol. **139**, 1589–1596 (1987)

van Olffen, R.W., Koning, N., van Gisbergen, K.P., Wensveen, F.M., Hoek, R.M., Boon, L., et al.: GITR triggering induces expansion of both effector and regulatory CD4+ T cells in vivo. J. Immunol. **182**, 7490–7500 (2009)

Vinay, D.S., Kwon, B.S.: Role of 4-1BB in immune responses. Semin. Immunol. **10**, 481–489 (1998)

Vinay, D.S., Kwon, B.S.: Immunotherapy of cancer with 4-1BB. Mol. Cancer Ther. **11**, 1062–1070 (2012)

Vitale, L.A., He, L.Z., Thomas, L.J., Widger, J., Weidlick, J., Crocker, A., et al.: Development of a human monoclonal antibody for potential therapy of CD27-expressing lymphoma and leukemia. Clin. Cancer Res. **18**, 3812–3821 (2012)

Voo, K.S., Bover, L., Harline, M.L., Vien, L.T., Facchinetti, V., Arima, K., et al.: Antibodies targeting human OX40 expand effector T cells and block inducible and natural regulatory T cell function. J. Immunol. **191**, 3641–3650 (2013)

Vu, M.D., Xiao, X., Gao, W., Degauque, N., Chen, M., Kroemer, A., et al.: OX40 costimulation turns off Foxp3+ Tregs. Blood **110**, 2501–2510 (2007)

Warzocha, K., Salles, G.: The tumor necrosis factor signaling complex: choosing a path toward cell death or cell proliferation. Leukemia & lymphoma. **29**, 81–92 (1998)

Watts, T.H.: TNF/TNFR family members in costimulation of T cell responses. Annu. Rev. Immunol. **23**, 23–68 (2005)

Weinberg, A.D., Bourdette, D.N., Sullivan, T.J., Lemon, M., Wallin, J.J., Maziarz, R., et al.: Selective depletion of myelin-reactive T cells with the anti-OX-40 antibody ameliorates autoimmune encephalomyelitis. Nat. Med. **2**, 183–189 (1996)

Weinberg, A.D., Wegmann, K.W., Funatake, C., Whitham, R.H.: Blocking OX-40/OX-40 ligand interaction in vitro and in vivo leads to decreased T cell function and amelioration of experimental allergic encephalomyelitis. J. Immunol. **162**, 1818–1826 (1999)

Weinberg, A.D., Rivera, M.M., Prell, R., Morris, A., Ramstad, T., Vetto, J.T., et al.: Engagement of the OX-40 receptor in vivo enhances antitumor immunity. J. Immunol. **164**, 2160–2169 (2000)

Wen, L., Zhuang, L., Luo, X., Wei, P.: TL1A-induced NF-kappaB activation and c-IAP2 production prevent DR3-mediated apoptosis in TF-1 cells. J. Biol. Chem. **278**, 39251–39258 (2003)

Wolf, D., Schreiber, T.H., Tryphonopoulos, P., Li, S., Tzakis, A.G., Ruiz, P., et al.: Tregs expanded in vivo by TNFRSF25 agonists promote cardiac allograft survival. Transplantation **94**, 569–574 (2012)

Xiao, X., Kroemer, A., Gao, W., Ishii, N., Demirci, G., Li, X.C.: OX40/OX40L costimulation affects induction of Foxp3+ regulatory T cells in part by expanding memory T cells in vivo. J. Immunol. **181**, 3193–3201 (2008)

Xiao, X., Gong, W., Demirci, G., Liu, W., Spoerl, S., Chu, X., et al.: New insights on OX40 in the control of T cell immunity and immune tolerance in vivo. J. Immunol. **188**, 892–901 (2012)

Yonezawa, A., Dutt, S., Chester, C., Kim, J., Kohrt, H.E.: Boosting cancer immunotherapy with anti-CD137 antibody therapy. Clin. Cancer Res. **21**, 3113–3120 (2015)

Zheng, G., Wang, B., Chen, A.: The 4-1BB costimulation augments the proliferation of CD4+CD25+ regulatory T cells. J. Immunol. **173**, 2428–2434 (2004)

Zhou, P., L'Italien, L., Hodges, D., Schebye, X.M.: Pivotal roles of CD4+ effector T cells in mediating agonistic anti-GITR mAb-induced-immune activation and tumor immunity in CT26 tumors. J. Immunol. **179**, 7365–7375 (2007)

Chapter 4
NK Cell Responses in Immunotherapy: Novel Targets and Applications

Russell Pachynski and Holbrook Kohrt

Abbreviations

ADAM17	A disintegrin and metalloprotease-17
ADCC	Antibody dependent cell mediated cytotoxicity
APC	Antigen presenting cell
CARs	Chimeric antigen receptors
DC	Dendritic cell
DNAM-1	DNAX accessory molecule 1
GSK3	Glycogen synthase kinase-3
HSCT	Hematopoietic stem cell transplants
IDO	Indoleamine 2,3-dioxygenase
IL	Interleukin
IRF1	IFN response factor 1
ITAM	Immunoreceptor tyrosine-based activation motifs
KIRs	Inhibitory killer immunoglobulin-like receptors
MDSC	Myeloid-derived suppressor cells
MMPs	Metalloproteinases
NCR	Natural cytotoxicity receptor
NKG2D	Natural killer group 2 member D

R. Pachynski (✉)
Division of Oncology, Washington University Medical School, St. Louis, MO 63110, USA
e-mail: rkpachynski@dom.wustl.edu

H. Kohrt (✉)
Division of Oncology, Stanford University Medical Center & School of Medicine, Stanford, CA 94305, USA
e-mail: kohrt@stanford.edu

P.D. Rennert (ed.), *Novel Immunotherapeutic Approaches to the Treatment of Cancer*, DOI 10.1007/978-3-319-29827-6_4

PAMP/DAMP	Pathogen or danger associated molecular patterns
TandAb	Tetravalent, bispecific antibody
TLR	Toll-like receptors
TME	Tumor Microenvironment

1 Introduction and NK Cell Basic Biology

NK cells are lymphoid cells in humans broadly defined by CD56 (NCAM) or CD16 (FcγRIII) along with the absence of CD3, the concurrent presence of which would define NKT cells (Godfrey et al. 2004; Lanier et al. 1989). In addition to the lack of CD56 expression, murine NK cells exhibit a number of important differences compared with human, the discussion of which is beyond the scope of this review. $CD16^{+}CD56^{dim}$ cells comprise ~90 % of human NK cells and have higher cytotoxic potential against tumor cells, while $CD16^{+}CD56^{bright}$ NK cells produce abundant cytokines and chemokines, but have little to no ability to kill tumor (Caligiuri 2008). Interestingly, several studies suggest the development of $CD56^{dim}$ NK cells directly from the $CD56^{bright}$ subset (Chan et al. 2007; Cooper et al. 2001; Romagnani et al. 2007), with evidence that activation of these $CD56^{bright}$ cells results in increased expression of receptors more characteristic of $CD56^{dim}$ subset (Ferlazzo et al. 2004).

Derived from CD34+ hematopoietic progenitor cells (HPCs) (Galy et al. 1995), NK cells represent ~10–20 % of peripheral blood lymphocytes, and have a relatively short half life (~1–2 weeks) in circulation (Zhang et al. 2007b). In humans, NK cell proliferation primarily occurs within the bone marrow (Galy et al. 1995), while NK cells can be found not only in the peripheral blood, but also skin, GI tract (gut and liver), uterus/placenta, lungs, and secondary lymphoid tissues in the homeostatic setting (Carrega and Ferlazzo 2012). Within the liver, NK cells comprise up to ~30–50 % of all lymphocytes and provide a key role in the hepatic immune system (Doherty and O'Farrelly 2000; Krueger et al. 2011). During pathophysiologic conditions, NK cells can be found in a variety of tissues as well. While the in vivo data in humans is somewhat limited, it appears that NK cell maturation can occur in both reactive secondary lymphoid tissues as well as inflamed tissues themselves (Carrega and Ferlazzo 2012). The local cytokine milieu can play a role in activation and maturation, and the trafficking of NK cells is then determined by their chemokine receptor repertoire (Maghazachi 2010).

NK cells are clinically important, and play varied key roles in host defense against infections, cancer, and autoimmunity (Orange 2013; Orange and Ballas 2006; Mamessier et al. 2011). Interestingly, one study found higher incidence of cancer in patients correlated with lower NK cell cytotoxicity (Imai et al. 2000), suggesting an important role in tumor immune surveillance in humans. And—as outlined in this review—NK cells can play critical roles in immunotherapeutic approaches to cancer.

2 NK Cell Receptors

NK cells have a multitude of activating and inhibitory receptors that help them distinguish target or "altered self" cells from normal tissue (Karre et al 1986; Moretta et al. 2004; Raulet and Held 1995), and ultimately help determine their activation state and functionality. In the context of immune surveillance and the distinction between "self" and "non-self," inhibitory killer immunoglobulin-like receptors (KIRs) are able to bind classical MHC I molecules (e.g., HLA-A,-B,-C), while other inhibitory receptors such as CD94/NKG2A are able to bind nonclassical MHC molecules (e.g., HLA-E) (O'Callaghan 2000; Braud et al. 1998). MHC class I molecules are also involved in the maturation or "licensing" of NK cells, allowing them to be functionally competent; the lack of interaction between MHC I and these receptors—or in NK cells lacking MHC-specific inhibitory receptors ("receptor-null")—results in functionally incompetent NK cells incapable of killing (Andrews et al. 2012; Yokoyama and Kim 2006; Valiante et al. 1997). Interestingly, these are the same receptors that block activation and effector function, as engagement with classical MHC I by inhibitory KIR can dominate over activating signals, thus abrogating NK effector responses towards MHC I expressing cells (Vivier et al. 2004).

With regards to activation, there are several receptors which can mediate such signals: NKG2D (natural killer group 2 member D), DNAM-1 (DNAX accessory molecule 1), NKp80, activating KIRs, CD94/NKG2C, and 2B4 (Koch et al. 2013; Bryceson et al. 2006a), for example. The natural cytotoxicity receptors (NCRs) are another major group of activating receptors that can help trigger and activate the NK cell immune response. NKp30 (CD337), NKp44 (CD336), and NKp46 (CD335) are in the type I membrane immunoglobulin superfamily, and are likely able to bind multiple cellular ligands, although there is limited data in this area. As they lack intracellular signaling domains, NCRs utilize adaptor proteins that interact with their transmembrane domains, for example, via ITAMs (immunoreceptor tyrosine-based activation motifs) to effect downstream signaling (Vivier et al. 2004). NKGD2 is one of the best-described activating receptors found on essentially all human NK cells, as well as various T cell subsets (Lanier 2015). Genes for several ligands have been described (e.g., MICA, MICB, RAET1E, RAET1G, RAET1H, RAET1I, RAET1L, and RAET1N), with these glycoprotein ligands typically absent on normal adult tissues. Induction of these ligands by "stress"—either pathogen infection, hyperproliferation or transformation—can then identify target cells that may then be susceptible to autologous NK cell killing (Lanier 2015; Gonzalez et al. 2006). Normally, however, differential affinities for MHC I ligands allow for the inhibitory receptors to dominate over activating receptors, thus preventing autoimmunity (Vales-Gomez et al. 1998).

Cytokines play a key role in modulating NK cell receptor expression and activity (Bryceson et al. 2006a). Various cytokines (e.g., IL1, IL-2, IL-7, IL-15, IL-21)—and typically IL-12—can induce receptor expression, stimulate activation, and/or enable NK cells to produce IFNγ. Signaling through CD16 (FcγRIIIa) or NKG2D can then result in NK release of IFNγ and other pro-inflammatory cytokines and chemokines. Other cytokines, however, can act to blunt activation by downregulation of NKG2D, such as IL-21, IFNβ1, and TGFβ (Castriconi et al. 2003; Lanier 2015). These cytokines can be produced during interactions with antigen presenting cells (APCs) such as dendritic cells (DC), which can occur quickly after engagement with APCs, thus hastening the innate immune response (Fehniger et al. 1999; Moretta et al. 2006). Such interactions typically take place in secondary lymphoid tissues, where reciprocal activation as well as additional cross-talk such as deletion of immature APCs can occur, further modulating antitumor immune responses (Jacobs and Ullrich 2012; Della Chiesa et al. 2003; Yu et al. 2006; Walzer et al. 2005).

Though more associated with pathogenic infections, NK cells express several toll-like receptors (TLRs) (e.g., TLR3, TLR4, TLR 7, TLR8, TLR9) that are able to provide costimulatory activating signals (Hart et al. 2005; Adib-Conquy et al. 2014). Various pathogen (PAMP) or danger associated molecular patterns (DAMP) can bind to TLRs and contribute to the NK cell's integration of activating/inhibitory signals. Tumor cells have been shown to release DAMPs in various settings (e.g., chemotherapy, radiation) (Apetoh et al. 2007; Tesniere et al. 2010), suggesting these receptors may play a relevant role in antitumor NK cell responses.

NK cell receptor diversity—and thus target specificity—is unlike T and B lymphocytes, where specificity is dependent on somatic rearrangement. Rather, NK diversity of response comes from a complex interplay between a wide variety of both activating and inhibitory receptors. In addition to having a large number of individual KIR molecules (Valiante et al. 1997)—which are variably expressed between individuals—KIR polymorphism and gene silencing via methylation may also play a role in modulating NK cell function through their interaction with ligands (Chan et al. 2003; Falco et al. 2013; Yokoyama and Kim 2006). Variations in spatial and temporal expression patterns of receptors also impact the outcome of the synapse between the NK cell and its target (Lanier 2008), providing further complexity and diversity of response.

3 The NK Cell Synapse and Cytotoxicity

Once stimulated and activated via the integration of activating and inhibitory receptor signals, NK cells are able to effectively kill their target cells mainly through two mechanisms: secretion of cytokines and direct cell killing (e.g., via perforin/granzyme and death receptors) (Romee et al. 2014). Formation of the NK cell "immunologic synapse" with its target cell is also critically important for optimal killing (Orange 2008). For example, blocking of the gap junction protein connexin 43—which is the main gap junction protein of the immune system—can significantly inhibit NK tumor killing via granzyme B (Tittarelli et al. 2014). Synapse formation happens following receptor recognition on target cells and determined again by the balance of inhibitory and activating signals. Exocytosis of granules containing perforin, granzymes, and other cytotoxic proteins into the synapse then occurs. Endocytosis of these mediators allows them to then effect a number of downstream toxicities, such as induction of apoptosis by granzyme-triggered caspase activity (Thiery et al. 2011). The NK-tumor synapse then also allows direct cell killing via surface receptors such as TRAIL and Fas ligand (Falschlehner et al. 2009).

Cytokines and chemokines released by activated NK cells in the tumor microenvironment also effect a number of downstream events. IFNγ is one of the best-studied cytokines in this context, and NK cells are a major source in the early innate immune response. IFNγ can act directly on tumor cells to increase MHC I expression, induce apoptosis, as well as inhibit angiogenesis. Indirectly, it can act on other immune cells to effect activation and differentiation/maturation, inducing a wide variety of downstream response genes via the JAK/STAT pathway and the transcription factor IFN response factor 1 (IRF1), which in turn activates a large number of secondary response genes (Zaidi and Merlino 2011). This has pleiotropic effects on the local immune environment, leading to favorable antitumor responses such as promoting NK cell migration, T cell activation, and Th1-type responses (Wendel et al. 2008; Wald et al. 2006; Carnaud et al. 1999). However, it can also lead to the development and maintenance of suppressive regulatory T cells (Tregs), myeloid-derived suppressor cells (MDSC) (Ostrand-Rosenberg and Sinha 2009), as well as induction of IDO by tumor cells (Brody et al. 2009), thus promoting immunosuppressive activity. Chemokines (e.g., CCL1, CCL3, CCL4, CCL5, CCL22, XCL1, and CXCL8) also produce release by NK cells can then not only activate, but recruit other immune cells such as APCs and T cells as well, further facilitating the transition to an adaptive immune response (Dorner et al. 2004; Salazar-Mather and Hokeness 2003).

Recent data has also shown that cytokines commonly secreted by NK cells (e.g., IFNγ and TNFα) can induce senescence in their target cells (Braumuller et al. 2013), providing an additional mechanism of killing. When such activation and killing occurs through engagement of CD16 (the FcγRIIIa receptor) by antibody on a target cell, it is then referred to as antibody-dependent cellular cytotoxicity, or ADCC. Engagement of CD16 and subsequent cross-linking requires a prior adaptive response, but is sufficient alone to effect cytokine release and cytotoxicity without the need for additional synergistic activating signals (Bryceson et al. 2006b). Thus, immunotherapeutic strategies that utilize monoclonal antibodies to take advantage of NK-mediated ADCC offer significant promise for cancer immunotherapy (Kohrt et al. 2012).

4 NK Cells and Feature of Adaptive Immunity

More recent studies have provided evidence that NK cells, although part of the innate immune system, share some features of the adaptive arm, perhaps suggesting an evolutionary link between the two (Sun and Lanier 2009). Work from Von Andrian's group provided the first evidence of NK cell antigen specific memory (O'Leary et al. 2006). Lanier and colleagues then produced further evidence of generation of antigen-specific memory NK cells that have the capacity to become reactivated more robustly than resting NK cells, undergoing vigorous secondary expansion (Nabekura and Lanier 2014; Sun et al. 2009). Importantly, work from the Fehniger lab showed the induction of memory-like function and properties in human NK cells after cytokine stimulation, suggesting possible strategies for inducing NK memory in the clinical setting (Romee et al. 2012).

5 NK Cell Migration into Tumors

During homeostasis, NK cells circulate mainly in the blood and often found in liver, bone marrow, and lymphoid tissues. Though there is robust NK cell accumulation at sites of pathogenic infection, there is wide variability in NK trafficking into human tumors (Gregoire et al. 2007; Platonova et al. 2011; Sconocchia et al. 2012; Rusakiewicz et al. 2013). Increased density and/or infiltration of NK cells in tumors have correlated with improved clinical outcomes in several cancers (Menard et al. 2009; Villegas et al. 2002; Sznurkowski et al. 2014; Ishigami et al. 2000), suggesting an important role for the trafficking of NK cells into the tumor microenvironment in addition to their activation/functional state. A number of factors control NK cell migration into tumors, including locally produced cytokines and chemokines, as well as NK-specific and chemokine receptors (Robertson 2002).

Chemokines and their receptors govern the migration and trafficking of leukocytes in both the homeostatic and inflammatory settings. There is substantial overlap between many chemokines and their receptors within this network, making the characterization of leukocyte subsets with distinct trafficking patterns difficult to elucidate (Zlotnik and Yoshie 2012). Work from Butcher and his colleagues found that most human NK cells express CXCR1, CXCR2, CXCR3, CXCR4, and CX3CR1 (Campbell et al. 2001). $CD56^{bright}CD16^{dim}$ cells express CCR7, and will undergo chemotactic migration towards CCL19 or CCL21 gradients which would allow them to traffic into peripheral lymph nodes (Campbell et al. 2001). Interestingly, human NK cells may acquire CCR7 expression via trogocytosis upon interactions with CCR7+ alloreactive cells, suggesting a potential mechanism for augmented trafficking of NK cells towards lymph nodes in the setting of hematopoietic stem cell transplants (HSCT) (Marcenaro et al. 2013).

Cytokines in the local tumor microenvironment can alter trafficking potential of NK cells. For example, TGFβ expressed by neuroblastoma cells has been shown to upregulate CXCR3 and CXCR4, while downregulating CX3CR1 in the $CD56^{dim}$ subset (Castriconi et al. 2013; Inngjerdingen et al. 2001), while activation with IL-2 or IL-15 can induce expression of CCR2, CCR4, CCR5, and CCR8 (Polentarutti et al. 1997; Inngjerdingen et al. 2001; Robertson 2002). IFNγ secreted by activated NK or T cells can lead to the production of CXCL9 and CXCL10, which can then lead to the recruitment of CXCR3+ NK cells. Preclinical models of adoptively transferred, activated CXCR3+ NK cells show increased migration of NK cells towards CXCL10-expressing tumors; local intratumoral administration of IFNγ upregulated CXCL10 expression augmenting NK infiltration, resulting in significantly reduced tumor burden and increased survival (Wennerberg et al. 2015). A number of chemokines themselves (e.g., CCL2, CCL3, CCL4, CCL5, CXCL10, CX3CL1) also have direct effects on NK cell cytotoxicity, promoting granule release during immunologic synapse formation (Taub et al. 1995; Nieto et al. 1998). Additional, novel chemoattractants may further tune the NK cell response. Thus, cytokines and chemokines not only control influx of NK cells into tumor sites, but can impact NK functionality as well, making them attractive targets of immunomodulation.

6 How Tumors Evade NK Cells

Tumors have developed a number of mechanisms that allow them to blunt the response of or avoid destruction by NK cells. In addition to immunosuppression within the tumor microenvironment, elimination of susceptible tumor cells by NK cells with outgrowth of escape clones (i.e., immunoediting) can also lead to progressive tumor growth (Vesely et al. 2011). Downregulation of NCRs on tumor cells can confer resistance to NK cell killing (Sivori et al. 1999; Elboim et al. 2010; Pietra et al. 2012). Alternative isoforms of NKp30 have been shown to increase the immunosuppressive cytokine IL-10 and reduce NK cell activation (Delahaye et al. 2011). NKG2D ligands can be released or proteolytically cleaved from the surface of target cells. Upon binding NKG2D on NK cells, they can modulate downregulation via internalization of receptors, thus blunting activation signals (Baragano Raneros et al. 2014). Additionally, TGFβ, often expressed at high levels in the tumor microenvironment, may also act to downregulate NKG2D as well as perforin, granzyme B, and TRAIL (Mamessier et al. 2011), and thus help evade NK mediated immunity (Castriconi et al. 2003; Groth et al. 2011). TGFβ may also effect the conversion of T cells into regulatory T cells, which can then further suppress the NK cell response (Ghiringhelli et al. 2005). Other immunosuppressive factors within the TME, such as prostaglandins, matrix metalloproteinases (MMPs), and indoleamine 2,3-dioxygenase (IDO) can also suppress NK function (Peng et al. 2014). Interestingly, a recent study supports the role of tumor hypoxia in suppressing NK cell function, with therapeutic hyperoxia resulting in significant improvement in antitumor immunity in preclinical models (Hatfield et al. 2015). As with other immune cells, NK cells may have dynamic plasticity within the context of the tumor microenvironment to not only have their activity suppressed, but in fact also have the ability to transform into immunosuppressive cells. Zitvogel and colleagues identified a subset of Kit+NK cells induced by tumor expressed IL-18 that are purportedly protumorigenic. This subset overexpresses PD-L1/B7-H1 and in preclinical models promotes tumor growth and mediates immuno-ablative functions (Terme et al. 2012). Other data also support the existence of such protumorigenic and/or proangiogenic NK cells, opening up a new area of investigation and opportunities for novel therapeutic targets (Bruno et al. 2014). Thus, tumors can utilize a variety of mechanisms to evade destruction by NK cells.

With the understanding of mechanisms involved in both NK cell activation and function, as well as evasion by tumor cells, several therapeutic immunomodulatory strategies have been undertaken, albeit with limited success to date.

7 Previous Human NK Cell Immunotherapies

As part of the innate immune system, NK cells are an essential component of the first line of defense against pathogen infection. They act quickly, efficiently, and with limited specificity for their target. Their ability to kill infected or abnormal (e.g., cancerous) cells without the need for selection or proliferation of specific clones certainly make them ideal candidates for immunosurveillance, but the question remains whether these cells can be effectively utilized as therapy against established tumors in humans. NK cells appear to be more effective at preventing metastases or treating small tumor inocula than primary or larger tumors in preclinical models (Glasner et al. 2012; Ljunggren and Karre 1990). And, as mentioned, there is variation in NK cell accumulation within tumors, with mounting evidence that the tumor microenvironment may suppress NK function even after migration and infiltration of NK cells into tumors (Platonova et al. 2011), suggesting that strategies that target multiple NK cell mechanisms will be needed to fully realize their therapeutic potential.

To date, several of these approaches have been studied and tested in humans, including cytokine therapy, immunomodulatory antibodies, and adoptive transfer/transplant.

8 Cytokines

Cytokines are critical mediators of NK cell activation and function, proliferation, and survival, and have been studied in this context in clinical trials with some promise. The major NK cell cytokines include IL-2, IL-12, IL15, IL-18, and IL-21 (Romee et al. 2014). A general approach for the utilization of these in clinical trials has been systemic administration, with alterations of dose and schedule to try and optimize effects on NK cell function.

Signaling through the shared IL-2/IL-5 beta and gamma common chain (βγc) receptor that is constitutively expressed on human NK cells, both IL-2 and Il-15 influence NK cell proliferation, homeostasis, and can enhance cytotoxic effector functions (Fehniger et al. 2002; Rodella et al. 2001). $CD56^{bright}$ NK cells constitutively express the IL-2Rα (CD25), which can heterotrimerize to form the high affinity IL-2R alpha and gamma common chain (αγc). This can be induced on both $CD56^{bright}$ and $CD56^{dim}$ cells following stimulation with a combination of IL-12, IL-15, and IL-18 (Leong et al. 2014). NK cells can then respond to picomolar concentrations of IL-2. This can result in significant expansion of the $CD56^{bright}CD16+$ population, with minimal toxicity (Caligiuri et al. 1991; Meropol et al. 1998). Although there was some initial hint of clinical activity when combined with antitumor monoclonal antibodies (Sondel and Hank 1997), subsequent studies showed an effect of IL-2 on regulatory T cell expansion and promotion, which can limit NK cell activity and promote tumor growth (Antony and Restifo 2005; Ahmadzadeh and Rosenberg 2006). While IL-2 was one of the first cytokines used in immunotherapy and remains an option in current practice for patients with metastatic melanoma and renal cell carcinoma (RCC), with durable response rates in the range of ~5–15 %, there are significant toxicities when given at high dose (Payne et al. 2014; Atkins et al. 1999; Fyfe et al. 1995). This high toxicity, which can include hypotension, cytopenias, acidosis, and capillary leak syndrome, unfortunately severely limits the use of this therapy in elderly or otherwise unfit patients. Future strategies utilizing IL-2 must take into account not only its toxicity, but its effects on regulatory immune cell subsets, and thus combination strategies aimed at limiting Treg expansion or function are likely to be more successful.

IL-15 shares many similarities to IL-2 in vivo, with subsequent signaling events that are similar to and in some cases identical to those of IL-2, given their shared IL-2/15βγc receptor. IL-15 is widely expressed and can be secreted from APCs as well as in the bone marrow (Blauvelt et al. 1996; Carson et al. 1995). The IL-15Rα chain subunit is primarily expressed on APCs, and can then present IL-15 to the IL-15Rβγc complex on NK cells. As with IL-2, IL-15 plays a role in NK cell stimulation, activation, but importantly also differentiation and maturation from CD34+ precursor cells. IL-15 aids in NK cell chemokine and cytokine production, cytotoxicity, and helps regulate interactions with APCs (Fehniger and Caligiuri 2001). Initial studies showed expansion of NK cells without concomitant Treg expansion, and low toxicity (Berger et al. 2009), thus suggesting promising clinical potential. In fact, rhIL-15 remains at the top of the NCI's Immunotherapy Agent Workshop list, with several ongoing studies utilizing it in multiple tumor types (AML, after NK cell adoptive transfer NCT01385423; RCC/melanoma: NCT01021059, NCT01369888; advanced cancers NCT01727076, NCT01572493).

While promising, rhIL-15 requires IL-15Rα for maximal stimulation of IL-2/15Rβγc, thus suggesting improved in vivo activity with a IL-15/IL-15Rα complex (Burkett et al. 2004; Stoklasek et al. 2006). To this end, a "superagonist" was developed, utilizing a fusion of a high affinity IL-15 variant to IL-15Rα and IgG1 Fc domains (ALT-803) (Han et al. 2011). Preclinical studies have been promising J Clin Oncol 31, 2013 (suppl 6; abstr 298), and several clinical trials are ongoing (advanced tumors: NCT01946789; melanoma: NCT01021059; and relapsed malignancies after allogeneic SCT: NCT01885897; multiple myeloma: NCT02099539; lymphoma with rituximab: NCT02384954; bladder cancer with BCG: NCT02138734).

IL-12 is a heterodimeric (alpha and beta chains) cytokine expressed primarily by APCs with ability to enhance NK cytotoxic activity (Adorini 1999). Its receptor, IL-12R, on NK cells and activated T cells then mediates increases in cytokine production, cytotoxicity, and proliferation via the JAK/STAT pathway (Ren et al. 1996). Resting NK cells can express IL-12R, which allows response in the early stages of inflammation without need for prior activation and upregulation (Wang et al. 2000). Preclinical tumor studies looked promising (Nastala et al. 1994; Brunda et al. 1993), however subsequent clinical studies in humans showed the potential for substantial toxicity (Atkins et al. 1997; Leonard et al. 1997), with limited clinical activity (Robertson et al. 1999; Motzer et al. 2001; Alatrash et al. 2004). Several studies have taken the approach of combination therapy using IL-12 with antitumor monoclonal antibodies (Parihar et al. 2004; Mani et al. 2009; Bekaii-Saab et al. 2009)—taking advantage of the ability of IL-12 to stimulate IFNγ production in the setting of antibody-coated tumor cells. An ongoing multicenter trial (head and neck: NCT01468896) will provide additional insight into IL-12 efficacy in the future.

IL-21 is another promising gamma-chain cytokine which can stimulate T, B, and NK cells through its receptor and JAK/STAT, MAPK, and PI3K pathways (Zeng et al. 2007). It can enhance maturation and cytotoxicity of NK and T cells, and has potent antitumor activity in preclinical models (Parrish-Novak et al. 2000; Wang et al. 2003; Di Carlo et al. 2004; Takaki et al. 2005; Andorsky and Timmerman 2008). In contrast to IL-2, IL-21 does not support Treg proliferation and function, and through its stimulation of CD4+CD25- T cells may counteract suppressive Treg functions (Peluso et al. 2007). Early phase human clinical trials have shown acceptable toxicity and reasonable clinical activity in RCC and melanoma (Hashmi and Van Veldhuizen 2010; Petrella et al. 2012). The ability of IL-21 to augment ADCC has been shown in vitro (Gowda et al. 2008; Roda et al. 2007), and promising clinical efficacy has been seen in colorectal cancer patients concurrently receiving the anti-EGFR antibody cetuximab, with 60 % of the patients showing stable disease (Steele et al. 2012), and in lymphoma patients in combination with rituximab with 42 % of the patients have clinical responses (Timmerman et al. 2012).

Several NK cell cytokines show promise in the clinical setting (Romee et al. 2014), and further investigation with these in the combination with more specific agents with fewer pleiotropic effects will likely secure their role in therapeutic immunomodulation of NK cells.

9 Adoptive Transfer

Adoptive transfer of NK cells has been used extensively in hematologic malignancies—mostly in the setting of hematopoietic stem cell transplantation—and in solid tumors with variable success (recently reviewed in (Eguizabal et al. 2014)). Early trials often utilized IL-2 that can stimulate Treg proliferation and function, or had poor persistence or function of transferred NK cells, and thus many of these trials resulted in disappointing clinical outcomes (Burns et al. 2003; Parkhurst et al. 2011; Geller et al. 2011). However, recent early phase studies in solid tumors utilizing NK cell infusions in combination with chemotherapy do show some potential clinical efficacy (Geller et al. 2011; Iliopoulou et al. 2010), suggesting there may be some beneficial immunomodulatory effects conferred by the addition of chemotherapy (Bracci et al. 2014). For example, metronomic cyclophosphamide can result in Treg suppression leading to improved innate killing activity (Ghiringhelli et al. 2007). Another approach that has been taken utilizes an NK cell line, NK-92, which has been initially shown to be safe with hints of efficacy. This is currently in clinical trials in advanced tumors (Arai et al. 2008), although still too early to fully assess its clinical efficacy.

Another approach to improve adoptive transfer therapy is to optimize the expansion and activation of ex vivo NK cells for adoptive transfer (Fujisaki et al. 2009; Lim et al. 2013). For example, expression of IL-15 and 4-1BBL on the leukemic K562 cell line has been shown to enhance human NK cell cytotoxicity during in vitro expansion of these cells (Fujisaki et al. 2009); this approach is currently being tested in a clinical trial to test the safety and tolerability of these cells (NCT02123836). Another approach utilizes the addition of a tumor-specific monoclonal antibody (e.g., anti-EGFR) during the ex vivo expansion, resulting in increased activation of and target-specific killing by the NK cells J Clin Oncol 33, 2015 (suppl; abstr e14017). Utilizing optimized combinations of cytokines and other targeted agents to expand NK cells ex vivo and/or aid in in vivo persistence after transfer may help to improve this therapeutic approach.

Of relevance to HSCT for hematologic malignancies, the concept of NK cell KIR ligand incompatibility or alloreactivity was initially described in patients with donor-reactive alloreactive NK cells in the setting of HSCT; from the human and murine data, Ruggeri et al. showed alloreactive NK could mediated GVL, reduced GVHD, and enhanced engraftment (Ruggeri et al. 2002). Other studies have also shown improved overall survival and reduced relapse in these KIR-mismatched transplants (Willemze et al. 2009). Haploidentical NK cells have also been transferred into AML patients in remission as a potential strategy for consolidative therapy (Moretta et al. 2014; Velardi 2012).

10 Genetically Modified NK Cells

With the clinical successes of chimeric antigen receptor (CAR) T cell therapy there has been significant interest in applying the same techniques to NK cells. CARs consist of a single-chain variable fragment (scFv) fused to a variety of costimulatory molecules, such as CD28, 41BB (CD137), or OX40. Tumor specificity is achieved by the scFV, and engagement of the CAR receptor allows for activation and proliferation of the CAR T cells (Jena et al. 2014; Kakarla and Gottschalk 2014). Unfortunately, there are a number of concerns with CAR T cells relating to potential on-target/off-tumor toxicity, as well as lack of persistence of these T cells, requiring additional infusions for recurrent or persistent disease. Applying this approach to NK cells has some potential advantages, as adoptive transfer of NK cells does not require HLA typing/matching, and NK cells can persist in patients up to months (Vivier et al. 2008).

Genetically modification of NK cells can utilize either NK cell lines (e.g., NK-92, NKG, HANK-1NK-YS, NKL) or donor-derived NK cells. NK-92 is probably the most studied to date, with several CAR constructs showing promising activity in preclinical models and potential in ongoing clinical trials (NCT00900809, NCT00990717) (Hermanson and Kaufman 2015). NK-92, however, lacks a number of key receptors found on donor-derived NK cells, such as CD16, NKp44, and NKp46 (Maki et al. 2001). Advanced generation CAR constructs include a variety of targeting (e.g., EpCAM, ErbB2, CS1) and signaling (e.g., CD3, OX40, CD28, CD137) domains that can increase their specificity and antitumor activity (Schonfeld et al. 2015; Topfer et al. 2015; Glienke et al. 2015). One approach utilizes NKG2D in concert with DAP10 and CD3zeta to improve NK cell efficacy. Transduction of the NKG2D-DAP10-CD3zeta construct increased NKG2D expression on NK cells and increased cytokine/chemokine secretion and cytotoxicity against target, but not control cells. Transduced NK cells with this construct demonstrated significant activity against multiple tumor lines and has potential for clinical benefit (Chang et al. 2013). Genetically modified NK cells have been used (Tonn et al. 2013) and continue to be tested in clinical trials (e.g., NCT00995137, NCT00900809, NCT00990717), the results of which should help inform additional strategies to optimize NK cell adoptive transfer.

11 Antibodies/ADCC

While adoptive transfer approaches hold some promise for NK cell therapy, there are a number of disadvantages with regards to cell source, in vitro manipulation, and administration, with resultant issues of cost, risk of infection, and need for good manufacturing practices. Utilizing therapeutic antibodies to improve NK cell function in vivo represents a more direct approach, and may provide equivalent if not superior clinical results. We review several of the antibodies/targets that are currently in clinical trials with promising results.

12 CD16 Ehancement

CD16 (the FcgRIIIα receptor) on NK cells mediates ADCC, and thus is a key component of antibody-directed therapies. Polymorphisms that affect CD16 have been correlated with differences in clinical efficacy (Zhang et al. 2007a; Weng and Levy 2003), suggesting optimization of the CD16/antibody interaction may improve ADCC. Additionally, fucosylation or glycosylation can influence the affinity and interaction of the Fc portion of antibodies with CD16 (Ferrara et al. 2011). Thus, one approach has been to enhance the affinity of therapeutic tumor-specific antibody for CD16, which can also be expressed on T cell subsets, monocytes, and macrophages. Ocaratuzumab (AME-133v, LY2469298), a humanized monoclonal antibody against CD20 with enhanced ADCC activity has been evaluated in clinical trials and was well-tolerated with promising results in heavily pretreated lymphoma patients, with approximately 64 % of patients have tumor shrinkage (Forero-Torres et al. 2012). Obinutuzuamb (GA101) is another glycol-engineered antibody currently in clinical development with enhanced ADCC activity via CD16, with promising clinical results in CD20+ malignancies (Herter et al. 2013; Goede et al. 2015).

13 Anti-KIR

Targeting KIR/KIR ligands represents an attractive approach at reducing the inhibition of NK cell cytotoxic activity. The first in this class and the most clinically advanced is lirilumab. Lirilumab (IPH2102/BMS-986015, formerly I-7F9) is a human IgG4 antibody that binds KIR2DL1/2/3/S1/S2 and blocks the interaction with KIRs on NK cells. It has shown promising efficacy in preclinical models, alone and in combination with tumor-specific monoclonal antibodies (Romagne et al. 2009; Kohrt et al. 2012, 2014b; Nijhof et al. 2015). Korht et al. utilized a KIR transgenic model to show significant enhancement of NK-cell mediated cytotoxicity against CD20+ lymphoma in combination with rituximab (Kohrt et al. 2014b). Recent results from a phase I trial of lirilumab showed it was well-tolerated with no DLTs and MTD not reached, with the ability to achieve full KIR occupancy for >4 weeks J Clin Oncol 33, 2015 (suppl; abstr 3065). Several clinical studies are now open and ongoing, evaluating lirilumab alone or in combination in both hematologic and solid malignancies (AML: NCT02399917, lymphoma and multiple myeloma (MM): NCT01592370, MM: NCT02252263, CLL: NCT02481297, advanced solid tumors: NCT01714739 NCT01750580, AML: NCT01687387) in order to assess the clinical efficacy of this therapeutic.

14 CD137

CD137 (4-1BB; TNFRS9) is an activation induced costimulatory molecule in T lymphocytes that was initially described by Kwon and colleagues (Kwon and Weissman 1989). Upon activation, a number of cells are able to upregulate and express CD137, including T and NK cells, and APCs. CD137 stimulation results in activation of multiple signaling cascades, eventually resulting in NF-κB activation and downstream immune effector responses. A number of responses to CD137 agonism have been described in various immune cells. Activation of CD137 can inhibit activation induced cell death (AICD), change production of IFNγ, TNFα, and other cytokines, upregulate B7 costimulatory molecules on APCs and promote APC maturation. Agonistic anti-CD137 antibodies have been used in a wide variety of preclinical tumor models, with variable reliance on T or NK cells for their antitumor efficacy (review in (Vinay and Kwon 2014)).

With respect to human NK cells, there is little to no expression of CD137 in resting NK cells, but CD137 can be upregulated after exposure to various stimuli including Fc interaction with Fc receptors (Lin et al. 2008). In isolated human NK cells, CD137 was significantly upregulated when exposed to antibody-coated tumor cell lines, with subsequent enhanced degranulation and cytotoxicity after exposure to an agonist CD137 antibody. In patients, an increase in CD137+ NK cells directly correlated to an increase in tumor-specific CD8+ T cells. This concept was tested in several preclinical tumor models resulting in significant activity (Kohrt et al. 2014a), and is now being evaluated in human clinical trials with promising results. A phase I trial of an anti-CD137 agonistic antibody (PF-05082566) in combination with rituximab in lymphoma patients (NCT01307267) showed the combination was well tolerated with no severe immune-related adverse events, and an overall response rate of 21 % (6/28). Interestingly, there were two complete responses both of which with durable responses of >2 years. This suggests there may be induction of long term memory responses. Several studies utilizing anti-CD137 agonistic antibodies (urelumab/BMS-663513 or PF-05082566) alone or in combination are now ongoing in several hematologic and solid tumor types. CD137 no doubt will continue to be a promising target to enhance NK cell cytotoxicity and efficacy in vivo.

15 TLR Agonists

TLRs are a class of single membrane spanning receptors primarily found on innate immune cells that are able to recognize a wide variety of viral and bacterial patterned molecules (PAMPs). While more often found on dendritic cells and monocytes/macrophages and less commonly on T cells, NK cells can express a number of TLRs, including TLR3, TLR7, and TLR8 (Hart et al. 2005). Activation of TLRs on NK cells can result in increased production of inflammatory cytokines such as IFNg, and augment their ability to mediate ADCC (Moga et al. 2008; Hart et al. 2005). Thus, TLR agonists represent a potential class of therapeutics that can target NK cells and improve their functionality.

Motolimod (VTX-2337) is one such TLR agonist currently in clinical trials. VTX-2337 was shown to stimulate NK cell activity in vitro likely through TLR8, although with likely contribution from additional stimulated cytokines such as IFNg and IL-18. In vitro studies with rituximab and trastuzumab showed that VTX-2337 significantly improved ADCC (Lu et al. 2012). A phase I trial in lymphoma and solid tumors has been published, and there are several ongoing or planned trials in combination with other agents (e.g., head and neck cancer with cetuximab/chemotherapy: NCT01836029; ovarian cancer with anti-PD1/chemotherapy: NCT02431559). The initial findings from the phase I trial show that VTX-2337 was well-tolerated, although with one dose-limiting toxicity of hypotension. Most of the adverse events were grade 1/2. Systemic increases in plasma levels of G-CSF, MCP-1, MIP-1β, and TNFα were seen, with 24 % of the patients achieving stable disease (Northfelt et al. 2014).

Given that various tumor cells can also express TLRs and utilize TLR signaling to their advantage (Kaczanowska et al. 2013), it will be important to select the appropriate tumor type and setting for such TLR agonists. For example, TLR7/8 can be expressed on human lung cancers and induce several factors, including chemokines associated with tumor cell migration, VEGFR2 (involved with angiogenesis), as well as anti-apoptotic protein Bcl-2 which resulted in increased tumor cell survival and resistance to chemotherapy (Cherfils-Vicini et al. 2010). However, TLR agonists may still provide yet another tool to increase the clinical efficacy of NK cells.

16 Checkpoint Inhibitors

While there has been substantial clinical activity with a number of monoclonal antibodies targeting various checkpoint molecules (e.g., CTLA-4, PD-1, PD-L1), the majority of research and focus has largely been on their effects on T cell activity. Anti-CTLA-4 and anti-PD-1 monoclonal antibodies are now FDA-approved for melanoma and lung cancer, with rapidly accelerating clinical development of anti-PD-L1 antibodies (Pardoll 2012). Multiple tumor types are being evaluated given the broad responses seen, and combinations of these checkpoint inhibitors are also moving forward quickly in clinical trials. The expression of CTLA-4 on NK cells is not well-studied, and there is no human data to suggest significant expression on NK cells. Interestingly, however, recent data shows that murine NK cells stimulated with IL-2 express CTLA-4, which can inhibit IFNγ release. Further, that tumor infiltrating NK cells respond to stimulation with recombinant B7-1, suggesting potential impact of anti-CTLA-4 antibodies on NK cell function (Stojanovic et al. 2014). PD-1 expression on human NK cells can be induced during chronic infection, or after long-term culture with IL-15, and associated with reduced NK cell proliferation (Norris et al. 2012). In multiple myeloma patients, PD-1 expression has been seen on NK cell with PD-L1 expression on primary tumor cells. An anti-PD-1 antibody (CT-011) enhanced NK cell function against tumor cells, with increased cytotoxicity against PD-L1+ tumor cells (Benson et al. 2010). These data suggest that in addition to well-known T cell-mediated mechanisms, checkpoint inhibitors may, in fact, impact NK cell function. To this end, ipilimumab (anti-CTLA-4) was recently shown to upregulate the IL-2Rα chain in human NK cells, with patients responding to ipilimumab having higher levels of IL-2Rα as well as improvements in cytotoxicity after exposure to IL-2 J Clin Oncol 33, 2015 (suppl; abstr 9065). Taken together, these data suggest NK cell likely have important—yet understudied—roles in clinical responses to checkpoint inhibitors, and should be further investigated and targeted for optimization.

17 OX40/OX40L

OX40/OX40L axis has been a major focus in the immunotherapy field, with several therapeutics targeting this pathway in clinical development (MOXR0916, MEDI6469, MEDI6383). OX40 is expressed on non-naïve T cells and stimulation through it results in increased cytotoxicity and activation (Croft 2010). Interestingly, both OX40 and OX40L have been shown to be expressed in human NK cells after stimulation (Zingoni et al. 2004; Takasawa et al. 2001). The OX40/OX40L pathway plays a number of important roles in T cell activation and function (Croft 2010), although the impact of this pathway is on human NK cell function is less studied. Stimulation via OX40/OX40L can augment NK cell function, however, at least in preclinical models, where signaling from OX40L on plasmacytoid DCs stimulated OX40+ NK cells to produce IFNγ (Liu et al. 2008). Thus, NK cells may be at least partially involved in the response to agents that target this pathway.

18 Elotuzumab

Elotuzumab (BMS-901608), formerly known as HuLuc63, is a humanized mAb targeting the surface glycoprotein CS1 (CD2 subest 1, SLAMF7, CRACC, CD319). CS1 is a member of the immunoglobulin gene superfamily and found at high levels on multiple myeloma cells, as well as NK, NKT, CD8 T, and activated monocytes and B cells. In preclinical models, elotuzumab induced NK-mediated killing of myeloma cells via ADCC, and had significant antitumor activity in several myeloma models (Palumbo and Sonneveld 2015; Balasa et al. 2015). CS1 expression on NK cells, where it acts as an activating receptor regulation cytolytic activity, enables elotuzumab-mediated activation and promotion of cytotoxicity against CD1+ myeloma cells (Collins et al. 2013).

Several clinical trials are ongoing with elotuzumab in multiple myeloma, the most advanced of which—ELOQUENT2 (NCT01239797)—compared the addition of elotuzumab/lenalidomide to lenalidomide in advanced multiple myeloma patients. There was a significantly improved overall response rate in the combination (79 %) compared to the control group (66 %), p=0.0002, with a clinically relevant 30 % reduction in risk of progression or death N Engl J Med. 2015 Aug 13;373(7):621-31. doi: 10.1056/NEJMoa1505654. Epub 2015 Jun 2. Given the ability of elotuzumab to stimulate NK-mediated cytotoxicity, it may have potential for use in other tumor types in combination with tumor-specific mAbs. Elotuzumab was recently (November 2015) approved by the FDA for use in combination with two other therapies to treat patients with relapsed or refractory multiple myeloma.

19 NK Bispecific Antibodies

Engineered bispecific antibodies have the advantage of tumor-targeting and bringing in close proximity and potentially activating effector immune cells. Several bispecific antibodies are in development targeting T cells as effectors (Baeuerle and Reinhardt 2009), with the first bispecific antibody (blinatumomab; CD19/CD3) recently approved by the FDA for ALL. In addition to T cells, bispecific antibodies targeting NK cells are currently in development as well. AFM13 is a tetravalent, bispecific antibody (TandAb,) designed to target CD30+ cancers. The bispecific antibody binds CD16a and is able to activate NK cells, albeit in a manner dependent on the presence of CD30+ target cells (Reusch et al. 2014). In a phase I dose finding study, patients with Hodgkin lymphoma were treated with increases doses of AFM13, although a MTD was not reached and was generally well tolerated. There was evidence of significant NK cell activation as well as a decrease in the biomarker sCD30. In heavily pretreated patients, the overall disease control rate was 61.5 %; impressively, in patients previously treated with brentuximab vedotin (anti-CD30 mAb), the disease control rate was 77 % (Rothe et al. 2015). Thus bispecific antibodies that target NK cells to tumors hold promise and should be evaluated in multiple tumor types.

20 Promising Preclinical Targets

20.1 ADAM17

CD16 expression in human NK cells is regulated on several levels, with rapid downregulation upon activation by various stimuli (Romee et al. 2013). ADAM17 (a disintegrin and metalloprotease-17) was shown to be the primary protease mediating CD16b cleavage (Wang et al. 2013). Inhibition of ADAM17 has been shown to enhance CD16-mediated NK cells function via its ability to mediate ADCC (Romee et al. 2013) Amino acid substitution identified cleavage sites and revealed that S197P effectively blocked CD16 cleavage in vitro. NK92 cell line or primary NK cells genetically engineered with CD16/S197P were resistant to CD16 cleavage ADAM17 (Jing et al. 2015). Inhibitors of ADAM17 or utilizing resistant CD16 constructs in adoptively transferred NK cells may offer a novel approach to increasing CD16 expression and augmenting ADCC.

20.2 Chemerin

Chemerin (*RARRES2*) is a novel leukocyte chemoattractant protein with structural similarities to cathelicidins (antibacterial peptides), cystatins (cysteine protease inhibitors), and kininogens (Wittamer et al. 2003). CMKLR1 (ChemR23) is its major chemotactic receptor, and is present on NK cells, in addition to macrophage and DC subsets. CMKLR1 has been shown to be co-expressed with CXCR1 and KIR receptors on CD56^{dim}CD16+ NK cells in the blood, and CMKLR1+ NK cells colocalized with chemerin expression in biopsies of human inflamed peripheral tissues (Parolini et al. 2007), suggesting a role for this axis in humans. Analysis of several human tumors revealed downregulation of chemerin, suggesting a possible mechanism of escape from NK cell mediated immunosurveillance. In preclinical tumor models, forced reexpression of chemerin in the tumor microenvironment resulted in increased infiltrating leukocytes and NK-dependent tumor regression (Pachynski et al. 2012). Targeting of this pathway could lead to increased NK cell trafficking into sites of tumor.

20.3 GSK3

Glycogen synthase kinase-3 (GSK3) is a serine–threonine kinase widely expressed in many tumors, and involved with multiple signaling pathways activated by various factors (e.g., Wnts, Hedgehog, EGF, insulin, etc) (Kaidanovich-Beilin and Woodgett 2011). Thus, GSK3 plays an important role in the proliferation and survival of cancer cells, and inhibitors to this enzyme have been extensively used to suppress the malignant proliferation (Mentlik James et al. 2013). Interestingly, inhibition of GSK3 in multiple myeloma cells resulted in significant upregulation of the NKGD2 ligand MICA, with little or no effects on MICB or DNAM-1. Increased NK degranulation and NK cell-mediated cytotoxicity was seen as well, with further enhancement of MICA expression with the addition of lenalidomide (Fionda et al. 2013). As GSK3 is active in multiple tumor types (McCubrey et al. 2014), it may prove useful to not only decrease tumor cell proliferation but induce sensitivity to NK cell killing.

21 Concluding Remarks

Despite 3 decades of investigation of natural killer cells' role in the antitumor immune response, today the search for the right therapeutic strategy to augment NK cell efficacy without exacerbating toxicity continues. Modulation of NK cell number by adoptive transfer and growth factors as well as modulation of NK cell phenotype by inhibiting inhibitory receptors (KIR) and activating stimulatory pathways will enhance the antitumor response including spontaneous NK cell cytotoxicity as well as NK cell ADCC. A continuously growing understanding of NK cell biology and NK cell subtypes provides a multitude of potential therapeutic targets yet to demonstrate the full therapeutic role of NK cells against cancer.

References

J. Clin. Oncol. **33**(suppl; abstr 3065) (2015)
J. Clin. Oncol. **33**(suppl; abstr 8508) (2015)
J. Clin. Oncol. **33**(suppl; abstr 9065) (2015)
J. Clin. Oncol. **33**(suppl; abstr e14017) (2015)
J. Immunother. Cancer **1**(Suppl 1), 40 (2013)
Adib-Conquy, M., Scott-Algara, D., Cavaillon, J.M., Souza-Fonseca-Guimaraes, F.: TLR-mediated activation of NK cells and their role in bacterial/viral immune responses in mammals. Immunol. Cell Biol. **92**, 256–262 (2014)
Adorini, L.: Interleukin-12, a key cytokine in Th1-mediated autoimmune diseases. Cell. Mol. Life Sci. **55**, 1610–1625 (1999)
Ahmadzadeh, M., Rosenberg, S.A.: IL-2 administration increases CD4+ CD25(hi) Foxp3+ regulatory T cells in cancer patients. Blood **107**, 2409–2414 (2006)
Alatrash, G., Hutson, T.E., Molto, L., Richmond, A., Nemec, C., Mekhail, T., Elson, P., Tannenbaum, C., Olencki, T., Finke, J., Bukowski, R.M.: Clinical and immunologic effects of subcutaneously administered interleukin-12 and interferon alfa-2b: phase I trial of patients with metastatic renal cell carcinoma or malignant melanoma. J. Clin. Oncol. **22**, 2891–2900 (2004)
Andorsky, D.J., Timmerman, J.M.: Interleukin-21: biology and application to cancer therapy. Expert Opin. Biol. Ther. **8**, 1295–1307 (2008)
Andrews, D.M., Sullivan, L.C., Baschuk, N., Chan, C.J., Berry, R., Cotterell, C.L., Lin, J., Halse, H., Watt, S.V., Poursine-Laurent, J., Wang, C.R., Scalzo, A.A., Yokoyama, W.M., Rossjohn, J., Brooks, A.G., Smyth, M.J.: Recognition of the nonclassical MHC class I molecule H2-M3 by the receptor Ly49A regulates the licensing and activation of NK cells. Nat. Immunol. **13**, 1171–1177 (2012)
Antony, P.A., Restifo, N.P.: CD4 + CD25+ T regulatory cells, immunotherapy of cancer, and interleukin-2. J. Immunother. **28**, 120–128 (2005)
Apetoh, L., Ghiringhelli, F., Tesniere, A., Obeid, M., Ortiz, C., Criollo, A., Mignot, G., Maiuri, M.C., Ullrich, E., Saulnier, P., Yang, H., Amigorena, S., Ryffel, B., Barrat, F.J., Saftig, P., Levi, F., Lidereau, R., Nogues, C., Mira, J.P., Chompret, A., Joulin, V., Clavel-Chapelon, F., Bourhis, J., Andre, F., Delaloge, S., Tursz, T., Kroemer, G., Zitvogel, L.: Toll-like receptor 4-dependent contribution of the immune system to anticancer chemotherapy and radiotherapy. Nat. Med. **13**, 1050–1059 (2007)
Arai, S., Meagher, R., Swearingen, M., Myint, H., Rich, E., Martinson, J., Klingemann, H.: Infusion of the allogeneic cell line NK-92 in patients with advanced renal cell cancer or melanoma: a phase I trial. Cytotherapy **10**, 625–632 (2008)

Atkins, M.B., Robertson, M.J., Gordon, M., Lotze, M.T., Decoste, M., Dubois, J.S., Ritz, J., Sandler, A.B., Edington, H.D., Garzone, P.D., Mier, J.W., Canning, C.M., Battiato, L., Tahara, H., Sherman, M.L.: Phase I evaluation of intravenous recombinant human interleukin 12 in patients with advanced malignancies. Clin. Cancer Res. **3**, 409–417 (1997)

Atkins, M.B., Lotze, M.T., Dutcher, J.P., Fisher, R.I., Weiss, G., Margolin, K., Abrams, J., Sznol, M., Parkinson, D., Hawkins, M., Paradise, C., Kunkel, L., Rosenberg, S.A.: High-dose recombinant interleukin 2 therapy for patients with metastatic melanoma: analysis of 270 patients treated between 1985 and 1993. J. Clin. Oncol. **17**, 2105–2116 (1999)

Baeuerle, P.A., Reinhardt, C.: Bispecific T-cell engaging antibodies for cancer therapy. Cancer Res. **69**, 4941–4944 (2009)

Balasa, B., Yun, R., Belmar, N.A., Fox, M., Chao, D.T., Robbins, M.D., Starling, G.C., Rice, A.G.: Elotuzumab enhances natural killer cell activation and myeloma cell killing through interleukin-2 and TNF-alpha pathways. Cancer Immunol. Immunother. **64**, 61–73 (2015)

Baragano Raneros, A., Suarez-Alvarez, B., Lopez-Larrea, C.: Secretory pathways generating immunosuppressive NKG2D ligands: new targets for therapeutic intervention. Oncoimmunology **3**, e28497 (2014)

Bekaii-Saab, T.S., Roda, J.M., Guenterberg, K.D., Ramaswamy, B., Young, D.C., Ferketich, A.K., Lamb, T.A., Grever, M.R., Shapiro, C.L., Carson 3RD, W.E.: A phase I trial of paclitaxel and trastuzumab in combination with interleukin-12 in patients with HER2/neu-expressing malignancies. Mol. Cancer Ther. **8**, 2983–2991 (2009)

Benson Jr., D.M., Bakan, C.E., Mishra, A., Hofmeister, C.C., Efebera, Y., Becknell, B., Baiocchi, R.A., Zhang, J., Yu, J., Smith, M.K., Greenfield, C.N., Porcu, P., Devine, S.M., Rotem-Yehudar, R., Lozanski, G., Byrd, J.C., Caligiuri, M.A.: The PD-1/PD-L1 axis modulates the natural killer cell versus multiple myeloma effect: a therapeutic target for CT-011, a novel monoclonal anti-PD-1 antibody. Blood **116**, 2286–2294 (2010)

Berger, C., Berger, M., Hackman, R.C., Gough, M., Elliott, C., Jensen, M.C., Riddell, S.R.: Safety and immunologic effects of IL-15 administration in nonhuman primates. Blood **114**, 2417–2426 (2009)

Blauvelt, A., Asada, H., Klaus-Kovtun, V., ALTMAN, D.J., Lucey, D.R., Katz, S.I.: Interleukin-15 mRNA is expressed by human keratinocytes Langerhans cells, and blood-derived dendritic cells and is downregulated by ultraviolet B radiation. J. Invest. Dermatol. **106**, 1047–1052 (1996)

Bracci, L., Schiavoni, G., Sistigu, A., Belardelli, F.: Immune-based mechanisms of cytotoxic chemotherapy: implications for the design of novel and rationale-based combined treatments against cancer. Cell Death Differ. **21**, 15–25 (2014)

Braud, V.M., Allan, D.S., O'callaghan, C.A., Soderstrom, K., D'andrea, A., Ogg, G.S., Lazetic, S., Young, N.T., Bell, J.I., Phillips, J.H., Lanier, L.L., Mcmichael, A.J.: HLA-E binds to natural killer cell receptors CD94/NKG2A, B and C. Nature **391**, 795–799 (1998)

Braumuller, H., Wieder, T., Brenner, E., Assmann, S., Hahn, M., Alkhaled, M., Schilbach, K., Essmann, F., Kneilling, M., Griessinger, C., Ranta, F., Ullrich, S., Mocikat, R., Braungart, K., Mehra, T., Fehrenbacher, B., Berdel, J., Niessner, H., Meier, F., van den Broek, M., Haring, H.U., Handgretinger, R., Quintanilla-Martinez, L., Fend, F., Pesic, M., Bauer, J., Zender, L., Schaller, M., Schulze-Osthoff, K., Rocken, M.: T-helper-1-cell cytokines drive cancer into senescence. Nature **494**, 361–365 (2013)

Brody, J.R., Costantino, C.L., Berger, A.C., Sato, T., Lisanti, M.P., Yeo, C.J., Emmons, R.V., Witkiewicz, A.K.: Expression of indoleamine 2,3-dioxygenase in metastatic malignant melanoma recruits regulatory T cells to avoid immune detection and affects survival. Cell Cycle **8**, 1930–1934 (2009)

Brunda, M.J., Luistro, L., Warrier, R.R., Wright, R.B., Hubbard, B.R., Murphy, M., Wolf, S.F., Gately, M.K.: Antitumor and antimetastatic activity of interleukin 12 against murine tumors. J. Exp. Med. **178**, 1223–1230 (1993)

Bruno, A., Ferlazzo, G., Albini, A., Noonan, D.M.: A think tank of TINK/TANKs: tumor-infiltrating/tumor-associated natural killer cells in tumor progression and angiogenesis. J. Natl. Cancer Inst. **106**, dju200 (2014)

Bryceson, Y.T., March, M.E., Ljunggren, H.G., Long, E.O.: Activation, coactivation, and costimulation of resting human natural killer cells. Immunol. Rev. **214**, 73–91 (2006a)

Bryceson, Y.T., March, M.E., Ljunggren, H.G., Long, E.O.: Synergy among receptors on resting NK cells for the activation of natural cytotoxicity and cytokine secretion. Blood **107**, 159–166 (2006b)

Burkett, P.R., Koka, R., Chien, M., Chai, S., Boone, D.L., Ma, A.: Coordinate expression and trans presentation of interleukin (IL)-15Ralpha and IL-15 supports natural killer cell and memory CD8+ T cell homeostasis. J. Exp. Med. **200**, 825–834 (2004)

Burns, L.J., Weisdorf, D.J., Defor, T.E., Vesole, D.H., Repka, T.L., Blazar, B.R., Burger, S.R., Panoskaltsis-Mortari, A., Keever-Taylor, C.A., Zhang, M.J., Miller, J.S.: IL-2-based immunotherapy after autologous transplantation for lymphoma and breast cancer induces immune activation and cytokine release: a phase I/II trial. Bone Marrow Transplant. **32**, 177–186 (2003)

Caligiuri, M.A.: Human natural killer cells. Blood **112**, 461–469 (2008)

Caligiuri, M.A., Murray, C., Soiffer, R.J., Klumpp, T.R., Seiden, M., Cochran, K., Cameron, C., Ish, C., Buchanan, L., Perillo, D., et al.: Extended continuous infusion low-dose recombinant interleukin-2 in advanced cancer: prolonged immunomodulation without significant toxicity. J. Clin. Oncol. **9**, 2110–2119 (1991)

Campbell, J.J., Qin, S., Unutmaz, D., Soler, D., Murphy, K.E., Hodge, M.R., Wu, L., Butcher, E.C.: Unique subpopulations of CD56+ NK and NK-T peripheral blood lymphocytes identified by chemokine receptor expression repertoire. J. Immunol. **166**, 6477–6482 (2001)

Carnaud, C., Lee, D., Donnars, O., Park, S.H., Beavis, A., Koezuka, Y., Bendelac, A.: Cutting edge: cross-talk between cells of the innate immune system: NKT cells rapidly activate NK cells. J. Immunol. **163**, 4647–4650 (1999)

Carrega, P., Ferlazzo, G.: Natural killer cell distribution and trafficking in human tissues. Front Immun. **3**, 347 (2012)

Carson, W.E., Ross, M.E., Baiocchi, R.A., Marien, M.J., Boiani, N., Grabstein, K., Caligiuri, M.A.: Endogenous production of interleukin 15 by activated human monocytes is critical for optimal production of interferon-gamma by natural killer cells in vitro. J. Clin. Invest. **96**, 2578–2582 (1995)

Castriconi, R., Cantoni, C., Della Chiesa, M., Vitale, M., Marcenaro, E., Conte, R., Biassoni, R., Bottino, C., Moretta, L., Moretta, A.: Transforming growth factor beta 1 inhibits expression of NKp30 and NKG2D receptors: consequences for the NK-mediated killing of dendritic cells. Proc. Natl. Acad. Sci. U. S. A. **100**, 4120–4125 (2003)

Castriconi, R., Dondero, A., Bellora, F., Moretta, L., Castellano, A., Locatelli, F., Corrias, M.V., Moretta, A., Bottino, C.: Neuroblastoma-derived TGF-beta1 modulates the chemokine receptor repertoire of human resting NK cells. J. Immunol. **190**, 5321–5328 (2013)

Chan, H.W., Kurago, Z.B., Stewart, C.A., Wilson, M.J., Martin, M.P., Mace, B.E., Carrington, M., Trowsdale, J., Lutz, C.T.: DNA methylation maintains allele-specific KIR gene expression in human natural killer cells. J. Exp. Med. **197**, 245–255 (2003)

Chan, A., Hong, D.L., Atzberger, A., Kollnberger, S., Filer, A.D., Buckley, C.D., Mcmichael, A., Enver, T., Bowness, P.: CD56bright human NK cells differentiate into CD56dim cells: role of contact with peripheral fibroblasts. J. Immunol. **179**, 89–94 (2007)

Chang, Y.H., Connolly, J., Shimasaki, N., Mimura, K., Kono, K., Campana, D.: A chimeric receptor with NKG2D specificity enhances natural killer cell activation and killing of tumor cells. Cancer Res. **73**, 1777–1786 (2013)

Cherfils-Vicini, J., Platonova, S., Gillard, M., Laurans, L., Validire, P., CALIANDRO, R., Magdeleinat, P., Mami-Chouaib, F., Dieu-Nosjean, M.C., Fridman, W.H., Damotte, D., Sautes-Fridman, C., Cremer, I.: Triggering of TLR7 and TLR8 expressed by human lung cancer cells induces cell survival and chemoresistance. J. Clin. Invest. **120**, 1285–1297 (2010)

Collins, S.M., Bakan, C.E., Swartzel, G.D., Hofmeister, C.C., Efebera, Y.A., Kwon, H., Starling, G.C., Ciarlariello, D., Bhaskar, S., Briercheck, E.L., Hughes, T., Yu, J., Rice, A., Benson Jr., D.M.: Elotuzumab directly enhances NK cell cytotoxicity against myeloma via CS1 ligation: evidence for augmented NK cell function complementing ADCC. Cancer Immunol. Immunother. **62**, 1841–1849 (2013)

Cooper, M.A., Fehniger, T.A., Turner, S.C., Chen, K.S., Ghaheri, B.A., Ghayur, T., Carson, W.E., Caligiuri, M.A.: Human natural killer cells: a unique innate immunoregulatory role for the CD56(bright) subset. Blood **97**, 3146–3151 (2001)

Croft, M.: Control of immunity by the TNFR-related molecule OX40 (CD134). Annu. Rev. Immunol. **28**, 57–78 (2010)

Delahaye, N.F., Rusakiewicz, S., Martins, I., Menard, C., Roux, S., Lyonnet, L., Paul, P., Sarabi, M., Chaput, N., Semeraro, M., Minard-Colin, V., Poirier-Colame, V., Chaba, K., Flament, C., Baud, V., Authier, H., Kerdine-Romer, S., Pallardy, M., Cremer, I., Peaudecerf, L., Rocha, B., Valteau-Couanet, D., Gutierrez, J.C., Nunes, J.A., Commo, F., Bonvalot, S., Ibrahim, N., Terrier, P., Opolon, P., Bottino, C., Moretta, A., Tavernier, J., Rihet, P., Coindre, J.M., Blay, J.Y., Isambert, N., Emile, J.F., Vivier, E., Lecesne, A., Kroemer, G., Zitvogel, L.: Alternatively spliced NKp30 isoforms affect the prognosis of gastrointestinal stromal tumors. Nat. Med. **17**, 700–707 (2011)

Della Chiesa, M., Vitale, M., Carlomagno, S., Ferlazzo, G., Moretta, L., Moretta, A.: The natural killer cell-mediated killing of autologous dendritic cells is confined to a cell subset expressing CD94/NKG2A, but lacking inhibitory killer Ig-like receptors. Eur. J. Immunol. **33**, 1657–1666 (2003)

di Carlo, E., Comes, A., Orengo, A.M., Rosso, O., Meazza, R., Musiani, P., Colombo, M.P., Ferrini, S.: IL-21 induces tumor rejection by specific CTL and IFN-gamma-dependent CXC chemokines in syngeneic mice. J. Immunol. **172**, 1540–1547 (2004)

Doherty, D.G., O'farrelly, C.: Innate and adaptive lymphoid cells in the human liver. Immunol. Rev. **174**, 5–20 (2000)

Dorner, B.G., Smith, H.R., French, A.R., Kim, S., Poursine-Laurent, J., Beckman, D.L., Pingel, J.T., Kroczek, R.A., Yokoyama, W.M.: Coordinate expression of cytokines and chemokines by NK cells during murine cytomegalovirus infection. J. Immunol. **172**, 3119–3131 (2004)

Eguizabal, C., Zenarruzabeitia, O., Monge, J., Santos, S., Vesga, M.A., Maruri, N., Arrieta, A., Rinon, M., Tamayo-Orbegozo, E., Amo, L., Larrucea, S., Borrego, F.: Natural killer cells for cancer immunotherapy: pluripotent stem cells-derived NK cells as an immunotherapeutic perspective. Front Immunol. **5**, 439 (2014)

Elboim, M., Gazit, R., Gur, C., Ghadially, H., Betser-Cohen, G., Mandelboim, O.: Tumor immunoediting by NKp46. J. Immunol. **184**, 5637–5644 (2010)

Falco, M., Moretta, L., Moretta, A., Bottino, C.: KIR and KIR ligand polymorphism: a new area for clinical applications? Tissue Antigens **82**, 363–373 (2013)

Falschlehner, C., Schaefer, U., Walczak, H.: Following TRAIL's path in the immune system. Immunology **127**, 145–154 (2009)

Fehniger, T.A., Caligiuri, M.A.: Interleukin 15: biology and relevance to human disease. Blood **97**, 14–32 (2001)

Fehniger, T.A., Shah, M.H., Turner, M.J., Vandeusen, J.B., Whitman, S.P., Cooper, M.A., Suzuki, K., Wechser, M., Goodsaid, F., Caligiuri, M.A.: Differential cytokine and chemokine gene expression by human NK cells following activation with IL-18 or IL-15 in combination with IL-12: implications for the innate immune response. J. Immunol. **162**, 4511–4520 (1999)

Fehniger, T.A., Cooper, M.A., Caligiuri, M.A.: Interleukin-2 and interleukin-15: immunotherapy for cancer. Cytokine Growth Factor Rev. **13**, 169–183 (2002)

Ferlazzo, G., Thomas, D., Lin, S.L., Goodman, K., Morandi, B., Muller, W.A., Moretta, A., Munz, C.: The abundant NK cells in human secondary lymphoid tissues require activation to express killer cell Ig-like receptors and become cytolytic. J. Immunol. **172**, 1455–1462 (2004)

Ferrara, C., Grau, S., Jager, C., Sondermann, P., Brunker, P., Waldhauer, I., Hennig, M., Ruf, A., Rufer, A.C., Stihle, M., Umana, P., Benz, J.: Unique carbohydrate-carbohydrate interactions are required for high affinity binding between FcgammaRIII and antibodies lacking core fucose. Proc. Natl. Acad. Sci. U. S. A. **108**, 12669–12674 (2011)

Fionda, C., Malgarini, G., Soriani, A., Zingoni, A., Cecere, F., Iannitto, M.L., Ricciardi, M.R., Federico, V., Petrucci, M.T., Santoni, A., Cippitelli, M.: Inhibition of glycogen synthase kinase-3 increases NKG2D ligand MICA expression and sensitivity to NK cell-mediated cytotoxicity in multiple myeloma cells: role of STAT3. J. Immunol. **190**, 6662–6672 (2013)

Forero-Torres, A., de Vos, S., Pohlman, B.L., Pashkevich, M., Cronier, D.M., Dang, N.H., Carpenter, S.P., Allan, B.W., Nelson, J.G., Slapak, C.A., Smith, M.R., Link, B.K., Wooldridge, J.E., Ganjoo, K.N.: Results of a phase 1 study of AME-133v (LY2469298), an Fc-engineered humanized monoclonal anti-CD20 antibody, in FcgammaRIIIa-genotyped patients with previously treated follicular lymphoma. Clin. Cancer Res. **18**, 1395–1403 (2012)

Fujisaki, H., Kakuda, H., Shimasaki, N., Imai, C., Ma, J., Lockey, T., Eldridge, P., Leung, W.H., Campana, D.: Expansion of highly cytotoxic human natural killer cells for cancer cell therapy. Cancer Res. **69**, 4010–4017 (2009)

Fyfe, G., Fisher, R.I., Rosenberg, S.A., Sznol, M., Parkinson, D.R., Louie, A.C.: Results of treatment of 255 patients with metastatic renal cell carcinoma who received high-dose recombinant interleukin-2 therapy. J. Clin. Oncol. **13**, 688–696 (1995)

Galy, A., Travis, M., Cen, D., Chen, B.: Human T, B, natural killer, and dendritic cells arise from a common bone marrow progenitor cell subset. Immunity **3**, 459–473 (1995)

Geller, M.A., Cooley, S., Judson, P.L., Ghebre, R., Carson, L.F., Argenta, P.A., Jonson, A.L., Panoskaltsis-Mortari, A., Curtsinger, J., Mckenna, D., Dusenbery, K., Bliss, R., Downs, L.S., Miller, J.S.: A phase II study of allogeneic natural killer cell therapy to treat patients with recurrent ovarian and breast cancer. Cytotherapy **13**, 98–107 (2011)

Ghiringhelli, F., Menard, C., Terme, M., Flament, C., Taieb, J., Chaput, N., Puig, P.E., Novault, S., Escudier, B., Vivier, E., Lecesne, A., Robert, C., Blay, J.Y., Bernard, J., Caillat-Zucman, S., Freitas, A., Tursz, T., Wagner-Ballon, O., Capron, C., Vainchencker, W., Martin, F., Zitvogel, L.: CD4+CD25+ regulatory T cells inhibit natural killer cell functions in a transforming growth factor-beta-dependent manner. J. Exp. Med. **202**, 1075–1085 (2005)

Ghiringhelli, F., Menard, C., Puig, P.E., Ladoire, S., Roux, S., Martin, F., Solary, E., le Cesne, A., Zitvogel, L., Chauffert, B.: Metronomic cyclophosphamide regimen selectively depletes CD4+CD25+ regulatory T cells and restores T and NK effector functions in end stage cancer patients. Cancer Immunol. Immunother. **56**, 641–648 (2007)

Glasner, A., Ghadially, H., Gur, C., Stanietsky, N., Tsukerman, P., Enk, J., Mandelboim, O.: Recognition and prevention of tumor metastasis by the NK receptor NKp46/NCR1. J. Immunol. **188**, 2509–2515 (2012)

Glienke, W., Esser, R., Priesner, C., Suerth, J.D., Schambach, A., Wels, W.S., Grez, M., Kloess, S., Arseniev, L., Koehl, U.: Advantages and applications of CAR-expressing natural killer cells. Front. Pharmacol. **6**, 21 (2015)

Godfrey, D.I., Macdonald, H.R., Kronenberg, M., Smyth, M.J., van Kaer, L.: NKT cells: what's in a name? Nat. Rev. Immunol. **4**, 231–237 (2004)

Goede, V., Klein, C., Stilgenbauer, S.: Obinutuzumab (GA101) for the treatment of chronic lymphocytic leukemia and other B-cell non-hodgkin's lymphomas: a glycoengineered type II CD20 antibody. Oncol Res Treat **38**, 185–192 (2015)

Gonzalez, S., Groh, V., Spies, T.: Immunobiology of human NKG2D and its ligands. Curr. Top. Microbiol. Immunol. **298**, 121–138 (2006)

Gowda, A., roda, J., Hussain, S.R., Ramanunni, A., Joshi, T., Schmidt, S., Zhang, X., Lehman, A., Jarjoura, D., Carson, W.E., Kindsvogel, W., Cheney, C., Caligiuri, M.A., Tridandapani, S., Muthusamy, N., Byrd, J.C.: IL-21 mediates apoptosis through up-regulation of the BH3 family member BIM and enhances both direct and antibody-dependent cellular cytotoxicity in primary chronic lymphocytic leukemia cells in vitro. Blood **111**, 4723–4730 (2008)

Gregoire, C., Chasson, L., Luci, C., TomasELLO, E., Geissmann, F., Vivier, E., Walzer, T.: The trafficking of natural killer cells. Immunol. Rev. **220**, 169–182 (2007)

Groth, A., Kloss, S., von Strandmann, E.P., Koehl, U., Koch, J.: Mechanisms of tumor and viral immune escape from natural killer cell-mediated surveillance. J. Innate Immun. **3**, 344–354 (2011)

Han, K.P., ZHU, X., Liu, B., Jeng, E., Kong, L., Yovandich, J.L., Vyas, V.V., MARCUS, W.D., Chavaillaz, P.A., Romero, C.A., Rhode, P.R., Wong, H.C.: IL-15:IL-15 receptor alpha superagonist complex: high-level co-expression in recombinant mammalian cells, purification and characterization. Cytokine **56**, 804–810 (2011)

Hart, O.M., Athie-Morales, V., O'connor, G.M., Gardiner, C.M.: TLR7/8-mediated activation of human NK cells results in accessory cell-dependent IFN-gamma production. J. Immunol. **175**, 1636–1642 (2005)

HASHMI, M.H., van Veldhuizen, P.J.: Interleukin-21: updated review of Phase I and II clinical trials in metastatic renal cell carcinoma, metastatic melanoma and relapsed/refractory indolent non-Hodgkin's lymphoma. Expert Opin. Biol. Ther. **10**, 807–817 (2010)

Hatfield, S.M., Kjaergaard, J., Lukashev, D., Schreiber, T.H., Belikoff, B., Abbott, R., Sethumadhavan, S., Philbrook, P., Ko, K., Cannici, R., Thayer, M., Rodig, S., Kutok, J.L., Jackson, E.K., Karger, B., Podack, E.R., Ohta, A., Sitkovsky, M.V.: Immunological mechanisms of the antitumor effects of supplemental oxygenation. Sci. Transl. Med. **7**, 277ra30 (2015)

Hermanson, D.L., Kaufman, D.S.: Utilizing chimeric antigen receptors to direct natural killer cell activity. Front. Immunol. **6**, 195 (2015)

Herter, S., Herting, F., Mundigl, O., Waldhauer, I., Weinzierl, T., Fauti, T., Muth, G., Ziegler-Landesberger, D., van Puijenbroek, E., Lang, S., Duong, M.N., Reslan, L., Gerdes, C.A., Friess, T., BAER, U., Burtscher, H., Weidner, M., Dumontet, C., Umana, P., Niederfellner, G., Bacac, M., Klein, C.: Preclinical activity of the type II CD20 antibody GA101 (obinutuzumab) compared with rituximab and ofatumumab in vitro and in xenograft models. Mol. Cancer Ther. **12**, 2031–2042 (2013)

Iliopoulou, E.G., Kountourakis, P., Karamouzis, M.V., Doufexis, D., Ardavanis, A., Baxevanis, C.N., Rigatos, G., Papamichail, M., PEREZ, S.A.: A phase I trial of adoptive transfer of allogeneic natural killer cells in patients with advanced non-small cell lung cancer. Cancer Immunol. Immunother. **59**, 1781–1789 (2010)

Imai, K., Matsuyama, S., Miyake, S., Suga, K., Nakachi, K.: Natural cytotoxic activity of peripheral-blood lymphocytes and cancer incidence: an 11-year follow-up study of a general population. Lancet **356**, 1795–1799 (2000)

Inngjerdingen, M., Damaj, B., Maghazachi, A.A.: Expression and regulation of chemokine receptors in human natural killer cells. Blood **97**, 367–375 (2001)

Ishigami, S., Natsugoe, S., Tokuda, K., Nakajo, A., Che, X., Iwashige, H., Aridome, K., Hokita, S., Aikou, T.: Prognostic value of intratumoral natural killer cells in gastric carcinoma. Cancer **88**, 577–583 (2000)

Jacobs, B., Ullrich, E.: The interaction of NK cells and dendritic cells in the tumor environment: how to enforce NK cell & DC action under immunosuppressive conditions? Curr. Med. Chem. **19**, 1771–1779 (2012)

Jena, B., Moyes, J.S., Huls, H., Cooper, L.J.: Driving CAR-based T-cell therapy to success. Curr. Hematol. Malig. Rep. **9**, 50–56 (2014)

Jing, Y., Ni, Z., Wu, J., Higgins, L., Markowski, T.W., Kaufman, D.S., Walcheck, B.: Identification of an ADAM17 cleavage region in human CD16 (FcgammaRIII) and the engineering of a non-cleavable version of the receptor in NK cells. PLoS One **10**, e0121788 (2015)

Kaczanowska, S., Joseph, A.M., Davila, E.: TLR agonists: our best frenemy in cancer immunotherapy. J. Leukoc. Biol. **93**, 847–863 (2013)

Kaidanovich-Beilin, O., Woodgett, J.R.: GSK-3: Functional Insights from Cell Biology and Animal Models. Front. Mol. Neurosci. **4**, 40 (2011)

Kakarla, S., Gottschalk, S.: CAR T cells for solid tumors: armed and ready to go? Cancer J. **20**, 151–155 (2014)

Karre, K., Ljunggren, H.G., Piontek, G., Kiessling, R.: Selective rejection of H-2-deficient lymphoma variants suggests alternative immune defence strategy. Nature **319**, 675–678 (1986)

Kiessling, R., Klein, E., Wigzell, H.: "Natural" killer cells in the mouse. I. Cytotoxic cells with specificity for mouse Moloney leukemia cells. Specificity and distribution according to genotype. Eur. J. Immunol. **5**, 112–117 (1975)

Koch, J., Steinle, A., Watzl, C., Mandelboim, O.: Activating natural cytotoxicity receptors of natural killer cells in cancer and infection. Trends Immunol. **34**, 182–191 (2013)

Kohrt, H.E., Houot, R., Marabelle, A., Cho, H.J., Osman, K., Goldstein, M., Levy, R., Brody, J.: Combination strategies to enhance antitumor ADCC. Immunotherapy **4**, 511–527 (2012)

Kohrt, H.E., Colevas, A.D., Houot, R., Weiskopf, K., Goldstein, M.J., Lund, P., Mueller, A., Sagiv-Barfi, I., Marabelle, A., Lira, R., Troutner, E., Richards, L., Rajapaska, A., Hebb, J., Chester, C., Waller, E., Ostashko, A., Weng, W.K., Chen, L., Czerwinski, D., Fu, Y.X., Sunwoo, J., Levy, R.: Targeting CD137 enhances the efficacy of cetuximab. J. Clin. Invest. **124**, 2668–2682 (2014a)

Kohrt, H.E., Thielens, A., Marabelle, A., Sagiv-Barfi, I., Sola, C., Chanuc, F., Fuseri, N., Bonnafous, C., Czerwinski, D., Rajapaksa, A., Waller, E., Ugolini, S., Vivier, E., Romagne, F., Levy, R., Blery, M., Andre, P.: Anti-KIR antibody enhancement of anti-lymphoma activity of natural killer cells as monotherapy and in combination with anti-CD20 antibodies. Blood **123**, 678–686 (2014b)

Krueger, P.D., Lassen, M.G., Qiao, H., Hahn, Y.S.: Regulation of NK cell repertoire and function in the liver. Crit. Rev. Immunol. **31**, 43–52 (2011)

Kwon, B.S., Weissman, S.M.: cDNA sequences of two inducible T-cell genes. Proc. Natl. Acad. Sci. U. S. A. **86**, 1963–1967 (1989)

Lanier, L.L.: Up on the tightrope: natural killer cell activation and inhibition. Nat. Immunol. **9**, 495–502 (2008)

Lanier, L.L.: NKG2D Receptor and Its Ligands in Host Defense. Cancer Immunol. Res. **3**, 575–582 (2015)

Lanier, L.L., Testi, R., Bindl, J., Phillips, J.H.: Identity of Leu-19 (CD56) leukocyte differentiation antigen and neural cell adhesion molecule. J. Exp. Med. **169**, 2233–2238 (1989)

Leonard, J.P., Sherman, M.L., Fisher, G.L., Buchanan, L.J., Larsen, G., Atkins, M.B., Sosman, J.A., Dutcher, J.P., Vogelzang, N.J., Ryan, J.L.: Effects of single-dose interleukin-12 exposure on interleukin-12-associated toxicity and interferon-gamma production. Blood **90**, 2541–2548 (1997)

Leong, J.W., Chase, J.M., Romee, R., Schneider, S.E., Sullivan, R.P., Cooper, M.A., Fehniger, T.A.: Preactivation with IL-12, IL-15, and IL-18 induces CD25 and a functional high-affinity IL-2 receptor on human cytokine-induced memory-like natural killer cells. Biol. Blood Marrow Transplant. **20**, 463–473 (2014)

Lim, S.A., Kim, T.J., Lee, J.E., Sonn, C.H., Kim, K., Kim, J., Choi, J.G., Choi, I.K., Yun, C.O., Kim, J.H., Yee, C., Kumar, V., Lee, K.M.: Ex vivo expansion of highly cytotoxic human NK cells by cocultivation with irradiated tumor cells for adoptive immunotherapy. Cancer Res. **73**, 2598–2607 (2013)

Lin, W., Voskens, C.J., Zhang, X., Schindler, D.G., Wood, A., Burch, E., Wei, Y., Chen, L., Tian, G., Tamada, K., Wang, L.X., Schulze, D.H., Mann, D., Strome, S.E.: Fc-dependent expression of CD137 on human NK cells: insights into "agonistic" effects of anti-CD137 monoclonal antibodies. Blood **112**, 699–707 (2008)

Liu, C., Lou, Y., Lizee, G., Qin, H., Liu, S., Rabinovich, B., Kim, G.J., Wang, Y.H., Ye, Y., Sikora, A.G., Overwijk, W.W., Liu, Y.J., Wang, G., Hwu, P.: Plasmacytoid dendritic cells induce NK cell-dependent, tumor antigen-specific T cell cross-priming and tumor regression in mice. J. Clin. Invest. **118**, 1165–1175 (2008)

Ljunggren, H.G., Karre, K.: In search of the 'missing self': MHC molecules and NK cell recognition. Immunol. Today **11**, 237–244 (1990)

Lu, H., Dietsch, G.N., Matthews, M.A., Yang, Y., Ghanekar, S., Inokuma, M., Suni, M., Maino, V.C., Henderson, K.E., Howbert, J.J., Disis, M.L., Hershberg, R.M.: VTX-2337 is a novel TLR8 agonist that activates NK cells and augments ADCC. Clin. Cancer Res. **18**, 499–509 (2012)

Maghazachi, A.A.: Role of chemokines in the biology of natural killer cells. Curr. Top. Microbiol. Immunol. **341**, 37–58 (2010)

Maki, G., Klingemann, H.G., Martinson, J.A., Tam, Y.K.: Factors regulating the cytotoxic activity of the human natural killer cell line, NK-92. J. Hematother. Stem Cell Res. **10**, 369–383 (2001)

Mamessier, E., Sylvain, A., Thibult, M.L., Houvenaeghel, G., Jacquemier, J., Castellano, R., Goncalves, A., Andre, P., Romagne, F., Thibault, G., Viens, P., Birnbaum, D., Bertucci, F., Moretta, A., Olive, D.: Human breast cancer cells enhance self tolerance by promoting evasion from NK cell antitumor immunity. J. Clin. Invest. **121**, 3609–3622 (2011)

Mani, A., Roda, J., Young, D., Caligiuri, M.A., Fleming, G.F., Kaufman, P., Brufsky, A., Ottman, S., Carson 3RD, W.E., Shapiro, C.L.: A phase II trial of trastuzumab in combination with low-dose interleukin-2 (IL-2) in patients (PTS) with metastatic breast cancer (MBC) who have previously failed trastuzumab. Breast Cancer Res. Treat. **117**, 83–89 (2009)

Marcenaro, E., Pesce, S., Sivori, S., Carlomagno, S., Moretta, L., Moretta, A.: KIR2DS1-dependent acquisition of CCR7 and migratory properties by human NK cells interacting with allogeneic HLA-C2+ DCs or T-cell blasts. Blood **121**, 3396–3401 (2013)

Mccubrey, J.A., Steelman, L.S., Bertrand, F.E., Davis, N.M., Sokolosky, M., Abrams, S.L., Montalto, G., D'assoro, A.B., Libra, M., Nicoletti, F., Maestro, R., Basecke, J., Rakus, D., Gizak, A., Demidenko, Z.N., Cocco, L., Martelli, A.M., Cervello, M.: GSK-3 as potential target for therapeutic intervention in cancer. Oncotarget **5**, 2881–2911 (2014)

Menard, C., Blay, J.Y., Borg, C., Michiels, S., Ghiringhelli, F., Robert, C., Nonn, C., Chaput, N., Taieb, J., Delahaye, N.F., Flament, C., Emile, J.F., le Cesne, A., Zitvogel, L.: Natural killer cell IFN-gamma levels predict long-term survival with imatinib mesylate therapy in gastrointestinal stromal tumor-bearing patients. Cancer Res. **69**, 3563–3569 (2009)

Mentlik James, A., Cohen, A.D., Campbell, K.S.: Combination immune therapies to enhance antitumor responses by NK cells. Front. Immunol. **4**, 481 (2013)

Meropol, N.J., Barresi, G.M., Fehniger, T.A., Hitt, J., Franklin, M., Caligiuri, M.A.: Evaluation of natural killer cell expansion and activation in vivo with daily subcutaneous low-dose interleukin-2 plus periodic intermediate-dose pulsing. Cancer Immunol. Immunother. **46**, 318–326 (1998)

Moga, E., Alvarez, E., Canto, E., Vidal, S., Rodriguez-Sanchez, J.L., Sierra, J., Briones, J.: NK cells stimulated with IL-15 or CpG ODN enhance rituximab-dependent cellular cytotoxicity against B-cell lymphoma. Exp. Hematol. **36**, 69–77 (2008)

Moretta, L., Bottino, C., Pende, D., Vitale, M., Mingari, M.C., Moretta, A.: Different checkpoints in human NK-cell activation. Trends Immunol. **25**, 670–676 (2004)

Moretta, L., Ferlazzo, G., Bottino, C., Vitale, M., Pende, D., Mingari, M.C., Moretta, A.: Effector and regulatory events during natural killer-dendritic cell interactions. Immunol. Rev. **214**, 219–228 (2006)

Moretta, L., Montaldo, E., Vacca, P., del Zotto, G., Moretta, F., Merli, P., Locatelli, F., Mingari, M.C.: Human natural killer cells: origin, receptors, function, and clinical applications. Int. Arch. Allergy Immunol. **164**, 253–264 (2014)

Motzer, R.J., Rakhit, A., Thompson, J.A., Nemunaitis, J., Murphy, B.A., Ellerhorst, J., Schwartz, L.H., Berg, W.J., Bukowski, R.M.: Randomized multicenter phase II trial of subcutaneous recombinant human interleukin-12 versus interferon-alpha 2a for patients with advanced renal cell carcinoma. J. Interferon Cytokine Res. **21**, 257–263 (2001)

Nabekura, T., Lanier, L.L.: Antigen-specific expansion and differentiation of natural killer cells by alloantigen stimulation. J. Exp. Med. **211**, 2455–2465 (2014)

Nastala, C.L., Edington, H.D., Mckinney, T.G., Tahara, H., Nalesnik, M.A., Brunda, M.J., Gately, M.K., Wolf, S.F., Schreiber, R.D., Storkus, W.J., et al.: Recombinant IL-12 administration induces tumor regression in association with IFN-gamma production. J. Immunol. **153**, 1697–1706 (1994)

Nieto, M., Navarro, F., Perez-Villar, J.J., del Pozo, M.A., Gonzalez-Amaro, R., Mellado, M., Frade, J.M., Martinez, A.C., Lopez-Botet, M., Sanchez-Madrid, F.: Roles of chemokines and receptor polarization in NK-target cell interactions. J. Immunol. **161**, 3330–3339 (1998)

Nijhof, I.S., van Bueren, J.J.L., van Kessel, B., Andre, P., Morel, Y., Lokhorst, H.M., van de Donk, N.W., Parren, P.W., Mutis, T.: Daratumumab-mediated lysis of primary multiple myeloma cells is enhanced in combination with the human anti-KIR antibody IPH2102 and lenalidomide. Haematologica **100**, 263–268 (2015)

Norris, S., Coleman, A., Kuri-Cervantes, L., Bower, M., Nelson, M., Goodier, M.R.: PD-1 expression on natural killer cells and CD8(+) T cells during chronic HIV-1 infection. Viral Immunol. **25**, 329–332 (2012)

Northfelt, D.W., Ramanathan, R.K., Cohen, P.A., von Hoff, D.D., WEISS, G.J., Dietsch, G.N., Manjarrez, K.L., Randall, T.D., Hershberg, R.M.: A phase I dose-finding study of the novel toll-like receptor 8 agonist VTX-2337 in adult subjects with advanced solid tumors or lymphoma. Clin. Cancer Res. **20**, 3683–3691 (2014)

O'callaghan, C.A.: Molecular basis of human natural killer cell recognition of HLA-E (human leucocyte antigen-E) and its relevance to clearance of pathogen-infected and tumour cells. Clin. Sci. (Lond.) **99**, 9–17 (2000)

O'leary, J.G., Goodarzi, M., Drayton, D.L., von Andrian, U.H.: T cell- and B cell-independent adaptive immunity mediated by natural killer cells. Nat. Immunol. **7**, 507–516 (2006)

Orange, J.S.: Formation and function of the lytic NK-cell immunological synapse. Nat. Rev. Immunol. **8**, 713–725 (2008)

Orange, J.S.: Natural killer cell deficiency. J. Allergy Clin. Immunol. **132**, 515–525 (2013). quiz 526

Orange, J.S., Ballas, Z.K.: Natural killer cells in human health and disease. Clin. Immunol. **118**, 1–10 (2006)

Ostrand-Rosenberg, S., Sinha, P.: Myeloid-derived suppressor cells: linking inflammation and cancer. J. Immunol. **182**, 4499–4506 (2009)

Pachynski, R.K., Zabel, B.A., Kohrt, H.E., Tejeda, N.M., Monnier, J., Swanson, C.D., Holzer, A.K., Gentles, A.J., Sperinde, G.V., Edalati, A., Hadeiba, H.A., Alizadeh, A.A., Butcher, E.C.: The chemoattractant chemerin suppresses melanoma by recruiting natural killer cell antitumor defenses. J. Exp. Med. **209**, 1427–1435 (2012)

Palumbo, A., Sonneveld, P.: Preclinical and clinical evaluation of elotuzumab, a SLAMF7-targeted humanized monoclonal antibody in development for multiple myeloma. Expert Rev. Hematol. **8**, 481–491 (2015)

Pardoll, D.M.: The blockade of immune checkpoints in cancer immunotherapy. Nat. Rev. Cancer **12**, 252–264 (2012)

Parihar, R., Nadella, P., Lewis, A., Jensen, R., de Hoff, C., Dierksheide, J.E., Vanbuskirk, A.M., Magro, C.M., Young, D.C., Shapiro, C.L., Carson 3RD, W.E.: A phase I study of interleukin 12 with trastuzumab in patients with human epidermal growth factor receptor-2-overexpressing malignancies: analysis of sustained interferon gamma production in a subset of patients. Clin. Cancer Res. **10**, 5027–5037 (2004)

Parkhurst, M.R., Riley, J.P., Dudley, M.E., Rosenberg, S.A.: Adoptive transfer of autologous natural killer cells leads to high levels of circulating natural killer cells but does not mediate tumor regression. Clin. Cancer Res. **17**, 6287–6297 (2011)

Parolini, S., Santoro, A., Marcenaro, E., Luini, W., Massardi, L., Facchetti, F., Communi, D., Parmentier, M., Majorana, A., Sironi, M., Tabellini, G., Moretta, A., Sozzani, S.: The role of chemerin in the colocalization of NK and dendritic cell subsets into inflamed tissues. Blood **109**, 3625–3632 (2007)

Parrish-Novak, J., Dillon, S.R., Nelson, A., Hammond, A., Sprecher, C., Gross, J.A., Johnston, J., Madden, K., Xu, W., West, J., Schrader, S., Burkhead, S., Heipel, M., Brandt, C., Kuijper, J.L., Kramer, J., Conklin, D., Presnell, S.R., Berry, J., Shiota, F., Bort, S., Hambly, K., Mudri, S., Clegg, C., Moore, M., Grant, F.J., Lofton-Day, C., Gilbert, T., Rayond, F., Ching, A., Yao, L., Smith, D., Webster, P., Whitmore, T., Maurer, M., Kaushansky, K., Holly, R.D., Foster, D.: Interleukin 21 and its receptor are involved in NK cell expansion and regulation of lymphocyte function. Nature **408**, 57–63 (2000)

Payne, R., Glenn, L., Hoen, H., Richards, B., Smith 2ND, J.W., Lufkin, R., Crocenzi, T.S., Urba, W.J., Curti, B.D.: Durable responses and reversible toxicity of high-dose interleukin-2 treatment of melanoma and renal cancer in a Community Hospital Biotherapy Program. J Immunother. Cancer **2**, 13 (2014)

Peluso, I., Fantini, M.C., Fina, D., Caruso, R., Boirivant, M., Macdonald, T.T., Pallone, F., Monteleone, G.: IL-21 counteracts the regulatory T cell-mediated suppression of human CD4+ T lymphocytes. J. Immunol. **178**, 732–739 (2007)

Peng, Y.P., Zhang, J.J., Liang, W.B., Tu, M., Lu, Z.P., Wei, J.S., Jiang, K.R., Gao, W.T., Wu, J.L., Xu, Z.K., Miao, Y., Zhu, Y.: Elevation of MMP-9 and IDO induced by pancreatic cancer cells mediates natural killer cell dysfunction. BMC Cancer **14**, 738 (2014)

Petrella, T.M., Tozer, R., Belanger, K., Savage, K.J., Wong, R., Smylie, M., Kamel-Reid, S., Tron, V., Chen, B.E., Hunder, N.N., Hagerman, L., Walsh, W., Eisenhauer, E.A.: Interleukin-21 has activity in patients with metastatic melanoma: a phase II study. J. Clin. Oncol. **30**, 3396–3401 (2012)

Pietra, G., Manzini, C., Rivara, S., Vitale, M., Cantoni, C., Petretto, A., Balsamo, M., Conte, R., Benelli, R., Minghelli, S., Solari, N., Gualco, M., Queirolo, P., Moretta, L., Mingari, M.C.: Melanoma cells inhibit natural killer cell function by modulating the expression of activating receptors and cytolytic activity. Cancer Res. **72**, 1407–1415 (2012)

Platonova, S., Cherfils-Vicini, J., Damotte, D., Crozet, L., Vieillard, V., Validire, P., Andre, P., Dieu-Nosjean, M.C., Alifano, M., Regnard, J.F., Fridman, W.H., Sautes-Fridman, C., Cremer, I.: Profound coordinated alterations of intratumoral NK cell phenotype and function in lung carcinoma. Cancer Res. **71**, 5412–5422 (2011)

Polentarutti, N., Allavena, P., Bianchi, G., Giardina, G., Basile, A., Sozzani, S., Mantovani, A., Introna, M.: IL-2-regulated expression of the monocyte chemotactic protein-1 receptor (CCR2) in human NK cells: characterization of a predominant 3.4-kilobase transcript containing CCR2B and CCR2A sequences. J. Immunol. **158**, 2689–2694 (1997)

Raulet, D.H., Held, W.: Natural killer cell receptors: the offs and ons of NK cell recognition. Cell **82**, 697–700 (1995)

Ren, X., Zhou, L., Jiang, H.: Molecular weight determination and protein analysis of GCF-5 antigens of giant cell tumor of bone. Zhonghua Wai Ke Za Zhi **34**, 57–60 (1996)

Reusch, U., Burkhardt, C., Fucek, I., le Gall, F., le Gall, M., Hoffmann, K., Knackmuss, S.H., Kiprijanov, S., Little, M., Zhukovsky, E.A.: A novel tetravalent bispecific TandAb (CD30/CD16A) efficiently recruits NK cells for the lysis of CD30+ tumor cells. MAbs **6**, 728–739 (2014)

Robertson, M.J.: Role of chemokines in the biology of natural killer cells. J. Leukoc. Biol. **71**, 173–183 (2002)

Robertson, M.J., Cameron, C., Atkins, M.B., Gordon, M.S., Lotze, M.T., Sherman, M.L., Ritz, J.: Immunological effects of interleukin 12 administered by bolus intravenous injection to patients with cancer. Clin. Cancer Res. **5**, 9–16 (1999)

Roda, J.M., Joshi, T., Butchar, J.P., Mcalees, J.W., Lehman, A., Tridandapani, S., Carson 3RD, W.E.: The activation of natural killer cell effector functions by cetuximab-coated, epidermal growth factor receptor positive tumor cells is enhanced by cytokines. Clin. Cancer Res. **13**, 6419–6428 (2007)

Rodella, L., Zamai, L., Rezzani, R., Artico, M., Peri, G., Falconi, M., Facchini, A., Pelusi, G., Vitale, M.: Interleukin 2 and interleukin 15 differentially predispose natural killer cells to apoptosis mediated by endothelial and tumour cells. Br. J. Haematol. **115**, 442–450 (2001)

Romagnani, C., Juelke, K., Falco, M., Morandi, B., D'agostino, A., Costa, R., Ratto, G., Forte, G., Carrega, P., Lui, G., Conte, R., Strowig, T., Moretta, A., Munz, C., Thiel, A., Moretta, L., Ferlazzo, G.: CD56brightCD16- killer Ig-like receptor- NK cells display longer telomeres and acquire features of CD56dim NK cells upon activation. J. Immunol. **178**, 4947–4955 (2007)

Romagne, F., Andre, P., Spee, P., Zahn, S., Anfossi, N., Gauthier, L., Capanni, M., Ruggeri, L., Benson Jr., D.M., Blaser, B.W., Della Chiesa, M., Moretta, A., Vivier, E., Caligiuri, M.A., Velardi, A., Wagtmann, N.: Preclinical characterization of 1-7F9, a novel human anti-KIR receptor therapeutic antibody that augments natural killer-mediated killing of tumor cells. Blood **114**, 2667–2677 (2009)

Romee, R., Schneider, S.E., Leong, J.W., Chase, J.M., Keppel, C.R., Sullivan, R.P., Cooper, M.A., Fehniger, T.A.: Cytokine activation induces human memory-like NK cells. Blood **120**, 4751–4760 (2012)

Romee, R., Foley, B., Lenvik, T., Wang, Y., Zhang, B., Ankarlo, D., Luo, X., Cooley, S., Verneris, M., Walcheck, B., Miller, J.: NK cell CD16 surface expression and function is regulated by a disintegrin and metalloprotease-17 (ADAM17). Blood **121**, 3599–3608 (2013)

Romee, R., Leong, J.W., Fehniger, T.A.: Utilizing cytokines to function-enable human NK cells for the immunotherapy of cancer. Scientifica (Cairo) **2014**, 205796 (2014)

Rothe, A., Sasse, S., Topp, M.S., Eichenauer, D.A., Hummel, H., Reiners, K.S., Dietlein, M., Kuhnert, G., Kessler, J., Buerkle, C., Ravic, M., Knackmuss, S., Marschner, J.P., von Strandmann, P.E., Borchmann, P., Engert, A.: A phase 1 study of the bispecific anti-CD30/CD16A antibody construct AFM13 in patients with relapsed or refractory Hodgkin lymphoma. Blood **125**, 4024–4031 (2015)

Ruggeri, L., Capanni, M., Urbani, E., Perruccio, K., Shlomchik, W.D., Tosti, A., Posati, S., Rogaia, D., Frassoni, F., Aversa, F., Martelli, M.F., Velardi, A.: Effectiveness of donor natural killer cell alloreactivity in mismatched hematopoietic transplants. Science **295**, 2097–2100 (2002)

Rusakiewicz, S., Semeraro, M., Sarabi, M., Desbois, M., Locher, C., Mendez, R., Vimond, N., Concha, A., Garrido, F., Isambert, N., Chaigneau, L., le Brun-Ly, V., Dubreuil, P., Cremer, I.,

Caignard, A., Poirier-Colame, V., Chaba, K., Flament, C., Halama, N., Jager, D., Eggermont, A., Bonvalot, S., Commo, F., Terrier, P., Opolon, P., Emile, J.F., Coindre, J.M., Kroemer, G., Chaput, N., le Cesne, A., Blay, J.Y., Zitvogel, L.: Immune infiltrates are prognostic factors in localized gastrointestinal stromal tumors. Cancer Res. **73**, 3499–3510 (2013)

Salazar-Mather, T.P., Hokeness, K.L.: Calling in the troops: regulation of inflammatory cell trafficking through innate cytokine/chemokine networks. Viral Immunol. **16**, 291–306 (2003)

Schonfeld, K., Sahm, C., Zhang, C., Naundorf, S., Brendel, C., Odendahl, M., Nowakowska, P., Bonig, H., Kohl, U., Kloess, S., Kohler, S., Holtgreve-Grez, H., Jauch, A., Schmidt, M., Schubert, R., Kuhlcke, K., Seifried, E., Klingemann, H.G., Rieger, M.A., Tonn, T., Grez, M., Wels, W.S.: Selective inhibition of tumor growth by clonal NK cells expressing an ErbB2/HER2-specific chimeric antigen receptor. Mol. Ther. **23**, 330–338 (2015)

Sconocchia, G., Arriga, R., Tornillo, L., Terracciano, L., Ferrone, S., Spagnoli, G.C.: Melanoma cells inhibit NK cell functions. Cancer Res. **72**, 5428–5429 (2012). author reply 5430

Sivori, S., Pende, D., Bottino, C., Marcenaro, E., Pessino, A., Biassoni, R., Moretta, L., Moretta, A.: NKp46 is the major triggering receptor involved in the natural cytotoxicity of fresh or cultured human NK cells. Correlation between surface density of NKp46 and natural cytotoxicity against autologous, allogeneic or xenogeneic target cells. Eur. J. Immunol. **29**, 1656–1666 (1999)

Sondel, P.M., Hank, J.A.: Combination therapy with interleukin-2 and antitumor monoclonal antibodies. Cancer J. Sci. Am. **3**(Suppl 1), S121–S127 (1997)

Steele, N., Anthony, A., Saunders, M., Esmarck, B., Ehrnrooth, E., Kristjansen, P.E., Nihlen, A., Hansen, L.T., Cassidy, J.: A phase 1 trial of recombinant human IL-21 in combination with cetuximab in patients with metastatic colorectal cancer. Br. J. Cancer **106**, 793–798 (2012)

Stojanovic, A., Fiegler, N., Brunner-Weinzierl, M., Cerwenka, A.: CTLA-4 is expressed by activated mouse NK cells and inhibits NK Cell IFN-gamma production in response to mature dendritic cells. J. Immunol. **192**, 4184–4191 (2014)

Stoklasek, T.A., Schluns, K.S., Lefrancois, L.: Combined IL-15/IL-15Ralpha immunotherapy maximizes IL-15 activity in vivo. J. Immunol. **177**, 6072–6080 (2006)

Sun, J.C., Lanier, L.L.: Natural killer cells remember: an evolutionary bridge between innate and adaptive immunity? Eur. J. Immunol. **39**, 2059–2064 (2009)

Sun, J.C., Beilke, J.N., Lanier, L.L.: Adaptive immune features of natural killer cells. Nature **457**, 557–561 (2009)

Sznurkowski, J.J., Zawrocki, A., Biernat, W.: Subtypes of cytotoxic lymphocytes and natural killer cells infiltrating cancer nests correlate with prognosis in patients with vulvar squamous cell carcinoma. Cancer Immunol. Immunother. **63**, 297–303 (2014)

Takaki, R., Hayakawa, Y., Nelson, A., Sivakumar, P.V., Hughes, S., Smyth, M.J., LANIER, L.L.: IL-21 enhances tumor rejection through a NKG2D-dependent mechanism. J. Immunol. **175**, 2167–2173 (2005)

Takasawa, N., Ishii, N., Higashimura, N., Murata, K., Tanaka, Y., Nakamura, M., Sasaki, T., Sugamura, K.: Expression of gp34 (OX40 ligand) and OX40 on human T cell clones. Jpn. J. Cancer Res. **92**, 377–382 (2001)

Taub, D.D., Sayers, T.J., Carter, C.R., Ortaldo, J.R.: Alpha and beta chemokines induce NK cell migration and enhance NK-mediated cytolysis. J. Immunol. **155**, 3877–3888 (1995)

Terme, M., Ullrich, E., Aymeric, L., Meinhardt, K., Coudert, J.D., Desbois, M., Ghiringhelli, F., Viaud, S., Ryffel, B., Yagita, H., Chen, L., Mecheri, S., Kaplanski, G., Prevost-Blondel, A., Kato, M., Schultze, J.L., Tartour, E., Kroemer, G., Degli-Esposti, M., Chaput, N., Zitvogel, L.: Cancer-induced immunosuppression: IL-18-elicited immunoablative NK cells. Cancer Res. **72**, 2757–2767 (2012)

Tesniere, A., Schlemmer, F., Boige, V., Kepp, O., Martins, I., Ghiringhelli, F., Aymeric, L., Michaud, M., Apetoh, L., Barault, L., Mendiboure, J., Pignon, J.P., Jooste, V., van Endert, P., Ducreux, M., Zitvogel, L., Piard, F., Kroemer, G.: Immunogenic death of colon cancer cells treated with oxaliplatin. Oncogene **29**, 482–491 (2010)

Thiery, J., Keefe, D., Boulant, S., Boucrot, E., Walch, M., Martinvalet, D., Goping, I.S., Bleackley, R.C., Kirchhausen, T., Lieberman, J.: Perforin pores in the endosomal membrane trigger the release of endocytosed granzyme B into the cytosol of target cells. Nat. Immunol. **12**, 770–777 (2011)

Timmerman, J.M., Byrd, J.C., Andorsky, D.J., Yamada, R.E., Kramer, J., Muthusamy, N., Hunder, N., Pagel, J.M.: A phase I dose-finding trial of recombinant interleukin-21 and rituximab in relapsed and refractory low grade B-cell lymphoproliferative disorders. Clin. Cancer Res. **18**, 5752–5760 (2012)

Tittarelli, A., Mendoza-Naranjo, A., Farias, M., Guerrero, I., Ihara, F., Wennerberg, E., Riquelme, S., Gleisner, A., Kalergis, A., Lundqvist, A., Lopez, M.N., Chambers, B.J., Salazar-Onfray, F.: Gap junction intercellular communications regulate NK cell activation and modulate NK cytotoxic capacity. J. Immunol. **192**, 1313–1319 (2014)

Tonn, T., Schwabe, D., Klingemann, H.G., Becker, S., Esser, R., Koehl, U., Suttorp, M., Seifried, E., Ottmann, O.G., Bug, G.: Treatment of patients with advanced cancer with the natural killer cell line NK-92. Cytotherapy **15**, 1563–1570 (2013)

Topfer, K., Cartellieri, M., Michen, S., Wiedemuth, R., Muller, N., Lindemann, D., Bachmann, M., Fussel, M., Schackert, G., Temme, A.: DAP12-based activating chimeric antigen receptor for NK cell tumor immunotherapy. J. Immunol. **194**, 3201–3212 (2015)

Vales-Gomez, M., Reyburn, H.T., Erskine, R.A., Strominger, J.: Differential binding to HLA-C of p50-activating and p58-inhibitory natural killer cell receptors. Proc. Natl. Acad. Sci. U. S. A. **95**, 14326–14331 (1998)

Valiante, N.M., Uhrberg, M., Shilling, H.G., Lienert-Weidenbach, K., Arnett, K.L., D'andrea, A., Phillips, J.H., Lanier, L.L., Parham, P.: Functionally and structurally distinct NK cell receptor repertoires in the peripheral blood of two human donors. Immunity **7**, 739–751 (1997)

Velardi, A.: Natural killer cell alloreactivity 10 years later. Curr. Opin. Hematol. **19**, 421–426 (2012)

Vesely, M.D., Kershaw, M.H., Schreiber, R.D., SMYTH, M.J.: Natural innate and adaptive immunity to cancer. Annu. Rev. Immunol. **29**, 235–271 (2011)

Villegas, F.R., Coca, S., Villarrubia, V.G., Jimenez, R., Chillon, M.J., Jareno, J., Zuil, M., Callol, L.: Prognostic significance of tumor infiltrating natural killer cells subset CD57 in patients with squamous cell lung cancer. Lung Cancer **35**, 23–28 (2002)

Vinay, D.S., Kwon, B.S.: 4-1BB (CD137), an inducible costimulatory receptor, as a specific target for cancer therapy. BMB Rep. **47**, 122–129 (2014)

Vivier, E., Nunes, J.A., Vely, F.: Natural killer cell signaling pathways. Science **306**, 1517–1519 (2004)

Vivier, E., Tomasello, E., Baratin, M., Walzer, T., Ugolini, S.: Functions of natural killer cells. Nat. Immunol. **9**, 503–510 (2008)

Wald, O., Weiss, I.D., Wald, H., Shoham, H., Bar-Shavit, Y., Beider, K., Galun, E., Weiss, L., Flaishon, L., Shachar, I., Nagler, A., Lu, B., Gerard, C., Gao, J.L., Mishani, E., Farber, J., Peled, A.: IFN-gamma acts on T cells to induce NK cell mobilization and accumulation in target organs. J. Immunol. **176**, 4716–4729 (2006)

Walzer, T., Dalod, M., Vivier, E., Zitvogel, L.: Natural killer cell-dendritic cell crosstalk in the initiation of immune responses. Expert Opin. Biol. Ther. **5**(Suppl 1), S49–S59 (2005)

Wang, K.S., Frank, D.A., Ritz, J.: Interleukin-2 enhances the response of natural killer cells to interleukin-12 through up-regulation of the interleukin-12 receptor and STAT4. Blood **95**, 3183–3190 (2000)

Wang, G., Tschoi, M., Spolski, R., Lou, Y., Ozaki, K., Feng, C., Kim, G., Leonard, W.J., Hwu, P.: In vivo antitumor activity of interleukin 21 mediated by natural killer cells. Cancer Res. **63**, 9016–9022 (2003)

Wang, Y., Wu, J., Newton, R., Bahaie, N.S., Long, C., Walcheck, B.: ADAM17 cleaves CD16b (FcgammaRIIIb) in human neutrophils. Biochim. Biophys. Acta **1833**, 680–685 (2013)

Wendel, M., Galani, I.E., Suri-Payer, E., Cerwenka, A.: Natural killer cell accumulation in tumors is dependent on IFN-gamma and CXCR3 ligands. Cancer Res. **68**, 8437–8445 (2008)

Weng, W.K., Levy, R.: Two immunoglobulin G fragment C receptor polymorphisms independently predict response to rituximab in patients with follicular lymphoma. J. Clin. Oncol. **21**, 3940–3947 (2003)

Wennerberg, E., Kremer, V., Childs, R., Lundqvist, A.: CXCL10-induced migration of adoptively transferred human natural killer cells toward solid tumors causes regression of tumor growth in vivo. Cancer Immunol. Immunother. **64**, 225–235 (2015)

Willemze, R., Rodrigues, C.A., Labopin, M., Sanz, G., Michel, G., Socie, G., Rio, B., Sirvent, A., Renaud, M., Madero, L., Mohty, M., Ferra, C., Garnier, F., Loiseau, P., Garcia, J., Lecchi, L., Kogler, G., Beguin, Y., Navarrete, C., Devos, T., Ionescu, I., Boudjedir, K., Herr, A.L., Gluckman, E., Rocha, V., Eurocord, N., Acute Leukaemia Working Party of The EbMT: KIR-ligand incompatibility in the graft-versus-host direction improves outcomes after umbilical cord blood transplantation for acute leukemia. Leukemia **23**, 492–500 (2009)

Wittamer, V., Franssen, J.D., Vulcano, M., Mirjolet, J.F., le Poul, E., Migeotte, I., Brezillon, S., Tyldesley, R., Blanpain, C., Detheux, M., Mantovani, A., Sozzani, S., Vassart, G., Parmentier, M., Communi, D.: Specific recruitment of antigen-presenting cells by chemerin, a novel processed ligand from human inflammatory fluids. J. Exp. Med. **198**, 977–985 (2003)

Yokoyama, W.M., Kim, S.: Licensing of natural killer cells by self-major histocompatibility complex class I. Immunol. Rev. **214**, 143–154 (2006)

Yu, J., Wei, M., Becknell, B., Trotta, R., Liu, S., Boyd, Z., Jaung, M.S., Blaser, B.W., Sun, J., Benson Jr., D.M., Mao, H., Yokohama, A., Bhatt, D., Shen, L., Davuluri, R., Weinstein, M., Marcucci, G., Caligiuri, M.A.: Pro- and antiinflammatory cytokine signaling: reciprocal antagonism regulates interferon-gamma production by human natural killer cells. Immunity **24**, 575–590 (2006)

Zaidi, M.R., Merlino, G.: The two faces of interferon-gamma in cancer. Clin. Cancer Res. **17**, 6118–6124 (2011)

Zeng, R., Spolski, R., Casas, E., Zhu, W., Levy, D.E., Leonard, W.J.: The molecular basis of IL-21-mediated proliferation. Blood **109**, 4135–4142 (2007)

Zhang, W., Gordon, M., Schultheis, A.M., Yang, D.Y., Nagashima, F., Azuma, M., Chang, H.M., Borucka, E., Lurje, G., Sherrod, A.E., Iqbal, S., Groshen, S., Lenz, H.J.: FCGR2A and FCGR3A polymorphisms associated with clinical outcome of epidermal growth factor receptor expressing metastatic colorectal cancer patients treated with single-agent cetuximab. J. Clin. Oncol. **25**, 3712–3718 (2007a)

Zhang, Y., Wallace, D.L., de Lara, C.M., Ghattas, H., Asquith, B., Worth, A., Griffin, G.E., Taylor, G.P., Tough, D.F., Beverley, P.C., Macallan, D.C.: In vivo kinetics of human natural killer cells: the effects of ageing and acute and chronic viral infection. Immunology **121**, 258–265 (2007b)

Zingoni, A., Sornasse, T., Cocks, B.G., Tanaka, Y., Santoni, A., Lanier, L.L.: Cross-talk between activated human NK cells and CD4+ T cells via OX40-OX40 ligand interactions. J. Immunol. **173**, 3716–3724 (2004)

Zlotnik, A., Yoshie, O.: The chemokine superfamily revisited. Immunity **36**, 705–716 (2012)

Chapter 5
Reversing T Cell Dysfunction for Tumor Immunotherapy

Lawrence P. Kane and Greg M. Delgoffe

Abbreviations

CTLA-4	Cytotoxic T lymphocyte-associated protein 4
ICR	Immune checkpoint receptor
LAG-3	Lymphocyte activation gene 3
LCMV	Lymphocytic choriomeningitis virus
PD-1	Programmed death 1
Tim-3	T cell (or transmembrane) immunoglobulin and mucin 3
Treg	Regulatory T cell

L.P. Kane (✉)
Department of Immunology, University of Pittsburgh School of Medicine,
BST E-1054, 200 Lothrop St., Pittsburgh, PA 15261, USA

Cancer Immunology Program, University of Pittsburgh School of Medicine,
Pittsburgh, PA 15261, USA
e-mail: lkane@pitt.edu

G.M. Delgoffe
Department of Immunology, University of Pittsburgh School of Medicine,
BST E-1054, 200 Lothrop St., Pittsburgh, PA 15261, USA

Cancer Immunology Program, University of Pittsburgh School of Medicine,
Pittsburgh, PA 15261, USA

Tumor Microenvironment Center, University of Pittsburgh School of Medicine,
Pittsburgh, PA 15261, USA

P.D. Rennert (ed.), *Novel Immunotherapeutic Approaches to the Treatment of Cancer*, DOI 10.1007/978-3-319-29827-6_5

1 T Cells and Tumor Rejection

It was suspected for many years that the human immune system possesses an inherent ability to recognize and eliminate transformed cells. Stretching back to the work of William Coley (1910, 1919, 1927, 1933, 1991), tremendous effort has been expended to understand whether and how an apparent association of certain infections resulted in rejection of a tumor. Despite tantalizing leads, however, these responses could not be consistently observed or enhanced. In fact, in the early days of cellular immunology, there was actually a healthy debate that raged around the question of whether immunological surveillance actually promoted or prevent tumor growth. One possible way to reconcile these disparate findings was the model that early in the development of a tumor, inflammation associated with an immune response to the tumor might promote growth of the tumor through secreted growth factors, but once the tumor was more established (and potentially more immunogenic) the immune response had a capacity to limit the growth of the same tumor. This is consistent with many elegant molecular studies performed in recent years, wherein it has been shown that inflammation associated with NF-κB induction can indeed increase the development of tumors in various tissues (reviewed in Karin et al. 2002). Conversely, from the perspective of the T cell, NF-κB is an important element of the costimulatory signaling that controls T cell activation (Kane et al. 2002).

Progress in this area awaited the definition of specific cell types that could mediate immune responses. NK cells in particular were identified early on as potent antitumor effectors, through their ability to recognize cells that were stressed and/or had downregulated MHC class I molecules. T cells (specifically the CD8+ cytotoxic variety) were also recognized as promising mediators of antitumor immunity. These advances led to attempts to "rev up" endogenous NK and T cell responses to tumors through the administration of the growth factor IL-2 (Ettinghausen et al. 1985; Paley and Wherry 2010; Okazaki et al. 2003; Paley et al. 2013; Woo et al. 2012; Lines et al. 2014). However, this approach was fraught with significant morbidity and mortality, due to the induction of serious side effects caused by the very large doses of IL-2 used (Le Mercier et al. 2014; Hamid et al. 2013; Huang and August 2015; Shi and Petrie 2012; Ishida et al. 1992). Many investigators have subsequently taken a more antigen-specific approach, which has yielded some promising leads, especially in cases where tumor neoantigens have been identified. The goal here is that tumor vaccines to such antigens will induce the formation of an effective immune response to the specific tumor, while sparing nontransformed host tissue. While tumor vaccines may turn out to be effective in some cases, this approach can still suffer from the negative effects of the tumor microenvironment, which is well known to be immunosuppressive. Thus, while tumor-specific T cells can be primed by the vaccine, the function of such T cells may be compromised by the tumor microenvironment, assuming they can enter the tumor. There are likely many reasons for this inhibition of T cell responses within a tumor, but here we will focus on one broad, and intrinsic, category of T cell dysfunction, i.e., T cell "exhaustion."

2 T Cell Exhaustion

The term T cell exhaustion refers to a cellular dysfunctional state, wherein an antigen-specific T cell that has been chronically stimulated through its T cell receptor (TCR) by antigen is eventually rendered refractory to restimulation through the TCR (Wherry 2011; Youngblood et al. 2012; Okazaki et al. 2013; Liao and Littman 1995). This state may show some functional overlap with the previously described phenomena of cellular senescence and clonal anergy. However, there is evidence that exhaustion is a distinct state of differentiation. Thus, senescence is usually associated with a history of extensive proliferation and telomere shortening (Akbar and Henson 2011). Clonal anergy, as applied to T cells, usually refers to a T cell that has received signals through the antigen receptor, in the absence of appropriate costimulation, which is usually provided by CD28/B7 interactions (Macian et al. 2004). Extensive molecular work has associated anergy with partial TCR signaling through calcium-dependent NFAT transcription factor induction, in the absence of accompanying Ras/MAPK-induced AP-1 transcription factor, which can dimerize, and cooperate, with NFAT. Recent work from Rao and colleagues has uncovered a possible molecular connection between anergy and exhaustion, although additional clarification will be needed to determine how faithfully the effects of constitutive NFAT monomers really model what is happening during T cell exhaustion.

The phenomenon of T cell exhaustion has been most extensively studied in the context of chronic viral infections, especially the powerful LCMV (lymphocytic choriomeningitis virus) system in mice. Thus, infection with certain acute strains of LCMV (e.g., Armstrong) results in a relatively rapid and effective T cell response, which clears the virus within 8 days, and also produces an effective pool of LCMV-specific memory T cells (Jamieson and Ahmed 1989; Jamieson et al. 1987; Lau et al. 1994). By contrast, a chronic strain of LCMV (Clone 13) is not completely cleared, although it does induce a specific T cell response, resulting in a chronic infection and a state of détente between the T cells and the virus (Wherry et al. 2003, 2007; Ahmed et al. 1984). This leads to chronic restimulation of LCMV-specific T cells that gradually lose their ability to respond effectively to stimulation and are thus thought to be exhausted. Existing tools for studying the response to LCMV in mice have enabled elegant cellular, molecular, and functional studies that have helped to define the nature of T cell exhaustion (Paley et al. 2012).

As demonstrated by several labs, the acquisition of T cell exhaustion appears to occur over the course of multiple, possibly distinct, stages. Along the way, T cells in the process of becoming exhausted gradually lose more of their effector functions, including production of various cytokines, cytotoxicity, and the ability to proliferate. In extreme cases, this may also lead to cell death, and deletion, of the exhausted clone during the so-called terminal stage of exhaustion. Of course, the ability to rescue T cell responses to tumors with checkpoint blockade therapies targeted at CTLA-4 (cytotoxic T lymphocyte-associated protein 4) or PD-1 (programmed death 1) (discussed below) demonstrates that if deletion is the eventual end point of this process that it does not occur at a high frequency or very rapidly, otherwise there would be a very low or absent steady state level of exhausted T cells from which to enhance a response to the tumor.

Since the first descriptions of T cell exhaustion, there have been a number of efforts to define the state of exhaustion at a molecular level. This has mainly taken the form of gene expression analyses, usually by microarray approaches—much of the data in this area have been reported by John Wherry and colleagues (Wherry et al. 2007; Crawford et al. 2014; Doering et al. 2012; Quigley et al. 2010). This topic has been reviewed in great detail elsewhere, most recently in Pauken and Wherry (2015). For the most part, these studies have so far failed to uncover an obvious inhibitory suppressive signature in the functionally exhausted T cell population, at least in the case of chronic viral infection. Rather, the elegant studies of Wherry and colleagues have revealed that exhausted T cells actually look a lot more like effector T cells, as opposed to those that would be considered memory or memory precursor T cells or even anergic T cells. Nonetheless, there is an interesting reciprocal relationship between the homologous transcription factors T-bet and Eomes in regulating terminal T cell effector fate. Thus, it now appears that continued expression of T-bet is important for sustaining CD8+ effector function and limiting PD-1 expression, while lower levels of T-bet are accompanied by increased Eomes, higher PD-1, and more profound exhaustion (Doering et al. 2012; Kao et al. 2011). Although these latter Eomes^{hi} cells appear to be derived from the T-bet^{hi} cells, they are not passive bystanders, since their elimination (as with the T-bet^{hi} cells) impairs viral control (Paley et al. 2012). As with many mechanistic aspects of T cell exhaustion first defined in chronic infection, it remains to be seen whether these observations with T-bet and Eomes hold true in tumors. However, there is some recent evidence that T-bet^{hi} and/or Eomes^{hi} cells in the tumor microenvironment are important for tumor immunity, depending on the system (Berrien-Elliott et al. 2015; Song et al. 2014). Clearly this is an area that requires further development, since it seems unlikely that T cell exhaustion will follow precisely the same rules in both chronic infection and cancer.

The observation of exhausted T cells in multiple diverse disease settings and animal models raises the question of why this functional state exists to begin with. This suggests that this process is at some level adaptive for the host, even thought it would appear to be mal-adaptive, particularly in the case of cancer. It is probably more instructive here to think about the setting of chronic infection. Thus, while the adaptive immune system has clearly evolved to fight off the advances of pathogens, overly vigorous immune responses can cause significant immune-mediated pathology that ends up doing more harm than good for host fitness. It is therefore logical that the adaptive immune system has evolved mechanisms to limit immune-mediated pathology in the case of infections that cannot be completely cleared. This seems to be most likely reason for the existence of immune exhaustion in mammals. As long as the immune system and the infectious agent reach some sort of détente, such an arrangement, while not being overtly adaptive, is at least not mal-adaptive for the host (or the pathogen, for that matter). As is often the case, the outgrowth and persistence of tumors appears to occur at least in part as an unwanted side effect of this phenomenon, since T cells within tumors are also often subject to persistent stimulation with antigen.

3 Metabolic Dysfunction and T Cell Exhaustion

The current era of molecular immunology has been dominated by study of signaling pathways and transcription factors, especially how they regulate lymphocyte activation and differentiation. Little thought was given to how cellular metabolic pathways were involved in these aspects of immunological regulation. In this regard, the work of Rathmell, Thompson, and colleagues was pioneering, in that it introduced concepts developed in cancer biology to the study of T cell activation and function (Fox et al. 2005). It has been known for a century that highly proliferative cancer cells ferment glucose into lactic acid, even under conditions of abundant oxygen, a phenomenon known as aerobic glycolysis or the "Warburg effect" (Kim and Dang 2006). While glycolysis generates relatively little ATP compared to pyruvate-driven TCA cycle and subsequent oxidative phosphorylation (OXPHOS), it is thought that aerobic glycolysis is used by highly proliferative cells to spare the mitochondria from catabolic damage, and to utilize TCA cycle intermediates and other mitochondrial products for biosynthesis of new proteins, nucleotides, and membranes (Dang 2012). However, this phenomenon is not unique to cancer cells, and in the 1970s it was shown that activated, highly proliferative lymphocytes participate in Warburg metabolism as well (Roos and Loos 1973).

Since these initial findings, it has become appreciated that metabolism has a critical and complex role in dictating T cell function and fate. As T cell activation and costimulatory pathways were discovered and dissected, key findings revealed that these pathways also influenced metabolism (Frauwirth and Thompson 2004). For instance, CD28 signaling, required for full T cell activation and differentiation away from tolerance, was shown to stimulate glucose uptake and promote glycolysis (Frauwirth et al. 2002). Akt signaling, downstream of CD28, seemed to be the dominant player in this immediate pathway (Rathmell et al. 2003; Cantrell 2002). However, other cytokines can stimulate Akt activation and its downstream targets to influence T cell metabolism (Wieman et al. 2007; Wofford et al. 2008). After these initial links were made, many studies revealed that Akt and the nutrient sensor mTOR both play critical roles in modulating T cell metabolism as well as influencing T cell fate, including critical differentiation events such as effector versus memory or helper versus regulatory cells (Delgoffe et al. 2009; Fruman 2004; Genot et al. 2000; Haxhinasto et al. 2008; O'Brien et al. 2011; Powell and Delgoffe 2010).

T cell activation is incredibly metabolically demanding. Few other cell types need to survive in extreme quiescence for a lifetime but, upon activation, initiate a 10- to 100,000-fold clonal expansion. Thus, it is not surprising that costimulatory molecules initiate altered metabolism and that nutrient sensors can dictate T cell fate: T cells must be able to interpret the environment to know if a commitment to activation is feasible. Indeed, the study of costimulatory and coinhibitory molecule signaling has revealed that many types of T cell dysfunction likely have metabolic underpinnings. T cell clonal anergy, a state of hyporesponsiveness induced when T cells receive antigenic stimulus in the absence of costimulation, interfaces heavily with metabolic signaling pathways (Schwartz 2003). Anergic T cells fail to upregulate metabolic machinery, but also starvation signals can trigger T cell anergy, even in the presence of costimulation (Powell et al. 1999; Zheng et al. 2009). Tolerized T cells stay unresponsive, in part, by rendering themselves metabolically inert.

In T cell exhaustion, however, the tables have turned. Unlike T cell anergy, which is a programmed response to minimal signaling, T cell exhaustion is hyporesponsiveness stemming from chronic stimulation, inflammatory cytokine environments, and coinhibitory molecule signaling (Wherry 2011). Indeed, coinhibitory molecule signaling (CTLA-4 and PD-1 being the most studied) can inhibit activation of Akt and mTOR, which thus may modulate metabolism (Chuang et al. 2000; Parry et al. 2005; Riley 2009; Francisco et al. 2009), and PD-1 signaling may directly influence glycolysis (Patsoukis et al. 2015; Staron et al. 2014). Exhausted T cells, prevalent in chronic viral infections and cancer, may be metabolically insufficient: chronic TCR signaling and inflammatory cytokines are driving their continual stimulation, but cannot energetically support their function. This may be at the level of nutrient sensing, nutrient uptake, intracellular trafficking, or mitochondrial function or mass. Given the recent clinical successes targeting T cell exhaustion (Topalian et al. 2015), future studies will seek to identify the precise mechanisms involved in the modulation of metabolism in T cell exhaustion.

4 Inhibitory Molecules in Antitumor T Cell Regulation

4.1 CTLA-4

The concept of immune checkpoint receptor (ICRs) modulation for cancer immunotherapy was initially demonstrated for the inhibitory coreceptor CTLA-4. Thus, CTLA-4 was discovered as an activation antigen on stimulated T cells. Pointing out a potential pitfall in this field, CTLA-4 was initially thought by many investigators to function as a positive regulator of T cell activation (Boussiotis et al. 1993; Freeman et al. 1993), but was eventually proven to be a negative regulator of T cell activation by Bluestone and colleagues (Walunas et al. 1994). Subsequent studies of CTLA-4 knockout mice demonstrated the powerful nature of this protein as a checkpoint in T cell activation (Waterhouse et al. 1995; Chambers et al. 1997). Soon after, work from Jim Allison and colleagues demonstrated that antibody blockade of CTLA-4 in mouse tumor models could dramatically enhance immune responses to these transplanted tumors (Leach et al. 1996).

Despite 20 or so years, there is still not complete agreement on how CTLA4 normally functions, nor how antibodies to CTLA-4 work to enhance T cell-dependent immune responses to tumors. Thus, it is clear that CTLA-4 can interact with the costimulatory ligands CD80 and CD86 (B71/B72), which themselves can also interact with the costimulatory molecule CD28, constitutively expressed on T cells. This binding of CTLA-4 with CD80/CD86 on APC's impairs T cell activation, and several mechanisms have been put forward for how this activity is mediated. One early model was that CTLA-4 can recruit inhibitory phosphatases (Lee et al. 1998; Marengere et al. 1996), but this now appears to be a minor activity (Nakaseko et al. 1999). CTLA-4 binding to CD80/CD86 is 10–20 times more avid that the binding of CD28 to these proteins (Linsley et al. 1991), so CTLA-4 may simply compete with CD28 for ligand binding. Elegant imaging and biochemical studies from Sansom and colleagues suggested CTLA-4 could actually remove CD80/CD86 from the surface of APC's, preventing further costimulation through CD28, in a process known as trans-endocytosis or trogocytosis (Qureshi et al. 2011, 2012). With regard to the therapeutic effects of CTLA-4 antibody, recent data suggest that at least a part of its in vivo activity might be due to FcR-dependent depletion of regulatory T cells (Tregs), due to the prominent expression of CTLA-4 on these cells (Bulliard et al. 2013; Simpson et al. 2013). This raises the possibility that otherCytotoxic T lymphocyte-associated protein 4 (CTLA-4) immune checkpoint therapies in development might function by a similar mechanism, something that has not been adequately explored up to this point. We discuss this point further below.

4.2 PD-1

Murine and human PD-1 were discovered by Honjo's lab in the early 1990s (Ishida et al. 1992). The cDNA for PD-1 was originally isolated by subtractive hybridization, focusing on genes that were induced upon apoptotic cell death, hence the name programmed death 1 (PD-1). In 2000, Honjo's lab also identified the first ligand for PD-1, a B7 family member that they termed PD-L1 (aka B7-H1), and showed that interaction of this ligand with PD-1 could inhibit T cell proliferation (Freeman et al. 2000). The following year, a second ligand—PD-L2/B7-DC was also shown to bind to PD-1, and the first biochemical evidence was presented that engagement of PD-1 led to the recruitment of an inhibitory phosphatase (SHP-2) to the cytoplasmic tail of PD-1 (Latchman et al. 2001). Thus, the stage was set to explore the ability of the PD-1/PD-L system to limit immune responses. This field has matured remarkably rapidly, prompted in part by the approval of the CTLA-4 antibody ipilimumab, and in 2014 two independent blocking antibodies for the PD-1/PD-L axis received FDA approval—pembrolizumab (for advanced treatment-refractory melanoma) and nivolumab (for melanoma or non-small cell lung carcinoma).

As discussed below with respect to Tim-3 (T cell (or transmembrane) immunoglobulin and mucin 3), it is important to keep in mind that expression of an exhaustion "marker," even one as well characterized as PD-1, is not sufficient to label a cell, or population of cells, as functionally exhausted. Thus, it is important to follow up such phenotypic characterization with functional assays, to more precisely define a state of exhaustion. For example, in at least one study, it was shown that the presence of PD-1+ cells at the tumor site correlated positively with an effective immune response to the tumor (Badoual et al. 2012; Gros et al. 2014).

5 Emerging Inhibitory Checkpoint Receptors: Tim-3

An emerging immunotherapy checkpoint target that has received a great amount of attention recently is the protein Tim-3. This protein was first described by Vijay Kuchroo's group, who identified it as a marker of Th1 T cells, while being absent from Th2 or naïve T cells (Monney et al. 2002). Further work from this group provided evidence for a negative regulatory role of Tim-3 in immune responses. Thus, in vivo administration of a Tim-3 mAb or a fusion protein containing the Tim-3 ecto domain fused to an IgG Fc domain (Tim3-Ig) resulted in the exacerbation of EAE, a common mouse model of MS (Monney et al. 2002; Sabatos et al. 2003; Sanchez-Fueyo et al. 2003). The Kuchroo group went on to identify a ligand for Tim-3, a lectin-like protein known as galectin-9 (Zhu et al. 2005), and showed that treatment of Th1 T cells with galectin-9 could induce cell death. This effect was linked at least in part to binding of galectin-9 to Tim-3, since there was preferential killing of Th1 T cells vs. Th2 T cells by galectin-9. Subsequent studies have complicated this picture somewhat. Thus, we and others showed that depending on the concentration used, galectin-9 could either enhance T cell activation (at low concentrations) or cause cell death (at high concentrations) (Su et al. 2010; Leitner et al. 2013). Furthermore, both of these effects could be observed in the absence of Tim-3, consistent with additional ligands for galectin-9 (Su et al. 2010; Leitner et al. 2013). Previous and subsequent studies have shown that galectin-9 could also bind to IgE and CD44, for example, so while we believe that galectin-9 does indeed interact with Tim-3, this is not an exclusive interaction in either direction (Bi et al. 2008; Niki et al. 2009; Wu et al. 2014).

Several ligands for Tim-3 itself have also now been identified, and these are a diverse group of protein and lipid moieties. The phospholipid phosphatidylserine (PS) is normally present on the inner leaflet of the plasma membrane of healthy cells. Upon stress, particularly that associated with programmed cell death, or apoptosis, PS is "flipped" out onto the outer surface of the cell. There, PS is recognized by a number of different receptors that can employ this PS recognition, along with other signals, to engage in uptake and clearance of the dying cell. At least three members of the TIM family, Tim-1, Tim-3, and Tim-4, have been shown to bind PS through the IgV domain in the TIM protein (Song et al. 2014; Waterhouse et al. 1995; DeKruyff et al. 2010; Kobayashi et al. 2007). In the case of Tim-4, this interaction was shown to mediate uptake of apoptotic cells in mice, as an important mechanism for maintaining self tolerance (Waterhouse et al. 1995). Tim-3 has also been shown to help mediate phagocytosis of apoptotic cells by DC's, which may facilitate the process of cross-presentation (i.e., presentation of peptides derived from extracellular sources on MHC Class I molecules) (Nakayama et al. 2009). It is important to keep in mind that PS can also be encountered in vivo through microvesicles, which often display significant amounts of PS on their surface (Frey and Gaipl 2011). Returning to Tim-3, it is not at all clear how interaction of Tim-3 with PS exposed either on the surface of cells or on vesicles, might modulate the function of Tim-3, including its interactions with other ligands. Another of these ligands is the danger-associated molecular pattern (DAMP) molecule known as HMGB1; this protein is normally sequestered in the nucleus of healthy cells, but can be released from dead or dying cells (Sims et al. 2010). Although it was previously shown to bind to the surface receptor RAGE (Sims et al. 2010), recent data demonstrated that it can also bind to Tim-3 expressed on myeloid dendritic cells, and inhibit the maturation of these cells (Chiba et al. 2012). This is in fact one of the few studies in which the ability of a Tim-3 Ab to block interaction with a ligand was shown. Of relevance for the broader discussion here, Tim3-expressing cells were found within tumor infiltrates in two different mouse models of transplantable tumors. This highlights the point that when assessing the effects of Tim-3 modulation in vivo, one cannot assume that the effects of such treatment occur exclusively through Tim-3-expressing T cells.

We have provided this extended discussion of Tim-3 ligands because we believe that it is an important issue to address in the context of Tim-3 as a target for checkpoint blockade immunotherapy. Many studies with Tim-3+ T cells of either murine or human origin have employed various Tim-3 antibodies in an attempt to reverse T cell dysfunction associated with chronic infection or tumors. However, in the majority of such studies it is not clear which (if any) Tim-3 ligands are being interfered with, despite persistent references in the literature to these antibodies as "blocking."

As discussed above for PD-1, expression of Tim-3 is not sufficient to define a T cell as functionally exhausted, even if it is believed that Tim-3 is expressed by the most-exhausted T cells more selectively, relative to expression of PD-1 or other markers alone. One early study in this area from Ponzio and colleagues assessed the ability of adoptively transferred Th1 (verified as Tim-3^{+}) or Th2 (Tim-3$^{lo/-}$) T cells to prevent the growth of transplanted or spontaneous tumors in mice (Simmons et al. 2005). Despite expressing high levels of Tim-3, these transferred T cells were able to colocalize with tumors and suppress their growth. Our own work has demonstrated an ability of Tim-3 to enhance TCR signaling and T cell activation, at least under acute conditions (Lee et al. 2011). As we discussed in a recent review, our results and those of several other groups call into question the simple model of Tim-3 as a dominant inhibitor of TCR signaling (Ferris et al. 2014). Indeed, bacterial infection studies using a Tim-3 knockout mouse model revealed less efficient CD8+ T cell responses (Gorman et al. 2014).

We have recently taken a different approach to more directly address the intrinsic effects of Tim-3 on T cells. To this end, we have generated a novel mouse model in which a Cre-inducible Tim-3 allele was knocked into the *Rosa26* locus. Using this model we have begun to address the effects of Tim-3 induction under circumstances where it is not normally expressed, importantly in the absence of other exhaustion markers. Despite the expression of high levels of Tim-3, driven by CD4-Cre, T cells from these mice do not appear to be exhausted (or anergic), but actually respond better to acute stimulation through the TCR (L. Avery and L.P.K. unpublished). Future studies will address the effects of enforced expression of Tim-3 on antitumor responses, as well as on responses to acute or chronic viral infection.

6 Other Emerging Checkpoint Receptors

Among the immunotherapy checkpoint targets that have not yet made it to market, LAG-3 is one of the most "mature." Thus several phase 1 clinical trials have been completed and several are still ongoing for various liquid and solid malignancies (Lesokhin et al. 2015). Although LAG-3 is a homologue of CD4 and can bind to Class II MHC molecules, this is unlikely to be the only factor in its regulation of exhausted T cells, since it appears to be a common marker for exhaustion of both CD8+ and CD4+ T cells (Goldberg and Drake 2011). While there is ample functional data at this point to continue developing LAG-3 as a target for checkpoint blockade, we still have a relatively poor understanding of the biochemical mechanisms underlying LAG-3 function on T cells. Early studies on murine LAG-3 showed that it can inhibit calcium mobilization downstream of the TCR (Hannier et al. 1998). The inhibitory function of LAG-3 does appear to depend on sequences in its cytoplasmic tail (Workman and Vignali 2003), suggesting that it can indeed deliver a negative signal to regulate T cell activation or function. However, the functional unit in the LAG-3 cytoplasmic tail seems to mainly consist of a "KIEELE" motif (Workman and Vignali 2003), which still leaves the question of how this motif might modulate T cell activation, as it does not conform to any previously described signaling motif in T cells. Regarding the in vivo blockade of LAG-3, it is also important to remember that LAG-3 interaction with Class II MHC molecules on dendritic (or other) cells may modulate the function of those cells as well (Andreae et al. 2003), although the impact of this activity in immunotherapy is not known.

As alluded to above, this is a rapidly progressing field, so there are a number of other emerging checkpoint receptors that have not yet reached the point of validation in clinical trials. These include proteins like TIGIT, 2B4, and VISTA, among others. Since these targets are not as well developed, we refer here to some recent reviews on these proteins (Pauken and Wherry 2014; Baksh and Weber 2015; Shin and Ribas 2015).

7 Positive Acting (Costimulatory) Checkpoint Receptors as Immunotherapy Targets

The flip side of immune checkpoint inhibitory receptors are the costimulatory receptors, which act to enhance T cell activation. The prototypical costimulatory molecule on T cells is CD28, which is constitutively expressed by essentially all α/β T cells. Engagement of CD28 by B7-1 or B7-2 is critical for the activation of naïve T cells. As a class, these targets have perhaps not yet received the same level of attention as the inhibitory checkpoint receptors, in part due to the very negative outcome of a phase 1 clinical trial with a so-called super agonist CD28 antibody (Suntharalingam et al. 2006). Nonetheless are now a large number of preclinical studies supporting the potential of several costimulatory molecules as therapeutic targets.

Many other costimulatory models are upregulated after T cell activation, and play important roles later in T cell responses, or upon restimulation. These represent possible targets for agonistic antibodies that enhance activation of previously stimulated T cells, which can include exhausted T cells. This would be a desired feature for a potential immunotherapy target, avoiding additional toxicity that might result from even broader enhancement of T cell activation, as in the case of CD28. Many of these upregulated costimulatory proteins are members of the tumor necrosis factor (TNF) receptor family. Two of these molecules in particular—OX-40 (CD134) and 4-1BB (CD137) have been explored in a large number of preclinical studies, either alone or in combination with other modalities, and there are now a number of phase 1 clinical trials underway for these targets (Croft et al. 2013; Croft 2003; Vinay and Kwon 2012). Phase 1 trials are also underway for additional TNF receptor family members, including CD40, CD27, and GITR (Croft et al. 2013).

8 Which Cells Are Being Targeted by ICR Blocking Antibodies?

As introduced above, there is still either a paucity of information, or disagreement, about the precise cell types targeted in vivo by ICR targeting therapies, even in the case of a well-characterized and clinically mature target such as CTLA-4. Assuming that the target of interest (like CTLA-4) is expressed exclusively by T cells, there are several possibilities to consider. First, the therapy in question, e.g., a proven blocking mAb, may be simply interfering with the interaction of a negative regulator with its ligand(s), and thereby preventing the delivery of an inhibitory signal to effector/exhausted T cells. Likewise, in the case of a positive acting checkpoint receptor (e.g., ICOS), a therapeutic mAb may crosslink the receptor and mimic the effect of ligand to deliver a positive costimulatory signal to effector and/or exhausted T cells.

Of course, many checkpoint receptors are expressed not only on effector/exhausted T cells, but also on Tregs. Thus, antibodies to positive or negative checkpoint receptors could modulate the function of Treg (either positively or negatively) through these receptors. Depending on the direction of the effect, checkpoint receptor engagement on Treg could either enhance or impair the desired effect of rejuvenating effector/exhausted T cells. An alternative possibility here is that binding of the checkpoint receptor mAb to Treg could cause Fc receptor (FcR)-dependent clearance of Treg. Such an effect might be particularly desirable if the checkpoint receptor in question is highly expressed on tumor-infiltrating Treg, compared with Treg in the peripheral T cell pool. Indeed evidence for Treg depletion has been published for CTLA-4 blocking antibody, in both mice and humans (Bulliard et al. 2013; Simpson et al. 2013; Furness et al. 2014). Intriguingly, a paper from Levy and colleagues provided evidence that local Treg depletion, i.e., in the tumor microenvironment, may be sufficient to unmask a more systemic antitumor immune response (Marabelle et al. 2013). In this case, the authors found preferential expression of CTLA-4 and OX-40 on Treg at the site of lymphomas in both mice humans. They then showed in the mouse model that local administration of depleting antibodies to these two molecules effectively depleted tumor-infiltrating Treg, and promoted systemic responses elicited by CpG therapy. Combining Treg depletion with immune checkpoint blockade is a potentially powerful approach, and there is precedent for reversing T cell exhaustion associated with chronic viral infection in mice using such an approach (Penaloza-MacMaster et al. 2014). Recent work has shown that Tim-3 can also be found on tumor-infiltrating Treg, and that these Treg appear to be a particularly suppressive population (Sakuishi et al. 2013).

For obvious reasons, there has been a great emphasis on the development of checkpoint receptor therapies that target molecules expressed primarily, if not exclusively, by T cells. In addition to the expression of many checkpoint receptors on both effector and Tregs, these receptors can be expressed by an even more diverse array of cell types, which may complicate their development as targets. For example, Tim-3 was shown some time ago to be expressed by many myeloid lineage cells, including some dendritic cells (DC) and macrophages (Chiba et al. 2012; Anderson et al. 2007; Maurya et al. 2014; Oikawa et al. 2006). However, the function of Tim-3 on these cells is still not entirely clear, with some studies pointing to a positive role (Anderson et al. 2007), and others suggesting an inhibitory role (Chiba et al. 2012). In addition, Tim-3 is highly expressed by mast cells, which has been demonstrated in bone marrow-derived mast cells from mice (Nakae et al. 2007) and cord blood (Wiener et al. 2006) and tissue (Huang et al. 2014) mast cells from patients. Our own recent work has confirmed that Tim-3 is a positive regulator of mast cell activation in mice, including studies with Tim-3 KO mice, in which there is a significant impairment of mast cell activation (Phong et al. 2015). In experiments with implications for Tim-3 function in T cells, we also found that Tim-3 acts at a point proximal to the FcεRI to enhance tyrosine kinase signaling downstream of this receptor (Phong et al. 2015).

9 Biomarkers for ICR Therapies

While approved checkpoint receptor therapies that target CTLA-4 or PD-1 have shown some very robust responses, there is still a substantial proportion of patients who remain refractory to these treatments (Callahan et al. 2014; Callahan and Wolchok 2013). There is thus a great need for the identification and implementation of effective biomarkers that would predict successful treatment. One of the strengths of the checkpoint receptor targeting approach is that many of the targets are expressed much more highly in the tumor microenvironment than in the general circulation. This fact should allow for more precise enhancement of immune responses to the tumor, as opposed to more general immune activation, which may lead to autoimmune sequellae. However, this can also hinder prioritization or monitoring of therapy, since the status of checkpoint receptor expression in the tumor cannot be easily monitored by, for example, a blood draw. The former problem is likely to become more acute in the coming years, as additional checkpoint therapies make their way into the clinic. Given the expense of these therapies and the potential cost to the patient of time spent treating patients with the "wrong" therapy, this is a critical issue to address in the near future. In cases where biopsies can be reasonably obtained, it is obviously preferable to obtain information about the phenotype of TILs at the tumor site. Identification of tumor-infiltrating T cells recognizing tumor neoantigens after checkpoint blockade therapy has been achieved, both in mouse models (Gubin et al. 2014) and in human patients (van Rooij et al. 2013). However, in cases where TIL cannot be readily isolated, it may eventually be possible to identify tumor-specific T cells in the circulating pool of lymphocytes. A major question here is: to what degree will emergent tumor antigens vary between patients on checkpoint blockade therapy, even when comparing those with the same type of tumor? This issue has yet to be addressed, but is likely to be in the near future, given the rapid pace of development in this space. If common neoantigens can be identified across patients responding to checkpoint blockade therapy, this may allow a priori development of adoptive T cell therapies to enhance the response of future patients. However, it seems likely that there will be considerable patient-to-patient variability in such epitopes, in which case implementation of this approach will be more challenging.

10 Summary

We are in the midst of an exciting period for tumor immunology and its application to clinical care. The current "embarrassment of riches" with regard to potential targets for checkpoint blockade suggests that we may even be on the cusp of a revolution in our ability to manipulate immune responses. However, some key fundamental questions will need to be addressed (see Box 5.1) in order for the further development and clinical implementation of these new targets to occur in a way that makes the best use of current resources.

Box 5.1. Key questions to be addressed in the future implementation of T cell-directed checkpoint modulation therapies for cancer

Key Questions

1. What are the phenotypic predictors of responsiveness to a particular T cell-directed immune checkpoint modulating therapeutic?
2. What are the phenotypic and functional correlates of effective responses to immune checkpoint therapies?
3. Which T cell subpopulations (effector, exhausted, regulatory) are the targets of each checkpoint therapy, and what is the functional effect of therapy on each subset?
4. What are the signaling and metabolic consequences of T cell exhaustion caused by specific checkpoint receptors (and combinations thereof), and how are these affected by checkpoint blockade?

References

Ahmed, R., Salmi, A., Butler, L.D., Chiller, J.M., Oldstone, M.B.: Selection of genetic variants of lymphocytic choriomeningitis virus in spleens of persistently infected mice. Role in suppression of cytotoxic T lymphocyte response and viral persistence. J. Exp. Med. **160**, 521–540 (1984)

Akbar, A.N., Henson, S.M.: Are senescence and exhaustion intertwined or unrelated processes that compromise immunity? Nat. Rev. Immunol. **11**, 289–295 (2011)

Anderson, A.C., Anderson, D.E., Bregoli, L., Hastings, W.D., Kassam, N., Lei, C., Chandwaskar, R., Karman, J., Su, E.W., Hirashima, M., Bruce, J.N., Kane, L.P., Kuchroo, V.K., Hafler, D.A.: Promotion of tissue inflammation by the immune receptor Tim-3 expressed on innate immune cells. Science **318**, 1141–1143 (2007)

Andreae, S., Buisson, S., Triebel, F.: MHC class II signal transduction in human dendritic cells induced by a natural ligand, the LAG-3 protein (CD223). Blood **102**, 2130–2137 (2003)

Badoual, C., Hans, S., Merillon, N., Van Ryswick, C., Ravel, P., Benhamouda, N., Levionnois, E., Nizard, M., Si-Mohamed, A., Besnier, N., Gey, A., Rotem-Yehudar, R., Pere, H., Tran, T., Guerin, C.L., Chauvat, A., Dransart, E., Alanio, C., Albert, S., Barry, B., Sandoval, F., Quintin-Colonna, F., Bruneval, P., Fridman, W.H., Lemoine, F.M., Oudard, S., Johannes, L., Olive, D., Brasnu, D., Tartour, E.: PD-1-expressing tumor-infiltrating T cells are a favorable prognostic biomarker in HPV associated head and neck cancer. Cancer Res. **73**(1), 128–138 (2012)

Baksh, K., Weber, J.: Immune checkpoint protein inhibition for cancer: preclinical justification for CTLA-4 and PD-1 blockade and new combinations. Semin. Oncol. **42**, 363–377 (2015)

Berrien-Elliott, M.M., Yuan, J., Swier, L.E., Jackson, S.R., Chen, C.L., Donlin, M.J., Teague, R.M.: Checkpoint blockade immunotherapy relies on T-bet but not Eomes to induce effector function in tumor-infiltrating CD8+ T cells. Cancer Immunol. Res. **3**, 116–124 (2015)

Bi, S., Earl, L.A., Jacobs, L., Baum, L.G.: Structural features of galectin-9 and galectin-1 that determine distinct T cell death pathways. J. Biol. Chem. **283**, 12248–12258 (2008)

Boussiotis, V.A., Freeman, G.J., Gribben, J.G., Daley, J., Gray, G., Nadler, L.M.: Activated human B lymphocytes express three CTLA-4 counterreceptors that costimulate T-cell activation. Proc. Natl. Acad. Sci. U. S. A. **90**, 11059–11063 (1993)

Bulliard, Y., Jolicoeur, R., Windman, M., Rue, S.M., Ettenberg, S., Knee, D.A., Wilson, N.S., Dranoff, G., Brogdon, J.L.: Activating Fc gamma receptors contribute to the antitumor activities of immunoregulatory receptor-targeting antibodies. J. Exp. Med. **210**, 1685–1693 (2013)

Callahan, M.K., Wolchok, J.D.: At the bedside: CTLA-4- and PD-1-blocking antibodies in cancer immunotherapy. J. Leukoc. Biol. **94**, 41–53 (2013)

Callahan, M.K., Postow, M.A., Wolchok, J.D.: CTLA-4 and PD-1 pathway blockade: combinations in the clinic. Front. Oncol. **4**, 385 (2014)

Cantrell, D.: Protein kinase B (Akt) regulation and function in T lymphocytes. Semin. Immunol. **14**, 19–26 (2002)

Chambers, C.A., Sullivan, T.J., Allison, J.P.: Lymphoproliferation in CTLA-4-deficient mice is mediated by costimulation-dependent activation of CD4+ T cells. Immunity **7**, 885–895 (1997)

Chiba, S., Baghdadi, M., Akiba, H., Yoshiyama, H., Kinoshita, I., Dosaka-Akita, H., Fujioka, Y., Ohba, Y., Gorman, J.V., Colgan, J.D., Hirashima, M., Uede, T., Takaoka, A., Yagita, H., Jinushi, M.: Tumor-infiltrating DCs suppress nucleic acid-mediated innate immune responses through interactions between the receptor TIM-3 and the alarmin HMGB1. Nat. Immunol. **13**, 832–842 (2012)

Chuang, E., Fisher, T.S., Morgan, R.W., Robbins, M.D., Duerr, J.M., Vander Heiden, M.G., Gardner, J.P., Hambor, J.E., Neveu, M.J., Thompson, C.B.: The CD28 and CTLA-4 receptors associate with the serine/threonine phosphatase PP2A. Immunity **13**, 313–322 (2000)

Coley, W.B.: The treatment of inoperable sarcoma by bacterial toxins (the mixed toxins of the Streptococcus erysipelas and the Bacillus prodigiosus). Proc. R. Soc. Med. **3**, 1–48 (1910)

Coley, W.B.: Further observations on the conservative treatment of sarcoma of the long bones. Ann. Surg. **70**, 633–660 (1919)

Coley, W.B.: Prognosis and treatment of giant-cell sarcoma: based on a further study of end results in sixty-nine cases. Ann. Surg. **86**, 641–665 (1927)

Coley, W.B.: The treatment of sarcoma of the long bones. Ann. Surg. **97**, 434–460 (1933)

Coley, W.B.: The treatment of malignant tumors by repeated inoculations of erysipelas. With a report of ten original cases. 1893. Clin. Orthop. Relat. Res. (262), 3–11 (1991)

Crawford, A., Angelosanto, J.M., Kao, C., Doering, T.A., Odorizzi, P.M., Barnett, B.E., Wherry, E.J.: Molecular and Transcriptional Basis of CD4 T Cell Dysfunction during Chronic Infection. Immunity **40**(2), 289–302 (2014)

Croft, M.: Costimulation of T cells by OX40, 4-1BB, and CD27. Cytokine Growth Factor Rev. **14**, 265–273 (2003)

Croft, M., Benedict, C.A., Ware, C.F.: Clinical targeting of the TNF and TNFR superfamilies. Nat. Rev. Drug Discov. **12**, 147–168 (2013)

Dang, C.V.: Links between metabolism and cancer. Genes Dev. **26**, 877–890 (2012)

DeKruyff, R.H., Bu, X., Ballesteros, A., Santiago, C., Chim, Y.L., Lee, H.H., Karisola, P., Pichavant, M., Kaplan, G.G., Umetsu, D.T., Freeman, G.J., Casasnovas, J.M.: T cell/transmembrane, Ig, and mucin-3 allelic variants differentially recognize phosphatidylserine and mediate phagocytosis of apoptotic cells. J. Immunol. **184**, 1918–1930 (2010)

Delgoffe, G.M., Kole, T.P., Zheng, Y., Zarek, P.E., Matthews, K.L., Xiao, B., Worley, P.F., Kozma, S.C., Powell, J.D.: The mTOR kinase differentially regulates effector and regulatory T cell lineage commitment. Immunity **30**, 832–844 (2009)

Doering, T.A., Crawford, A., Angelosanto, J.M., Paley, M.A., Ziegler, C.G., Wherry, E.J.: Network analysis reveals centrally connected genes and pathways involved in CD8+ T cell exhaustion versus memory. Immunity **37**, 1130–1144 (2012)

Ettinghausen, S.E., Lipford III, E.H., Mule, J.J., Rosenberg, S.A.: Systemic administration of recombinant interleukin 2 stimulates in vivo lymphoid cell proliferation in tissues. J. Immunol. **135**, 1488–1497 (1985)

Ferris, R.L., Lu, B., Kane, L.P.: Too much of a good thing? Tim-3 and TCR signaling in T cell exhaustion. J. Immunol. **193**, 1525–1530 (2014)

Fox, C.J., Hammerman, P.S., Thompson, C.B.: Fuel feeds function: energy metabolism and the T-cell response. Nat. Rev. Immunol. **5**, 844–852 (2005)

Francisco, L.M., Salinas, V.H., Brown, K.E., Vanguri, V.K., Freeman, G.J., Kuchroo, V.K., Sharpe, A.H.: PD-L1 regulates the development, maintenance, and function of induced regulatory T cells. J. Exp. Med. **206**, 3015–3029 (2009)

Frauwirth, K.A., Thompson, C.B.: Regulation of T lymphocyte metabolism. J. Immunol. (Baltimore, Md. 1950) **172**, 4661–4665 (2004)

Frauwirth, K.A., Riley, J.L., Harris, M.H., Parry, R.V., Rathmell, J.C., Plas, D.R., Elstrom, R.L., June, C.H., Thompson, C.B.: The CD28 signaling pathway regulates glucose metabolism. Immunity **16**, 769–777 (2002)

Freeman, G.J., Gribben, J.G., Boussiotis, V.A., Ng, J.W., Restivo Jr., V.A., Lombard, L.A., Gray, G.S., Nadler, L.M.: Cloning of B7-2: a CTLA-4 counter-receptor that costimulates human T cell proliferation. Science **262**, 909–911 (1993)

Freeman, G.J., Long, A.J., Iwai, Y., Bourque, K., Chernova, T., Nishimura, H., Fitz, L.J., Malenkovich, N., Okazaki, T., Byrne, M.C., Horton, H.F., Fouser, L., Carter, L., Ling, V., Bowman, M.R., Carreno, B.M., Collins, M., Wood, C.R., Honjo, T.: Engagement of the PD-1 immunoinhibitory receptor by a novel B7 family member leads to negative regulation of lymphocyte activation. J. Exp. Med. **192**, 1027–1034 (2000)

Frey, B., Gaipl, U.S.: The immune functions of phosphatidylserine in membranes of dying cells and microvesicles. Semin. Immunopathol. **33**, 497–516 (2011)

Fruman, D.A.: Phosphoinositide 3-kinase and its targets in B-cell and T-cell signaling. Curr. Opin. Immunol. **16**, 314–320 (2004)

Furness, A.J., Vargas, F.A., Peggs, K.S., Quezada, S.A.: Impact of tumour microenvironment and Fc receptors on the activity of immunomodulatory antibodies. Trends Immunol. **35**, 290–298 (2014)
Genot, E.M., Arrieumerlou, C., Ku, G., Burgering, B.M., Weiss, A., Kramer, I.M.: The T-cell receptor regulates Akt (protein kinase B) via a pathway involving Rac1 and phosphatidylinositide 3-kinase. Mol. Cell. Biol. **20**, 5469–5478 (2000)
Goldberg, M.V., Drake, C.G.: LAG-3 in cancer immunotherapy. Curr. Top. Microbiol. Immunol. **344**, 269–278 (2011)
Gorman, J.V., Starbeck-Miller, G., Pham, N.L., Traver, G.L., Rothman, P.B., Harty, J.T., Colgan, J.D.: Tim-3 directly enhances CD8 T cell responses to acute Listeria monocytogenes infection. J. Immunol. **192**, 3133–3142 (2014)
Gros, A., Robbins, P.F., Yao, X., Li, Y.F., Turcotte, S., Tran, E., Wunderlich, J.R., Mixon, A., Farid, S., Dudley, M.E., Hanada, K., Almeida, J.R., Darko, S., Douek, D.C., Yang, J.C., Rosenberg, S.A.: PD-1 identifies the patient-specific CD8+ tumor-reactive repertoire infiltrating human tumors. J. Clin. Invest. **124**, 2246–2259 (2014)
Gubin, M.M., Zhang, X., Schuster, H., Caron, E., Ward, J.P., Noguchi, T., Ivanova, Y., Hundal, J., Arthur, C.D., Krebber, W.J., Mulder, G.E., Toebes, M., Vesely, M.D., Lam, S.S., Korman, A.J., Allison, J.P., Freeman, G.J., Sharpe, A.H., Pearce, E.L., Schumacher, T.N., Aebersold, R., Rammensee, H.G., Melief, C.J., Mardis, E.R., Gillanders, W.E., Artyomov, M.N., Schreiber, R.D.: Checkpoint blockade cancer immunotherapy targets tumour-specific mutant antigens. Nature **515**, 577–581 (2014)
Hamid, O., Robert, C., Daud, A., Hodi, F.S., Hwu, W.J., Kefford, R., Wolchok, J.D., Hersey, P., Joseph, R.W., Weber, J.S., Dronca, R., Gangadhar, T.C., Patnaik, A., Zarour, H., Joshua, A.M., Gergich, K., Elassaiss-Schaap, J., Algazi, A., Mateus, C., Boasberg, P., Tumeh, P.C., Chmielowski, B., Ebbinghaus, S.W., Li, X.N., Kang, S.P., Ribas, A.: Safety and tumor responses with lambrolizumab (anti-PD-1) in melanoma. N. Engl. J. Med. **369**, 134–144 (2013)
Hannier, S., Tournier, M., Bismuth, G., Triebel, F.: CD3/TCR complex-associated lymphocyte activation gene-3 molecules inhibit CD3/TCR signaling. J. Immunol. **161**, 4058–4065 (1998)
Haxhinasto, S., Mathis, D., Benoist, C.: The AKT-mTOR axis regulates de novo differentiation of CD4+Foxp3+ cells. J. Exp. Med. **205**, 565–574 (2008)
Huang, W., August, A.: The signaling symphony: T cell receptor tunes cytokine-mediated T cell differentiation. J. Leukoc. Biol. **97**, 477–485 (2015)
Huang, S., Lu, F., Li, J., Lan, T., Huang, B., Yin, X., Jin, H.: Quantification of tryptase-TIM-3 double-positive mast cells in human chronic periodontitis. Arch. Oral Biol. **59**, 654–661 (2014)
Ishida, Y., Agata, Y., Shibahara, K., Honjo, T.: Induced expression of PD-1, a novel member of the immunoglobulin gene superfamily, upon programmed cell death. EMBO J. **11**, 3887–3895 (1992)
Jamieson, B.D., Ahmed, R.: T cell memory. Long-term persistence of virus-specific cytotoxic T cells. J Exp Med **169**, 1993–2005 (1989)
Jamieson, B.D., Butler, L.D., Ahmed, R.: Effective clearance of a persistent viral infection requires cooperation between virus-specific Lyt2+ T cells and nonspecific bone marrow-derived cells. J. Virol. **61**, 3930–3937 (1987)
Kane, L.P., Lin, J., Weiss, A.: It's all Rel-ative: NF-kappaB and CD28 costimulation of T-cell activation. Trends Immunol. **23**, 413–420 (2002)
Kao, C., Oestreich, K.J., Paley, M.A., Crawford, A., Angelosanto, J.M., Ali, M.A., Intlekofer, A.M., Boss, J.M., Reiner, S.L., Weinmann, A.S., Wherry, E.J.: Transcription factor T-bet represses expression of the inhibitory receptor PD-1 and sustains virus-specific CD8+ T cell responses during chronic infection. Nat. Immunol. **12**, 663–671 (2011)
Karin, M., Cao, Y., Greten, F.R., Li, Z.W.: NF-kappaB in cancer: from innocent bystander to major culprit. Nat. Rev. Cancer **2**, 301–310 (2002)
Kim, J.W., Dang, C.V.: Cancer's molecular sweet tooth and the Warburg effect. Cancer Res. **66**, 8927–8930 (2006)
Kobayashi, N., Karisola, P., Pena-Cruz, V., Dorfman, D.M., Jinushi, M., Umetsu, S.E., Butte, M.J., Nagumo, H., Chernova, I., Zhu, B., Sharpe, A.H., Ito, S., Dranoff, G., Kaplan, G.G., Casasnovas, J.M., Umetsu, D.T., Dekruyff, R.H., Freeman, G.J.: TIM-1 and TIM-4 glycoproteins bind phosphatidylserine and mediate uptake of apoptotic cells. Immunity **27**, 927–940 (2007)

Latchman, Y., Wood, C.R., Chernova, T., Chaudhary, D., Borde, M., Chernova, I., Iwai, Y., Long, A.J., Brown, J.A., Nunes, R., Greenfield, E.A., Bourque, K., Boussiotis, V.A., Carter, L.L., Carreno, B.M., Malenkovich, N., Nishimura, H., Okazaki, T., Honjo, T., Sharpe, A.H., Freeman, G.J.: PD-L2 is a second ligand for PD-1 and inhibits T cell activation. Nat. Immunol. **2**, 261–268 (2001)

Lau, L.L., Jamieson, B.D., Somasundaram, T., Ahmed, R.: Cytotoxic T-cell memory without antigen. Nature **369**, 648–652 (1994)

Le Mercier, I., Chen, W., Lines, J.L., Day, M., Li, J., Sergent, P., Noelle, R.J., Wang, L.: VISTA regulates the development of protective antitumor immunity. Cancer Res. **74**, 1933–1944 (2014)

Leach, D.R., Krummel, M.F., Allison, J.P.: Enhancement of antitumor immunity by CTLA-4 blockade. Science **271**, 1734–1736 (1996)

Lee, K.M., Chuang, E., Griffin, M., Khattri, R., Hong, D.K., Zhang, W., Straus, D., Samelson, L.E., Thompson, C.B., Bluestone, J.A.: Molecular basis of T cell inactivation by CTLA-4. Science **282**, 2263–2266 (1998)

Lee, J., Su, E.W., Zhu, C., Hainline, S., Phuah, J., Moroco, J.A., Smithgall, T.E., Kuchroo, V.K., Kane, L.P.: Phosphotyrosine-dependent coupling of Tim-3 to T-cell receptor signaling pathways. Mol. Cell. Biol. **31**, 3963–3974 (2011)

Leitner, J., Rieger, A., Pickl, W.F., Zlabinger, G., Grabmeier-Pfistershammer, K., Steinberger, P.: TIM-3 does not act as a receptor for galectin-9. PLoS Pathog. **9**, e1003253 (2013)

Lesokhin, A.M., Callahan, M.K., Postow, M.A., Wolchok, J.D.: On being less tolerant: enhanced cancer immunosurveillance enabled by targeting checkpoints and agonists of T cell activation. Sci Transl Med **7**, 280sr281 (2015)

Liao, X.C., Littman, D.R.: Altered T cell receptor signaling and disrupted T cell development in mice lacking Itk. Immunity **3**, 757–769 (1995)

Lines, J.L., Pantazi, E., Mak, J., Sempere, L.F., Wang, L., O'Connell, S., Ceeraz, S., Suriawinata, A.A., Yan, S., Ernstoff, M.S., Noelle, R.: VISTA is an immune checkpoint molecule for human T cells. Cancer Res. **74**, 1924–1932 (2014)

Linsley, P.S., Brady, W., Urnes, M., Grosmaire, L.S., Damle, N.K., Ledbetter, J.A.: CTLA-4 is a second receptor for the B cell activation antigen B7. J. Exp. Med. **174**, 561–569 (1991)

Macian, F., Im, S.H., Garcia-Cozar, F.J., Rao, A.: T-cell anergy. Curr. Opin. Immunol. **16**, 209–216 (2004)

Marabelle, A., Kohrt, H., Sagiv-Barfi, I., Ajami, B., Axtell, R.C., Zhou, G., Rajapaksa, R., Green, M.R., Torchia, J., Brody, J., Luong, R., Rosenblum, M.D., Steinman, L., Levitsky, H.I., Tse, V., Levy, R.: Depleting tumor-specific Tregs at a single site eradicates disseminated tumors. J. Clin. Invest. **123**, 2447–2463 (2013)

Marengere, L.E., Waterhouse, P., Duncan, G.S., Mittrucker, H.W., Feng, G.S., Mak, T.W.: Regulation of T cell receptor signaling by tyrosine phosphatase SYP association with CTLA-4. Science **272**, 1170–1173 (1996)

Maurya, N., Gujar, R., Gupta, M., Yadav, V., Verma, S., Sen, P.: Immunoregulation of dendritic cells by the receptor T cell Ig and mucin protein-3 via Bruton's tyrosine kinase and c-Src. J. Immunol. **193**, 3417–3425 (2014)

Monney, L., Sabatos, C.A., Gaglia, J.L., Ryu, A., Waldner, H., Chernova, T., Manning, S., Greenfield, E.A., Coyle, A.J., Sobel, R.A., Freeman, G.J., Kuchroo, V.K.: Th1-specific cell surface protein Tim-3 regulates macrophage activation and severity of an autoimmune disease. Nature **415**, 536–541 (2002)

Nakae, S., Iikura, M., Suto, H., Akiba, H., Umetsu, D.T., Dekruyff, R.H., Saito, H., Galli, S.J.: TIM-1 and TIM-3 enhancement of Th2 cytokine production by mast cells. Blood **110**, 2565–2568 (2007)

Nakaseko, C., Miyatake, S., Iida, T., Hara, S., Abe, R., Ohno, H., Saito, Y., Saito, T.: Cytotoxic T lymphocyte antigen 4 (CTLA-4) engagement delivers an inhibitory signal through the membrane-proximal region in the absence of the tyrosine motif in the cytoplasmic tail. J. Exp. Med. **190**, 765–774 (1999)

Nakayama, M., Akiba, H., Takeda, K., Kojima, Y., Hashiguchi, M., Azuma, M., Yagita, H., Okumura, K.: Tim-3 mediates phagocytosis of apoptotic cells and cross-presentation. Blood **113**(16), 3821–3830 (2009)

Niki, T., Tsutsui, S., Hirose, S., Aradono, S., Sugimoto, Y., Takeshita, K., Nishi, N., Hirashima, M.: Galectin-9 is a high affinity IgE-binding lectin with anti-allergic effect by blocking IgE-antigen complex formation. J. Biol. Chem. **284**, 32344–32352 (2009)

O'Brien, T.F., Gorentla, B.K., Xie, D., Srivatsan, S., McLeod, I.X., He, Y.W., Zhong, X.P.: Regulation of T-cell survival and mitochondrial homeostasis by TSC1. Eur. J. Immunol. **41**, 3361–3370 (2011)

Oikawa, T., Kamimura, Y., Akiba, H., Yagita, H., Okumura, K., Takahashi, H., Zeniya, M., Tajiri, H., Azuma, M.: Preferential involvement of Tim-3 in the regulation of hepatic CD8+ T cells in murine acute graft-versus-host disease. J. Immunol. **177**, 4281–4287 (2006)

Okazaki, T., Tanaka, Y., Nishio, R., Mitsuiye, T., Mizoguchi, A., Wang, J., Ishida, M., Hiai, H., Matsumori, A., Minato, N., Honjo, T.: Autoantibodies against cardiac troponin I are responsible for dilated cardiomyopathy in PD-1-deficient mice. Nat. Med. **9**, 1477–1483 (2003)

Okazaki, T., Chikuma, S., Iwai, Y., Fagarasan, S., Honjo, T.: A rheostat for immune responses: the unique properties of PD-1 and their advantages for clinical application. Nat. Immunol. **14**, 1212–1218 (2013)

Paley, M.A., Wherry, E.J.: TCF-1 flips the switch on Eomes. Immunity **33**, 145–147 (2010)

Paley, M.A., Kroy, D.C., Odorizzi, P.M., Johnnidis, J.B., Dolfi, D.V., Barnett, B.E., Bikoff, E.K., Robertson, E.J., Lauer, G.M., Reiner, S.L., Wherry, E.J.: Progenitor and terminal subsets of CD8+ T cells cooperate to contain chronic viral infection. Science **338**, 1220–1225 (2012)

Paley, M.A., Gordon, S.M., Bikoff, E.K., Robertson, E.J., Wherry, E.J., Reiner, S.L.: Technical advance: fluorescent reporter reveals insights into eomesodermin biology in cytotoxic lymphocytes. J. Leukoc. Biol. **93**, 307–315 (2013)

Parry, R.V., Chemnitz, J.M., Frauwirth, K.A., Lanfranco, A.R., Braunstein, I., Kobayashi, S.V., Linsley, P.S., Thompson, C.B., Riley, J.L.: CTLA-4 and PD-1 receptors inhibit T-cell activation by distinct mechanisms. Mol. Cell. Biol. **25**, 9543–9553 (2005)

Patsoukis, N., Bardhan, K., Chatterjee, P., Sari, D., Liu, B., Bell, L.N., Karoly, E.D., Freeman, G.J., Petkova, V., Seth, P., Li, L., Boussiotis, V.A.: PD-1 alters T-cell metabolic reprogramming by inhibiting glycolysis and promoting lipolysis and fatty acid oxidation. Nat. Commun. **6**, 6692 (2015)

Pauken, K.E., Wherry, E.J.: TIGIT and CD226: tipping the balance between costimulatory and coinhibitory molecules to augment the cancer immunotherapy toolkit. Cancer Cell **26**, 785–787 (2014)

Pauken, K.E., Wherry, E.J.: Overcoming T cell exhaustion in infection and cancer. Trends Immunol. **36**, 265–276 (2015)

Penaloza-MacMaster, P., Kamphorst, A.O., Wieland, A., Araki, K., Iyer, S.S., West, E.E., O'Mara, L., Yang, S., Konieczny, B.T., Sharpe, A.H., Freeman, G.J., Rudensky, A.Y., Ahmed, R.: Interplay between regulatory T cells and PD-1 in modulating T cell exhaustion and viral control during chronic LCMV infection. J. Exp. Med. **211**, 1905–1918 (2014)

Phong, B.L., Avery, L., Sumpter, T.L., Gorman, J.V., Watkins, S.C., Colgan, J.D., Kane, L.P.: Tim-3 enhances FcεRI-proximal signaling to modulate mast cell activation. J Exp Med **212**(13), 2289–304 (2015)

Powell, J.D., Delgoffe, G.M.: The mammalian target of rapamycin: linking T cell differentiation, function, and metabolism. Immunity **33**, 301–311 (2010)

Powell, J.D., Lerner, C.G., Schwartz, R.H.: Inhibition of cell cycle progression by rapamycin induces T cell clonal anergy even in the presence of costimulation. J. Immunol. (Baltimore, Md. 1950) **162**, 2775–2784 (1999)

Quigley, M., Pereyra, F., Nilsson, B., Porichis, F., Fonseca, C., Eichbaum, Q., Julg, B., Jesneck, J.L., Brosnahan, K., Imam, S., Russell, K., Toth, I., Piechocka-Trocha, A., Dolfi, D., Angelosanto, J., Crawford, A., Shin, H., Kwon, D.S., Zupkosky, J., Francisco, L., Freeman, G.J., Wherry, E.J., Kaufmann, D.E., Walker, B.D., Ebert, B., Haining, W.N.: Transcriptional analysis of HIV-specific CD8+ T cells shows that PD-1 inhibits T cell function by upregulating BATF. Nat. Med. **16**, 1147–1151 (2010)

Qureshi, O.S., Zheng, Y., Nakamura, K., Attridge, K., Manzotti, C., Schmidt, E.M., Baker, J., Jeffery, L.E., Kaur, S., Briggs, Z., Hou, T.Z., Futter, C.E., Anderson, G., Walker, L.S., Sansom, D.M.: Trans-endocytosis of CD80 and CD86: a molecular basis for the cell-extrinsic function of CTLA-4. Science **332**, 600–603 (2011)

Qureshi, O.S., Kaur, S., Hou, T., Jeffery, L.E., Poulter, N.S., Briggs, Z., Kenefeck, R., Willox, A.K., Royle, S.J., Rappoport, J.Z., Sansom, D.M.: Constitutive clathrin-mediated endocytosis of CTLA-4 persists during T cell activation. J. Biol. Chem. **287**(12), 9429–9440 (2012)

Rathmell, J.C., Elstrom, R.L., Cinalli, R.M., Thompson, C.B.: Activated Akt promotes increased resting T cell size, CD28-independent T cell growth, and development of autoimmunity and lymphoma. Eur. J. Immunol. **33**, 2223–2232 (2003)

Riley, J.L.: PD-1 signaling in primary T cells. Immunol. Rev. **229**, 114–125 (2009)

Roos, D., Loos, J.A.: Changes in the carbohydrate metabolism of mitogenically stimulated human peripheral lymphocytes. II. Relative importance of glycolysis and oxidative phosphorylation on phytohaemagglutinin stimulation. Exp. Cell Res. **77**, 127–135 (1973)

Sabatos, C.A., Chakravarti, S., Cha, E., Schubart, A., Sanchez-Fueyo, A., Zheng, X.X., Coyle, A.J., Strom, T.B., Freeman, G.J., Kuchroo, V.K.: Interaction of Tim-3 and Tim-3 ligand regulates T helper type 1 responses and induction of peripheral tolerance. Nat. Immunol. **4**, 1102–1110 (2003)

Sakuishi, K., Ngiow, S.F., Sullivan, J.M., Teng, M.W., Kuchroo, V.K., Smyth, M.J., Anderson, A.C.: TIM3FOXP3 regulatory T cells are tissue-specific promoters of T-cell dysfunction in cancer. Oncoimmunology **2**, e23849 (2013)

Sanchez-Fueyo, A., Tian, J., Picarella, D., Domenig, C., Zheng, X.X., Sabatos, C.A., Manlongat, N., Bender, O., Kamradt, T., Kuchroo, V.K., Gutierrez-Ramos, J.C., Coyle, A.J., Strom, T.B.: Tim-3 inhibits T helper type 1-mediated auto- and alloimmune responses and promotes immunological tolerance. Nat. Immunol. **4**, 1093–1101 (2003)

Schwartz, R.H.: T cell anergy. Annu. Rev. Immunol. **21**, 305–334 (2003)

Shi, J., Petrie, H.T.: Activation kinetics and off-target effects of thymus-initiated cre transgenes. PLoS One **7**, e46590 (2012)

Shin, D.S., Ribas, A.: The evolution of checkpoint blockade as a cancer therapy: what's here, what's next? Curr. Opin. Immunol. **33**, 23–35 (2015)

Simmons, W.J., Koneru, M., Mohindru, M., Thomas, R., Cutro, S., Singh, P., Dekruyff, R.H., Inghirami, G., Coyle, A.J., Kim, B.S., Ponzio, N.M.: Tim-3+ T-bet+ tumor-specific Th1 cells colocalize with and inhibit development and growth of murine neoplasms. J. Immunol. **174**, 1405–1415 (2005)

Simpson, T.R., Li, F., Montalvo-Ortiz, W., Sepulveda, M.A., Bergerhoff, K., Arce, F., Roddie, C., Henry, J.Y., Yagita, H., Wolchok, J.D., Peggs, K.S., Ravetch, J.V., Allison, J.P., Quezada, S.A.: Fc-dependent depletion of tumor-infiltrating regulatory T cells co-defines the efficacy of anti-CTLA-4 therapy against melanoma. J. Exp. Med. **210**, 1695–1710 (2013)

Sims, G.P., Rowe, D.C., Rietdijk, S.T., Herbst, R., Coyle, A.J.: HMGB1 and RAGE in inflammation and cancer. Annu. Rev. Immunol. **28**, 367–388 (2010)

Song, C., Sadashivaiah, K., Furusawa, A., Davila, E., Tamada, K., Banerjee, A.: Eomesodermin is required for antitumor immunity mediated by 4-1BB-agonist immunotherapy. Oncoimmunology **3**, e27680 (2014)

Staron, M.M., Gray, S.M., Marshall, H.D., Parish, I.A., Chen, J.H., Perry, C.J., Cui, G., Li, M.O., Kaech, S.M.: The transcription factor FoxO1 sustains expression of the inhibitory receptor PD-1 and survival of antiviral CD8(+) T cells during chronic infection. Immunity **41**, 802–814 (2014)

Su, E.W., Bi, S., Kane, L.P.: Galectin-9 regulates T helper cell function independently of Tim-3. Glycobiology **21**(10), 1258–1265 (2010)

Suntharalingam, G., Perry, M.R., Ward, S., Brett, S.J., Castello-Cortes, A., Brunner, M.D., Panoskaltsis, N.: Cytokine storm in a phase 1 trial of the anti-CD28 monoclonal antibody TGN1412. N. Engl. J. Med. **355**, 1018–1028 (2006)

Topalian, S.L., Drake, C.G., Pardoll, D.M.: Immune checkpoint blockade: a common denominator approach to cancer therapy. Cancer Cell **27**, 450–461 (2015) van Rooij, N., van Buuren, M.M., Philips, D., Velds, A., Toebes, M., Heemskerk, B., van Dijk, L.J., Behjati, S., Hilkmann, H., El Atmioui, D., Nieuwland, M., Stratton, M.R., Kerkhoven, R.M., Kesmir, C., Haanen, J.B., Kvistborg, P., Schumacher, T.N.: Tumor exome analysis reveals neoantigen-specific T-cell reactivity in an ipilimumab-responsive melanoma. J Clin. Oncol. **31**, e439–e442 (2013)

Vinay, D.S., Kwon, B.S.: Immunotherapy of cancer with 4-1BB. Mol. Cancer Ther. **11**, 1062–1070 (2012)

Walunas, T.L., Lenschow, D.J., Bakker, C.Y., Linsley, P.S., Freeman, G.J., Green, J.M., Thompson, C.B., Bluestone, J.A.: CTLA-4 can function as a negative regulator of T cell activation. Immunity **1**, 405–413 (1994)

Waterhouse, P., Penninger, J.M., Timms, E., Wakeham, A., Shahinian, A., Lee, K.P., Thompson, C.B., Griesser, H., Mak, T.W.: Lymphoproliferative disorders with early lethality in mice deficient in Ctla-4. Science **270**, 985–988 (1995)

Wherry, E.J.: T cell exhaustion. Nat. Immunol. **12**, 492–499 (2011)

Wherry, E.J., Blattman, J.N., Murali-Krishna, K., van der Most, R., Ahmed, R.: Viral persistence alters CD8 T-cell immunodominance and tissue distribution and results in distinct stages of functional impairment. J. Virol. **77**, 4911–4927 (2003)

Wherry, E.J., Ha, S.J., Kaech, S.M., Haining, W.N., Sarkar, S., Kalia, V., Subramaniam, S., Blattman, J.N., Barber, D.L., Ahmed, R.: Molecular signature of CD8+ T cell exhaustion during chronic viral infection. Immunity **27**, 670–684 (2007)

Wieman, H.L., Wofford, J.A., Rathmell, J.C.: Cytokine stimulation promotes glucose uptake via phosphatidylinositol-3 kinase/Akt regulation of Glut1 activity and trafficking. Mol. Biol. Cell **18**, 1437–1446 (2007)

Wiener, Z., Kohalmi, B., Pocza, P., Jeager, J., Tolgyesi, G., Toth, S., Gorbe, E., Papp, Z., Falus, A.: TIM-3 is expressed in melanoma cells and is upregulated in TGF-beta stimulated mast cells. J. Invest. Dermatol. **127**(4), 906–914 (2006)

Wofford, J.A., Wieman, H.L., Jacobs, S.R., Zhao, Y., Rathmell, J.C.: IL-7 promotes Glut1 trafficking and glucose uptake via STAT5-mediated activation of Akt to support T-cell survival. Blood **111**, 2101–2111 (2008)

Woo, S.R., Turnis, M.E., Goldberg, M.V., Bankoti, J., Selby, M., Nirschl, C.J., Bettini, M.L., Gravano, D.M., Vogel, P., Liu, C.L., Tangsombatvisit, S., Grosso, J.F., Netto, G., Smeltzer, M.P., Chaux, A., Utz, P.J., Workman, C.J., Pardoll, D.M., Korman, A.J., Drake, C.G., Vignali, D.A.: Immune inhibitory molecules LAG-3 and PD-1 synergistically regulate T-cell function to promote tumoral immune escape. Cancer Res. **72**, 917–927 (2012)

Workman, C.J., Vignali, D.A.: The CD4-related molecule, LAG-3 (CD223), regulates the expansion of activated T cells. Eur. J. Immunol. **33**, 970–979 (2003)

Wu, C., Thalhamer, T., Franca, R.F., Xiao, S., Wang, C., Hotta, C., Zhu, C., Hirashima, M., Anderson, A.C., Kuchroo, V.K.: Galectin-9-CD44 interaction enhances stability and function of adaptive regulatory T cells. Immunity **41**, 270–282 (2014)

Youngblood, B., Wherry, E.J., Ahmed, R.: Acquired transcriptional programming in functional and exhausted virus-specific CD8 T cells. Curr. Opin. HIV AIDS **7**, 50–57 (2012)

Zheng, Y., Delgoffe, G.M., Meyer, C.F., Chan, W., Powell, J.D.: Anergic T cells are metabolically anergic. J. Immunol. (Baltimore, Md. 1950) **183**, 6095–6101 (2009)

Zhu, C., Anderson, A.C., Schubart, A., Xiong, H., Imitola, J., Khoury, S.J., Zheng, X.X., Strom, T.B., Kuchroo, V.K.: The Tim-3 ligand galectin-9 negatively regulates T helper type 1 immunity. Nat. Immunol. **6**, 1245–1252 (2005)

Chapter 6
Immunomodulation Within a Single Tumor Site to Induce Systemic Antitumor Immunity: In Situ Vaccination for Cancer

Linda Hammerich and Joshua D. Brody

Abbreviations

APC	Antigen-presenting cell
CNS	Central nervous system
CTL	Cytotoxic T-lymphocyte
CTLA-4	Cytotoxic T-lymphocyte-associated protein 4
DC	Dendritic cell
ECM	Extracellular matrix
EGFR	Epidermal growth factor receptor
FLT3L	Fms-like tyrosine kinase 3 ligand
GM-CSF	Granulocyte-macrophage colony-stimulating factor
HSPs	Heat shock proteins
IFN	Interferon
IL	Interleukin
LPS	Lipopolysaccharide
PD-1	Programmed death 1
Rb	Retinoblastoma
TAA	Tumor-associated antigen
TLR	Toll-like receptor

L. Hammerich, Ph.D.
Division of Hematology and Medical Oncology, Icahn School of Medicine at Mount Sinai, New York, NY, USA

J.D. Brody, M.D. (✉)
Lymphoma Immunotherapy Program, Division of Hematology and Medical OncologyIcahn School of Medicine at Mount Sinai, New York, NY 10029, USA
e-mail: joshuabrody@gmail.com

P.D. Rennert (ed.), *Novel Immunotherapeutic Approaches to the Treatment of Cancer*, DOI 10.1007/978-3-319-29827-6_6

TNF	Tumor necrosis factor
VEGF	Vascular endothelial growth factor
VSV	Vesicular stomatitis virus

1 Introduction

Prophylactic vaccinations have been one of the greatest advances in modern medicine, both eradicating disease and reducing mortality. The translation of this advance into cancer therapy has been challenging and dates back to the turn of the twentieth century (Currie 1972). Cancer cells, derived from an aberrant clone, bear predominantly self-antigens and thus avoid alerting the immune system. In addition, the tumor microenvironment can be severely immunosuppressive; adding an extra layer of protection against the host immune response. Tumor cells can actively suppress immune responses through the downregulation of antigen presentation and the production of membrane-bound and secreted immuneregulatory molecules (Upadhyay et al. 2015). To overcome such obstacles, a successful cancer vaccine must be able to induce a powerful immune response against tumor-associated antigens (TAAs) while avoiding normal host cells. This strategy has proven difficult because TAAs are highly variable in their immunogenicity and undergo immune editing to escape recognition. In addition, they can differ between tumor types and more importantly between individuals (Escors 2014). The presence of antigen-presenting cells (APCs) is generally low in the tumor microenvironment. Some efficacy in the treatment of cancer has been demonstrated by the use of autologous dendritic cells (DCs) pulsed with tumor cell lysates containing a whole array of antigens as well as single TAAs (Reichardt et al. 2004). DC can be differentiated and expanded from peripheral blood ex vivo, and a resected tumor mass can be used to subsequently load the DC with TAAs. These strategies, while successful in developing a patient-specific vaccine, are labor and time intensive limiting the ability to experiment with numerous iterations to optimize the approach.

"In situ vaccination" represents an alternative approach in which the cancer vaccine is generated in vivo without the need to previously identify and isolate the TAA. Herein, in situ vaccination refers to any approach which exploits TAA available at a tumor site to induce a TAA-specific adaptive immune response. TAAs are commonly released upon tumor cell death and may be subsequently processed and presented by APCs. This can be augmented by stimulating tumor cell death leading to release of TAAs and subsequent presentation by APCs while at the same time administering immunomodulators to enhance particular steps of the process. Such an approach allows for the development of vaccines in patients themselves, thereby minimizing the resource allocation required for ex vivo processing. Furthermore, this strategy can take advantage of the complete antigenic repertoire of a tumor and not be limited to a single TAA. In order to elicit a strong memory antitumor immune response, an in situ vaccine should ideally be able to induce immunogenic cancer cell death, facilitate the release of TAAs, as well as enhance antigen uptake by, and

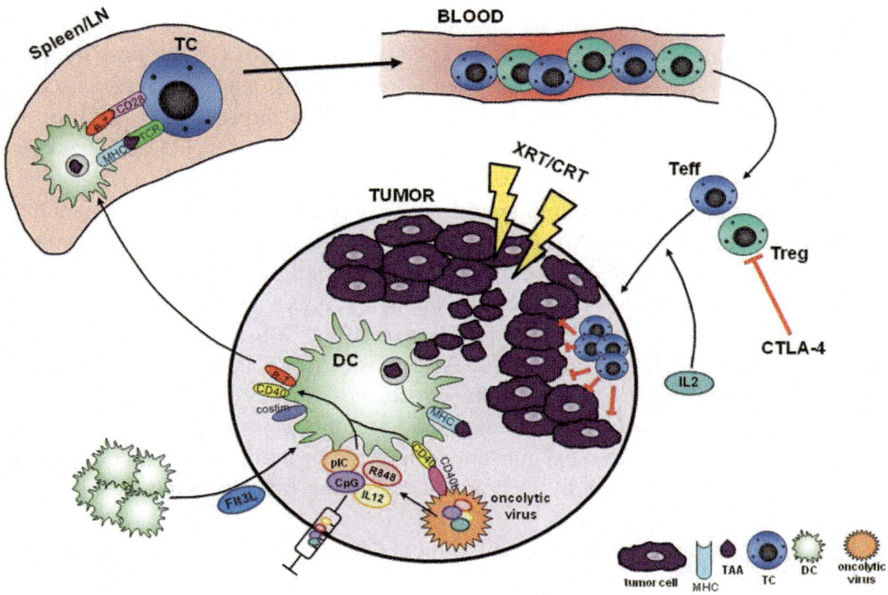

Fig. 6.1 Effective in situ vaccination uses local or intratumoral immunomodulation to produce abundant, highly activated, antigen-presenting cells such as dendritic cells (DC) able to present the full repertoire of tumor-associated antigens (TAAs) to tumor-reactive T cells which, in turn, mount a systemic antitumor immune response. Optimally, this approach occurs through: (1) increasing intratumoral DC populations, by recruitment or local proliferation (e.g., with intratumoral Flt3L administration); (2) inducing immunogenic tumor cell death locally or systemically to release TAA (e.g., with radiotherapy, chemotherapy, or oncolytic virus); (3) enhancing TAA uptake, processing and presentation, or cross-presentation by DC (e.g., with heat shock proteins or using prime-boost oncolytic viral strategies); (4) promoting antigen-loaded DC to trafficking to secondary lymphoid tissue; (5) presentation or cross-presentation to antigen-specific T cells; (6) trafficking of T cells to tumor sites systemically; and (7) inhibition of multiple levels of immunosuppression, including cells and molecules suppressing T cells both at the vaccine site as well as distant tumor sites (e.g., with intratumoral or systemic checkpoint blockade)

activation of, APCs to induce antitumor T-cell responses that will result in systemic antitumor immunity (Fig. 6.1). The generation of potent antitumor T cells at one tumor site should allow them to also attack distant tumor lesions since fully activated effector T cells do not need a costimulatory signal to kill their target cells and are less susceptible to inhibitory signals (Suresh et al. 2001; London et al. 2000; Gudmundsdottir et al. 1999). Therefore, effective development of an in situ vaccination will result in a systemic response in the setting of localized treatment similar to the abscopal effect that is described in radiation therapy and likely driven by a T-cell response (Formenti and Demaria 2009).

One tool which can be part of in situ vaccination, oncolytic viruses—viruses that preferentially infect and kill cancer cells—are being explored for the treatment of various malignancies (Nemunaitis 1999). They display either a natural or engineered tumor tropism and are able to kill tumor cells via direct and indirect mechanisms (Elsedawy and Russell 2013; Bartlett et al. 2013). The host immune system directly kills viral protein-expressing tumor cells, leading to regression in infected tumors. Uninfected cells are indirectly killed through cross-priming of cytotoxic T-lymphocytes (CTLs) and disruption of the tumor vasculature. However, the antitumor efficacy of naturally occurring viruses has been limited, suggesting that the degree of the induced immune response depends on several factors, including the particular virus used, the tumor burden, and the immunogenicity (Elsedawy and Russell 2013). An advantage of killing tumor cells with virus is their abundance of innately immunostimulatory components, e.g., viral proteins and nucleic acid sequences which have been shown to activate Toll-like receptors (TLRs) expressed on APC (Zhu et al. 2007a; Appledorn et al. 2008; Banchereau et al. 2014). Another advantage of oncolytic viruses is that they can be engineered to express transgenes which can influence the antitumoral immune responses. This includes (a) enhancing the cross-presentation of tumor antigens, (b) increasing the maturation of APCs, especially DC, and (c) reducing immune suppression in the tumor microenvironment.

Herein, we examine preclinical and clinical data of in situ vaccination strategies and their emerging role in the treatment of cancer as well as new developments in tumor immunology that will continue to drive translational research.

2 Manipulation of Intratumoral Myeloid Cells

2.1 Increasing the Number of APC at the Tumor Site

2.1.1 Autologous DC

Increasing the number of effective APC within the tumor microenvironment yields greater capacity for cross-presentation of TAA to CD8+ T cells, potentially augmenting the immune response against malignant cells. As a result, several studies have recently focused on strategies to increase the number of DC at the tumor site through administration of DC growth/differentiation factors or local administration of DC themselves. In mice with subcutaneous colon cancer or lymphoma, systemic chemotherapy followed by intratumoral injection of immature DC resulted in complete regression of treated and distant tumors and protected mice from rechallenge with the same tumor cells (Tong et al. 2001; Song and Levy 2005). This effect was also observed when mice with the same colon cancer were treated with photodynamic therapy and injection of naïve DC (Saji et al. 2006). In patients with advanced melanoma, treatment with local hyperthermia and injection of autologous DC reduced tumor growth and increased infiltration of CD8+ T cells, but overall survival was not improved (Guo et al. 2007). However, in patients with stage III/IV treatment naïve or relapsed follicular lymphoma local radiotherapy followed by intranodal injection of autologous DC, low-dose rituximab, and granulocyte-macrophage colony-stimulating factor (GM-CSF) caused durable remission in a subset of patients. Clinical response correlated closely with evidence of an immune response to autologous tumor (Kolstad et al. 2015). A phase I/II clinical trial is currently investigating the intratumoral injection of autologous DC for the treatment of solid tumors (NCT01882946). Similar studies are combining intratumoral administration of autologous DC combined with chemotherapy for patients with breast cancer (NCT02018458) and combined with local cryotherapy for patients with prostate cancer (NCT02423928).

2.1.2 Allogeneic DC

Preclinically, it has been shown that allogeneic leukocyte cocultures generate immature DC-recruiting chemokines and proinflammatory cytokines which induce CD40 upregulation, increase IL-12 production, and deviate T-cell responses toward Th1 (Wallgren et al. 2005). Additionally, allogeneic DC-based vaccines demonstrated induction of melanoma-protective immunity in multiple animal models (Siders et al. 2009).

In an early phase clinical trial, allogeneic DC activated with a formulation including TLRa and IFNγ (COMBIG) were administered intratumorally (INTUVAK) in 12 patients with metastatic renal cell cancer (RCC) prior to nephrectomy. At the time of nephrectomy, a marked infiltration of CD8+ T cells was demonstrated and a majority of patients exhibited an increase in circulating tumor-specific T cells after vaccination. Median overall survival in patients with poor prognosis compared favorably with historical controls (http://meetinglibrary.asco.org/content/126079-144). The approach has progressed to an ongoing randomized trial of post-nephrectomy sunitinib with or without pre-nephrectomy INTUVAK (NCT02432846) as well as an ongoing phase I study in patients with hepatoma (NCT01974661).

2.1.3 GM-CSF

Granulocyte-macrophage colony-stimulation factor (GM-CSF), a hematopoietic growth factor that increases DC differentiation, maturation, and function has been administered intratumorally to promote the number of DC and stimulating DC activation at the tumor site. A seminal study compared antitumor immunity of melanoma cells transduced with a panel of immunostimulatory genes including IL-2, IL-4, IL-5, IL-6, GM-CSF, IFNγ, IL1-RA, ICAM, CD2, and TNFα. GM-CSF-expressing tumors showed the greatest effects and induced systemic tumor rejection. Treatment also protected mice from rechallenge with nontransduced melanoma cells (Dranoff et al. 1993). Using a related approach, mice with colon cancer received macrophages engineered to express GM-CSF intratumorally and developed antitumor immunity (Yizhi et al. 1998). Vaccination of melanoma patients with irradiated autologous tumor cells engineered to express GM-CSF also resulted in tumor destruction. Those with tumor response were found to have profound infiltration of activated T cells. Three of the 11 patients who responded had continued response at 20–36 months, which was an improvement over dacarbazine therapy—the standard of care at that time (Serrone et al. 2000). The number of CD+ in GM-CSF-expressing tumor lesions was significantly increased in both mice and patients (Mach et al. 2000). In patients with melanoma, intratumoral or peritumoral injection of recombinant GM-CSF has been investigated with mixed results. While some demonstrated tumor regression in a majority of patients, including some complete responses, others reported only partial responses in a minority of patients (Si et al. 1996; Nasi et al. 1999; Hoeller et al. 2001). Regardless of response rate or degree of response, all three studies observed an increase of DC in tumor lesions. As described earlier, GM-CSF also has promising results when combined with autologous DC and a monoclonal ab in the treatment of low-grade follicular lymphoma (Kolstad et al. 2015). As described, GM-CSF has therapeutic potential as both a monotherapy and in combination with other immune modulating agents stimulating DC activation, immune response, and systemic tumor regressions.

2.1.4 Flt3L

Fms-like tyrosine kinase 3 ligand (Flt3L) is a crucial growth factor in DC development (Shortman and Naik 2007) and particularly important in the development of the DC2 subset—remarkably capable CD8 T-cell stimulators whose intratumoral proportion correlates with patient clinical outcomes (Broz et al. 2014; Salmon 2016). Subcutaneous injection of Flt3L stimulates mobilization of DC to the peripheral blood of patients with melanoma or colon cancer (Marroquin et al. 2002; Morse et al. 2000). Expansion of DC is observed in mice treated with adenovirally expressed or recombinant Flt3L in colon cancer or leukemia, respectively (Pawlowska et al. 2001; Riediger et al. 2013). However, while vaccination with Flt3L prior to tumor challenge is able to prevent tumor development in both models, therapeutic application of Flt3L could not eliminate established tumors. In contrast, the combination of intratumoral adeno-Flt3L with systemic chemotherapy inhibits the growth and induces complete remissions of murine hepatoma and colon cancer (Hou et al. 2007). Similarly, systemic administration of Flt3L followed by intranodal injection of antigen-encoding naked RNA—thereby delivering an antigen as well as TLR stimulation—resulted in significantly enhanced tumor clearance and survival in mice with melanoma (Kreiter et al. 2011). When combined with cytotoxic therapies or DC activation, Flt3L-induced DC expansion leads to clinical response as opposed to the administration of Flt3L alone. Several clinical trials combining Flt3L with cytotoxic and/or other concomitant treatments are currently underway (NCT02129075, NCT01811992, NCT01976585). The latter study combining intratumoral injection of recombinant Flt3L and poly-ICLC in combination with low-dose radiotherapy has reported increased DC numbers, partial and complete remissions of treated and untreated tumor sites in patients with advanced-stage follicular lymphoma (Bhardwaj et al. 2014). In this study, cell killing appeared to be tumor-specific since concomitant with malignant B-cell clearing from peripheral blood, nonmalignant B cells actually increased with time. This is in contrast to standard lymphoma therapies such anti-CD20 antibodies which induce B-cell aplasia (Maloney et al. 1994) and prompts inquiry into what TAA might be targeted by T cells which spare nonmalignant B cells. Preliminary results report only mild adverse effects from such therapy suggesting that Flt3L-primed in situ vaccination is safe as well as immunologically and clinically active.

2.1.5 Oncolytic Viruses that Increase the Number of APC at the Tumor Site

The most extensively studied cytokine for this purpose is GM-CSF. A vaccinia virus engineered to express GM-CSF, JX-594, selectively replicates in tumor cells as compared to normal cells (Parato et al. 2012) and has demonstrated antitumor efficacy in preclinical models and several early phase clinical trials. Rabbits and rats with liver cancer have improved survival and decreased metastatic burden when treated with JX-594 systemically *or* intratumorally. These models reveal increased infiltration of T cells into the tumor microenvironment (Kim et al. 2006) and disruption of tumor-associated vasculature in mice and humans, leading to reduced blood flow, ischemia, and rapid necrosis of tumor cells (Breitbach et al. 2011, 2013). Again, this effect is tumor specific as endothelial cells of normal blood vessels are not affected. Clinical trials in liver cancer and melanoma demonstrate that intratumoral treatment with JX-594 is well tolerated and results in encouraging survival times and overall response of treated and untreated tumors (Heo et al. 2013; Park et al. 2008; Hwang et al. 2011; Breitbach et al. 2015; Cripe et al. 2015).

Similarly promising results have been observed with an oncolytic herpes simplex virus (HSV) deleted for genes that block antigen presentation on MHC molecules or support viral replication in normal cells. This HSV strain specifically replicates in tumor cells with high oncolytic potential enhancing antitumor efficacy. Immunogenicity was enhanced by inserting GM-CSF into the viral genome (Liu et al. 2003). Liu et al. have demonstrated that intratumoral administration in murine lymphoma tumors results in tumor shrinkage and antitumor immunity in both treated tumors and distant, noninjected tumors. In addition, it protects mice against rechallenge with tumor cells after the primary tumor has been cured. Clinical studies using the same HSV strain referred to as talimogene laherparepvec or T-VEC (previously OncoVEX-GM-CSF) have shown durable response rates and increases survival time in patients with melanoma, head and neck cancer, and other metastatic cancers (Harrington et al. 2010; Hu et al. 2006; Senzer et al. 2009; Kaufman et al. 2010). A recent phase III study in patients with advanced-stage melanoma, T-VEC demonstrates superior durable response rate compared to GM-CSF and a trend toward improvement in overall survival ($p=0.051$) (Andtbacka et al. 2015b). In concordance with the preclinical studies, treated patients appear to develop systemic antitumor immunity associated with an increase in tumor-specific T cells resulting responses at both injected tumors and distant sites (Kaufman et al. 2010;

Senzer et al. 2009). Clinical investigation of combining intratumoral virotherapy with systemic cytotoxic T-lymphocyte-associated protein 4 (CTLA-4) blockade for melanoma is currently ongoing (NCT01740297) with preliminary report of overall response rate of 41 %, higher than historical results with ipilimumab alone (Puzanov et al. 2014) and studies combining T-VEC with systemic programmed death 1 (PD-1) blockade are currently accruing (NCT02263508).

2.2 Activation of APC

2.2.1 TLR9

TLRs are a class of pattern recognition receptors expressed primarily by leukocytes, and especially by APCs, including DC and macrophages. They bind to pathogen-associated molecular patterns (e.g., lipopolysaccharide (LPS), CpG-enriched DNA, double-stranded RNA), and their ligation results in APC activation, enhanced presentation to T cells and initiation of immune responses. In addition, they can have a direct influence on tumor cells themselves when expressing TLRs. B-cell lymphomas are derived from mature B cells—a potential APC population—and therefore can express multiple TLR, including TLR9 (Bourke et al. 2003). As a result, hypomethylated CG-enriched oligonucleotides (CpG) resembling prokaryotic DNA can activate TLR9 and increase expression of costimulatory molecules on lymphoma cells in vitro (Jahrsdörfer et al. 2001; Li et al. 2007), though differentially amongst different lymphoma subtypes (Jahrsdorfer et al. 2005). At the same time, CpG inhibited proliferation of these cells (Li et al. 2007). Furthermore, systemic chemotherapy combined with intratumoral vaccination with CpG-induced tumor-reactive, memory CD8 T cells and tumor regression at both local and distant sites in a murine lymphoma model. Both local and systemic antitumor response depended on CD8+ T cells (Li et al. 2007). Interestingly, this effect was seen in mice with TLR9 deficiency, carrying TLR9-expressing tumors. This finding suggests that antigen presentation by tumor cells, not host APC, may be sufficient to induce potent immune responses. This therapy could be further enhanced by transferring splenocytes from vaccinated mice into lymphodepleted mice (immunotransplantation) bearing the same tumor cell line, demonstrating that transferred CD8 T cells were both necessary and sufficient (Brody et al. 2009). Regulatory T cells (T_{reg}) cells could also be depleted locally by intratumoral injection of anti-CTLA-4 and anti-OX-40 during CpG vaccination, generating a systemic antitumor immune response able to cure disseminated disease (Marabelle et al. 2013). Mice were cured in the absence of systemic chemotherapy, validating the potency of combination treatment (Houot and Levy 2009).

In a murine glioma model, intratumoral injection of CpG also resulted in tumor regression. Again increased T-cell infiltration was seen and cured mice were protected from rechallenge with tumor cells (Grauer et al. 2008). In contrast to the lymphoma model, TLR9 expression is required in nontumor host cells since GL261 glioma cells are negative for TLR9. Furthermore, beneficial effects of intratumoral CpG are also observed in mice with mesothelioma, breast cancer, or melanoma tumors (Stone et al. 2009a; Sharma et al. 2008; Furumoto et al. 2004). In breast cancer models, CpG injection even leads to tumor regression in old mice—an effect not observed with other TLR agonists used in the study (Sharma et al. 2008). In the case of B16 melanoma, CpG injection alone is not sufficient to induce tumor regression but results in antitumor immunity when combined with CCL20-mediated accumulation of DC within the tumor (Furumoto et al. 2004). Of note, a different synthetic TLR9 agonist (with modified CpG motifs) reduced tumor growth and increased survival in a murine lung cancer model when combined with local tumor irradiation (Zhang et al. 2012). Since these modified CpG motifs use a 3′-3′-attached structure and a dCp7-deaza-dG have shown greater potency in murine and human studies, they may be incorporated into future in situ approaches.

Type B TLR9 agonists preferentially activate B cells (versus plasmacytoid DC). The type B TLR9 agonist Agatolimod (PF-3512676) has been used in the greatest number of clinical trials, including three trials using a combination of low-dose irradiation and intratumoral CpG administration showing promising results in 60 patients with low-grade B-cell lymphoma and mycosis fungoides including partial and complete remissions, lasting up to >4 years (Brody et al. 2010; Kim et al. 2012; Kohrt et al. 2014). A study of intracerebral (intratumoral) infusion of another type B TLR9 agonist Litenimod (CpG-28) in 34 patients with recurrent glioblastoma multiforme also showed efficacy in controlling disease burden yielding 1 and 2 year survival rates higher than historical controls (Carpentier et al. 2010). Type C TLR9 agonists—by contrast—comparably activate B cells and plasmacytoid DC, thus inducing higher amounts of both IFNα and IFNλ. One such molecule—SD-101—is currently being studied for the treatment of relapsed or refractory, low-grade lymphoma in combination with radiotherapy and/or intratumoral CTLA-4 blockade (NCT02266147, NCT01745354, NCT02254772). In the completed clinical trials, treatment was generally well tolerated, with a dose-related incidence of injection site reactions and the approaches warrant further studies on the use of this in situ vaccination for the treatment of human cancer.

2.2.2 TLR7/8

TLR7 agonists such as imiquimod (an imidazoquinolinamine derivative) were first investigated in the context of cutaneous viral infections, due to their induction of type I interferon (IFNα/β). Imiquimod can be applied topically and is approved for the treatment of genital warts, actinic keratoses, and basal cell carcinoma (Miller et al. 1999). Beginning in the early 1990s, systemic treatment with imiquimod had been assessed in the treatment of various murine cancers, with oral treatment leading to significant inhibition of growth in colon carcinoma and more modest effects in lung carcinoma and sarcoma. This effect was mediated by IFN induction and could be further enhanced when combined with cyclophosphamide (Sidky et al. 1992). More recently, imiquimod has been investigated as a potential adjuvant for in situ cancer vaccination for metastatic disease. In case reports and prospective series of melanoma and superficial breast cancer metastases, topical application of imiquimod induces a proimmunogenic tumor microenvironment with histologic tumor regression (Adams et al. 2012; Henriques et al. 2014; Smyth et al. 2011). Similarly, numerous case reports and series have demonstrated antitumor effects of imiquimod in cutaneous T-cell (Calista et al. 2015; Didona et al. 2004; Ehst et al. 2008; Ariffin and Khorshid 2006; Dummer et al. 2003; Suchin et al. 2002; Chong et al. 2004; Deeths et al. 2005; Ardigo et al. 2006) and B-cell (Richmond et al. 2008; Stavrakoglou et al. 2007; Coors et al. 2006; Spaner et al. 2005) lymphomas. In a murine model of cutaneous breast cancer, topical application of imiquimod combined with local radiotherapy resulted in complete regression of locally treated tumors and inhibited growth at untreated sites. This response is associated with increase in T-cell infiltration into tumor lesions, and the effect depended on CD8+ T cells. Pretreatment with low-dose cyclophosphamide augments the antitumor effect and protects the mice from tumor rechallenge, suggesting that a long-term memory response against the tumor was induced (Dewan et al. 2012). Similar results have been observed with R848/resiquimod, another imidazoquinolinamine derivative, in mouse models of lymphoma. Systemic delivery of R848 combined with local tumor irradiation induces durable antitumor immune responses leading to clearance of T- and B-cell lymphomas and improved survival (Dovedi et al. 2013). Combined therapy also increased tumor antigen-specific CD8+ T cells and protected mice from tumor rechallenge after clearance of the primary tumor. A novel injectable imidazoquinoline, 3M-052, formulated in a lipid-based vehicle to allow tissue retention has been shown to suppress melanoma growth in mice, both of injected and distant untreated sites. This antitumor effect was enhanced by CTLA-4 or PD-L1 blockade, even in tumor models in which systemic checkpoint blockade was ineffective as monotherapy (Singh et al. 2014).

2.2.3 TLR3

TLR3 has an important role in host defense against viruses by recognizing dsRNA, activating IRF-3, and ultimately increasing the production of type I interferons. Polyinosinic:polycytidylic acid (poly-IC) is a synthetic TLR3 and MDA-5 agonist due to its structural similarity to double-stranded RNA (Gitlin et al. 2006) and can be stabilized with poly-lysine and carboxymethylcellulose (poly-ICLC) for in vivo use. Poly-ICLC has been shown to be a promising vaccine adjuvant because it promotes type 1 immune responses (Salem et al. 2005, 2006). There is a significant set of clinical and preclinical studies of in situ vaccination with TLR3 agonists. Several peptide-based vaccine studies on brain cancer (Zhu et al. 2007b, 2010; Rosenfeld et al. 2010) suggest that poly-ICLC might also have positive effects in the context of in situ vaccination. When used as an adjuvant for an intratumoral HPV peptide-based vaccine, poly-IC is able to significantly improve therapeutic antitumor effects and increase the proportion of tumor-specific T cells (Wu et al. 2010). Additionally, in murine melanoma, intratumoral injection of poly-IC markedly reduced tumor growth and prolonged survival, leading to complete eradication of tumors when combined with transfer of tumor-peptide-specific T cells, CD40L-expressing plasmids, or systemic Flt3L.(Amos et al. 2011; Fujimura et al. 2006; Stone et al. 2009b; Salmon 2015) There is also preclinical data to suggest that it may augment anti-EGFR antibody therapy of head and neck cancer indicating potential for near-term clinical translation (Ming Lim et al. 2013). In a case report of a patient with an advanced facial rhabdomyosarcoma, treatment with intratumoral injections of poly-ICLC resulted in tumor inflammation and necrosis followed by marked tumor regression (Salazar et al. 2014); such results have prompted an ongoing phase II study investigating this approach in patients with advanced, unresectable solid tumors (NCT01984892). Additionally, the above described study combining intratumoral FLt3L and poly-ICLC with radiotherapy for low-grade lymphoma demonstrated that the poly-ICLC induced order-of-magnitude increase in intratumoral, activated APCs while having minimal effect on systemic APC activation status (Marron et al. 2014).

2.2.4 TLR4

Bacterial LPS is the primary ligand for TLR4 and ligation of TLR4 leads to activation of DC with improved processing and presentation of antigens and consequently the production of various proinflammatory cytokines (Lu et al. 2008; Blander and Medzhitov 2006). While systemically administered LPS has antitumor effects in mice and humans (Berendt et al. 1978; Goto et al. 1996; Otto et al. 1996), it also leads to cytokine storm with clinical symptoms of fevers, chills, hypotension, hepatic, and hematologic effects (Engelhardt et al. 1990). Intratumoral administration of LPS maintains antitumor efficacy while avoiding significant toxicity. Mice with subcutaneous glioblastoma or rats with subcutaneous glioma tumors treated with intratumoral LPS experience partial and complete tumor regression and these responses are lessened in T-cell deficient animals (Chicoine et al. 2001; Won et al. 2003; Mariani et al. 2007). Similarly, intratumoral injection of LPS in B16 melanoma mice results in tumor regression in those mice with increased activation of DC and T cells (Maito et al. 2012). By contrast, another study on the same model reported that LPS only reduced tumor growth when given in the context of a GM-CSF-expressing whole-cell vaccine (Davis et al. 2011). This treatment regimen is, however, sufficient to induce regression of CT26 colon carcinomas and protected mice from tumor rechallenge. Another approach using Glucopyranosyl Lipid A (GLA-SE), a small synthetic TLR4 agonist, is currently being studied by intratumoral injection in patients with Merkel cell carcinoma (NCT02035657) and sarcoma used in combination with radiotherapy (NCT02180698). A different TLR4 agonist (OK-432/Picibanil) is currently being investigated in clinical trials for treatment of pancreatic adenocarcinoma in combination with intratumoral DC injection (NCT00795977) and for treatment of head and neck cancer in combination with chemotherapy and DC transfer (NCT01149902).

2.2.5 Live Bacteria

Clostridia—as gram-positive bacteria—are able to activate DC via TLR2 (and likely other mechanisms) (Kashiwagi et al. 2015) and—as an anaerobe—are well suited to proliferate and disseminate in the hypoxic environment within tumors. *C. novyi* are endospore-forming, obligate anaerobic gram-positive bacteria closely related to *C. botulinum* and a genetically engineered, lethal-toxin deficient strain, has demonstrated CD8 T-cell-mediated antitumor effects in preclinical tumor renal, colon, and anaplastic squamous cell carcinoma models (Agrawal et al. 2004). Further studies demonstrated that intratumoral *C. novyi* induced tumor regressions in rat glioma tumors, spontaneously occurring canine sarcomas, and—in early, preliminary report from an ongoing clinical trial (NCT01924689)—marked tumor regression associated with fevers and local tissue necrosis, requiring intravenous narcotic analgesics, and antibiotics (Roberts et al. 2014).

2.2.6 Anti-CD40 Monoclonal Antibody

DC signaling pathways downstream of CD40 include recruitment of TNF Receptor-Associated Factor family of proteins (TRAFs)—particularly TRAF6 (Kobayashi et al. 2003)—followed by p38 MAPK, JNK (Pullen et al. 1999), and NF-κB and culminate in cytokine production, and costimulatory molecule (e.g., CD80/CD86) upregulation (Ma and Clarke 2009). Overall, DC signaling nodes downstream of CD40 are similar to TLRs and RANK–RANKL pathways, but are sufficiently distinct that activation of multiple pathways can lead to synergistic DC activation (Kerkmann et al. 2003).

In numerous small trials of systemic agonistic anti-CD40 mAb, there have been data demonstrating immune activation but with *some* concerns of toxicity or pro-tumorigenic effects (Vonderheide and Glennie 2013) though a preclinical model of local anti-CD40 mAb showed decrease in liver inflammation compared to systemic therapy (Fransen et al. 2011) A recently developed agonistic mAb with high affinity for CD40—ADC-1013—has been tested intratumorally in human and murine in vitro models and in vivo bladder cancer models, inducing DC activation and IL12 secretion as well as antigen-specific T-cell proliferation and long-term tumor-specific immunity (Mangsbo et al. 2015) and have led to an ongoing study of intratumoral ADC-1013 for patients with solid tumors (NCT02379741).

2.3 Oncolytic Viruses That Enhance the Cross-presentation of tumor Antigens

Under conditions of cellular stress, heat shock proteins (HSPs) are produced and function as molecular chaperones mediating the folding and refolding of proteins. When HSP–peptide complexes are released by dying tumor cells, they are taken up by APC via receptor-mediated endocytosis, leading to cross-presentation of tumor peptides on MHC class I molecules (Singh-Jasuja et al. 2000; Noessner et al. 2002). Though HSP-autologous tumor derived peptide complexes have shown limited success (Wood et al. 2008) recent preclinical and clinical studies of oncolytic adenoviruses, expressing HSP70 or heat shock transcription factor 1 (HSF1), have shown encouraging results. Intratumoral injection of these viruses eradicated primary tumors in mice, induced tumor-specific immune responses that inhibited metastatic tumor growth, and protected mice from tumor rechallenge (Huang et al. 2003; Fan et al. 2012; Wang et al. 2010). A phase I clinical study demonstrated that intratumoral administration of recombinant oncolytic adenovirus expressing HSP70 is safe and exhibited promising clinical antitumor activity (Li et al. 2009).

One potential obstacle with these approaches is that oncolytic viruses can drive an antiviral immune response which may divert the immune system from tumor-specific antigens; a process called "immunodominance" (Alemany 2014). Immunodominance occurs because the large numbers of viral peptides introduced into the patient overwhelm the APC system, thereby diverting APCs from TAAs. Immunodominant viral epitopes also have the ability to induce neutralizing antibodies which preclude subsequent booster vaccinations with the same vector. A "prime-boost" approach is an elegant method to address both of these issues; this refers to a vaccination using two different virus strains expressing the same tumor antigen in sequence. Priming with vesicular stomatitis virus (VSV) expressing a melanoma-associated antigen followed by a booster immunization with adenovirus expressing the same antigen (or vice versa) significantly increased tumor-specific T-cell responses in B16 murine melanoma (Bridle et al. 2009). Furthermore, this combination approach shifted the immune response from viral antigens to tumor antigens and reduced viral replication in normal tissues, thereby increasing efficacy as well as safety (Bridle et al. 2010). A clinical trial using intratumoral fowlpox administration has been completed (Kaufman et al. 2014) and randomized trials of prime-boost strategies are ongoing (NCT02285816).

Even intratumorally administered oncolytic viruses may also be cytotoxic to healthy cells which might drive an immune response to self-antigens. Increasing viral specificity for tumor cells may be an important way to increase the proportion of TAA presented on local APC. Several approaches in viral engineering have worked toward tumor-specific infection or lysis.

An adenovirus engineered to replicate in retinoblastoma (Rb)-deficient cells and with increased binding for $\alpha V\beta 3$ and $\alpha V\beta 5$ integrins demonstrated induction of antitumor immunity in preclinical glioma model. In a phase 1 study, high grade glioma patients received a single intratumoral injection of DNX-2401 followed by tumor resection 2 weeks later (and repeat DNX-2401 injection into the surgical site). Complete responses were observed in 3 or 25 treated patients, all of whom are experienced prolonged (>1.5 years) remission. Resected tumor demonstrated abundant macrophages and CD8 T cells and—amongst the clinical responders—serum concentrations of IL-12p70 were increased 10- to 10,000-fold (Lang et al. 2014). Ongoing trials are investigating combination of DNX-2401 with temozolomide (NCT01956734) and IFNγ (NCT02197169).

A modified herpesvirus, HSV-1716—because of genetic deletion of ICP34.5—is unable to maintain protein translation in terminally differentiated cells and thus replicates selectively in tumor tissue. Infection by HSV-1716 induces high levels of viral glycoprotein B and D expression and HSP70 in ovarian cancer cells which are efficiently phagocytosed by DC, upregulating DC costimulatory molecules and migration (Benencia et al. 2008). Intratumoral HSV-1716 injection induces IFNγ expression and increase in intratumoral activated NK and CD8+ T cells (Benencia et al. 2005). HSV-1716 administered intratumorally in five melanoma patients yielded microscopic evidence of tumor necrosis (MacKie et al. 2001) and in 12 glioma patients confirmed that viral replication can occur at the tumor site and possibly within distant tumors (Papanastassiou et al. 2002). Ongoing studies in high grade glioma (NCT02031965) and solid tumors (NCT00931931) will further assess the efficacy of the approach. More recently, additional genetic modifications of HSV-1716 have incorporated the enzyme nitroreductase (which converts the prodrug CB1954 into an active alkylating agent) (Braidwood et al. 2009) or selected a clone which expresses inhibitor of growth 4 (Ing4) (a tumor suppressor protein) (Conner and Braidwood 2012) significantly augmenting its oncolytic potency.

2.4 Oncolytic Viruses That Increase the Maturation of APCs

As previously described, TLR agonists activate APC functions and through this mechanism can initiate antitumor immune responses hence their study as potential vaccine adjuvants and cancer immunotherapies. Oncolytic viruses enriched for CpG motifs, a TLR9 agonist, have shown higher antitumor activity than their parental viral strains. Raykov et al. demonstrated that the oncolytic parvovirus H-1PV enriched for CpG motifs is a potent anticancer vaccine when used in a metastatic lung cancer rat model (Raykov et al. 2008). Compared to the original virus, subcutaneous injection of tumor cells with CpG-enriched virus leads to increased immune responses and decrease in metastatic disease burden. This clinical and immune response correlates with high levels of IFNγ and activated DC in the tumor-draining lymph nodes. Similar effects were observed by Cerrullo et al. when utilizing a CpG-enriched adenovirus in murine lung cancer and melanoma (Cerullo et al. 2012). Intratumoral administration of the enriched virus led to a reduction in tumor growth in both models, with increased numbers of tumor-specific T cells in tumors and spleen. In a related approach using the same melanoma model, Rommelfanger et al. combined intratumoral injection of VSV with subsequent injection of a TLR4 agonist. As compared to treatment with the virus alone, this approach led to improvement in survival and increased numbers of tumor-specific T cells in the tumors and draining lymph nodes (Rommelfanger et al. 2013).

Engaging costimulatory molecules such as CD40 on the surface of the APC, which provide a secondary stimulus for activation is a different approach to increasing their capacity to present TAA. Oncolytic adenovirus expressing CD40 ligand (CD40L, CD154) has shown significant antitumor effect in mice as well as patients with solid tumors (Diaconu et al. 2012; Pesonen et al. 2012). Intratumoral injection of the virus led to increases in tumor cell apoptosis and delayed tumor growth in murine melanoma and bladder cancer. Treatment was also associated with enhanced recruitment of APC and CD8+ T cells to tumor lesions locally and systemically (Diaconu et al. 2012). An early phase study of nine solid tumor patients received intratumoral injections of CD40L-encoding adenovirus and demonstrated the induction of IFN-γ-producing survivin-specific (as well as adenovirus-specific) T in the peripheral blood. Some patients experienced prolonged stable disease in addition to regression of untreated tumors and clearance of serum tumor markers (e.g., the breast cancer marker Ca15-3) (Pesonen et al. 2012). Similar results have been observed with oncolytic herpes simplex or adenovirus encoding CD80, a costimulatory ligand for CD28 on T cells, resulting in enhanced T-cell activation and antitumor immune responses (Fukuhara et al. 2005; Ino et al. 2006; Todo et al. 2001; Lee et al. 2006; Choi et al. 2006).

Another approach has been the intratumoral administration of coxsackie virus A21 which binds intercellular adhesion molecule (ICAM-1) and decay-accelerating factor (DAF)—molecules that are frequently upregulated on malignant melanoma cells. This genetically unmodified, wild-type, common cold-producing human enterovirus (CAVATAK™) has demonstrated oncolytic activity in preclinical and early phase clinical studies and induces immune cell infiltration in melanoma (Andtbacka et al. 2015a). A recently reported phase II study (NCT01227551) demonstrated responses in 16 of 57 evaluable and median duration of response not reached after 17 months (Andtbacka et al. 2015c). Biomarker analyses have shown an association of serum IL8 and IFNγ with systemic responses and preclinical melanoma models have demonstrated marked synergy between intratumoral CAVATAK and PD-1 blockade (Shafren et al. 2014).

3 Manipulation of Intratumoral Lymphocytes

3.1 Activation of T Cells

3.1.1 Interleukin-12

Interleukin-12 (IL-12) is a cytokine with an important role in the regulation of adaptive T-cell responses (Colombo and Trinchieri 2002). It is released by various immune cells—particularly myeloid APC such as monocytes (D' Andrea et al. 1992) upon stimulation by infection or inflammation to induce differentiation of type 1 helper T cells; thus increasing activity of CTLs as well as IFNγ production. For more than two decades, IL-12 has been known to have potent antitumor activity (Brunda et al. 1993) and has been extensively investigated for use in cancer treatments. In murine transplantable tumors, IL-12 antitumor activity is dependent on a variety of factors, including tumor type, dose, and route of injection (Colombo and Trinchieri 2002). Clinical studies have used systemic administration of IL-12 in patients with melanoma, RCC and colon cancer, unfortunately this approach was associated with considerable hepatic and hematologic toxicity with only modest efficacy at doses tested (Atkins et al. 1997; Leonard et al. 1997). Intratumoral administration of IL-12 is associated with less toxicity and has shown to cause partial or complete tumor regression at the locally injected tumor site, but little to no response at distant sites (Rook et al. 1999; Sangro et al. 2004; Mahvi et al. 2007; Zapała et al. 2013). By contrast, when IL-12 is encapsulated into polymer microspheres, which release their contents over an extended period of time, regression of primary and secondary murine tumors as well as regression of metastasis lesions has been achieved (Egilmez et al. 2000). In glioblastoma models, complete regression can also be achieved by combining intratumoral IL-12 administration with systemic immune checkpoint blockade using an antibody against CTLA-4 (Vom Berg et al. 2013).

IL-12 is also under investigation with oncolytic viruses for the development of cancer vaccines. In preclinical murine cancer models including prostate, colon, liver, and brain cancer, viruses modified to express IL-12 induce strong antitumor immune responses with reduced tumor growth and increased survival (Toda et al. 1998; Bennett et al. 2001; Varghese et al. 2006; Zhang et al. 2013; Cheema et al. 2013).

Early phase clinical studies are currently investigating the use of intratumoral IL-12 plasmid electroporation for the treatment of cutaneous lymphoma (NCT01579318) and advanced melanoma (NCT01502293) and have demonstrated no grade 3/4 drug-related AEs, a doubling of intratumoral NK, activation of circulating NK cells, clinical response in 9 of 28 patients and regression of noninjected lesions in 13 of 21 evaluable patients (Soiffer et al. 1998). A related approach is the use of lipopolymer to increase plasmid delivery into cells which has been administered intra- or peritumorally by intraperitoneal delivery in patients with ovarian cancer in an early study of 13 patients, demonstrating increase IL-12 and IFNγ levels in peritoneal fluid (but not serum) and a minority of patients with treatment-related decrease in serum CA-125 levels (Anwer et al. 2010). More recently this approach has been combined with systemic liposomal doxorubicin resulting in partial remissions and stable disease in two and four of the seven patients in the highest-dose cohort, warranting further study of the combination (Thaker et al. 2015).

Adenovirally delivered IL-12 is being investigated for the treatment of glioblastoma (NCT02026271), breast cancer (NCT01703754, NCT02423902), and melanoma (NCT01397708). Because of the variable persistence of adenoviral vectors and potential toxicity of IL-12, an elegant approach has been the development of vectors incorporating an ecdysone-inducible expression system with a goal of titrating IL-12 levels after administration. Preliminary report on intratumoral administration of Ad-RTS-hIL-12 in 38 patients with breast cancer or melanoma followed by increasing doses of veledimex (an orally administered ecdysone analog) resulted in a veledimex dose-dependent increases in intratumoral and serum IL-12 transcript and protein as well as serum IFNγ levels. A minority of patients experienced partial remission or subclinical tumor regressions and a small number of patients had grade ≥3 adverse events (e.g., hepatic or hematologic), but—perhaps the most significant proof of principle—was the rapid reversibility of adverse events with the discontinuation of veledimex (Nemunaitis et al. 2014).

3.1.2 Interleukin-2

Interleukin-2 (IL-2) is important in the development of adaptive immune response as it mediates expansion of T cells and differentiation into effector lymphocytes and has been amongst the most thoroughly investigated cancer immunotherapies. Systemic administration of IL-2 is FDA approved for the treatment of RCC and melanoma (Fyfe et al. 1995; Atkins et al. 1999), though systemic treatment is associated with significant toxicity, prompting the investigation of intratumoral IL-2 therapies. Intratumoral injections of soluble IL-2 result in increased infiltration of CD8+ T cells, reduced tumor growth, and increased survival in mice bearing transplantable tumors (Fiszer-Maliszewska et al. 1998; Jackaman et al. 2003). The clinical and immune response can be further accentuated by using expression vectors encoding IL-2 to allow prolonged production of the cytokine (Horton et al. 1999; Slos et al. 2001). Intratumoral injection of an adenovirally encoded IL-2 also inhibits growth of distant, untreated tumors, and protects mice from rechallenge with the same tumor type (Slos et al. 2001). This effect is also observed with a slow-release, liposomal formulation of IL-2 in mice with a nonimmunogenic B16 melanoma tumor, inducing systemic immune responses not observed with injections of soluble IL-2 (Neville et al. 2001). In mice with lung or hepatocellular carcinoma, using a combined treatment with microparticles encapsulating IL-2 and microwave coagulation to induce tumor cell death results in a systemic tumor-specific immune response (Kuang et al. 2005). Clinical trials reveal promising results in patients with RCC or melanoma who received intratumoral treatment with IL-2 encoding plasmids or recombinant IL-2, respectively. Compared to systemic treatment, this treatment modality generally resulted in low toxicity. While plasmid treatment of RCC led to a low number of responses (Hoffman and Figlin 2000; Galanis et al. 1999), injection of recombinant IL-2 into melanoma metastases induced high response rates as measured by tumor regression (Radny et al. 2003; Weide et al. 2010; Gutwald et al. 1994). However, although most injected lesions regressed and did not recur, this treatment failed to cause complete regression of untreated melanoma lesions or prevent subsequent development of metastases (Radny et al. 2003; Weide et al. 2010). Clinical studies investigating the combination of intratumoral IL-2 and systemic or intratumoral treatment with anti-CTLA-4 are currently ongoing (NCT02076633, NCT01672450, NCT01480323).

3.1.3 T-Cell Activating Oncolytic Viruses

Intratumorally administered modified herpesvirus has been shown to induce CD8-dependent tumor lysis and regression of untreated tumors in preclinical models (Meshii et al. 2013) and early phase clinical trials in patients with pancreatic (Nakao et al. 2011) and breast cancer (Kimata et al. 2006; Sahin et al. 2012) have yielded local tumor regressions. Recent preclinical studies have demonstrated incremental benefit of HF10 herpesvirus combination with agonistic monoclonal antibody for murine glucocorticoid-induced tumor necrosis factor receptor (Ishihara et al. 2014), the anti-VEGF mAb bevacizumab (Tan et al. 2015), and GM-CSF (Goshima et al. 2014).

3.2 Intratumoral Checkpoint Blockade

Immune checkpoint molecules, such as CTLA-4 or PD-1, are receptors expressed on T cells and down regulate their activity. In normal homeostatic settings, these molecules protect the host from auto-immunopathology due to unchecked immune responses. However, in the tumor microenvironment, they contribute to TAA tolerance. Toxicity associated with systemic CTLA-4 blockade (Hodi et al. 2010; Robert et al. 2011; Postow et al. 2015) has been avoided in preclinical models of intratumoral anti-CTLA4 antibody, along an increase in the CTL:T_{reg} ratio within tumors (Tuve et al. 2007; Simmons et al. 2008). Similarly, in a mouse model of colon cancer, peritumoral injection of anti-CTLA-4 in a slow-release formulation induced regression of treated as well as untreated nodules (Fransen et al. 2013). In addition, checkpoint blockade antibodies can be delivered intratumorally by using oncolytic viruses encoding these antibodies. As described in Sect. 2.3, adenovirus or measles virus encoding anti-CTLA-4 have shown encouraging antitumor efficacy in murine models of colon cancer and melanoma (Engeland et al. 2014; Du et al. 2014).

Finally, intratumoral injection of anti-CTLA-4 also depletes T_{reg} at the injected site, and combination treatment with anti-OX40 and CpG results in eradication of disseminated central nervous system (CNS) lymphoma (Marabelle et al. 2013). An ongoing phase I/II clinical trial is investigating the combination of local irradiation and intratumoral injection of ipilimumab for the treatment of melanoma, lymphoma, colon, and rectal cancer (NCT01769222) as well as using combined intratumoral ipilimumab and IL-2 (NCT01672450).

3.3 Oncolytic Viruses to Reduce Immune Suppression in the Tumor Microenvironment

As a result of the immunosuppressive nature of tumors, effective therapy requires not only the induction of immune responses, but also the downregulation of immune inhibitory mechanisms. Therefore, oncolytic viruses are being used in combination with agents that inhibit the induction of immunosuppressive cells—i.e., regulatory T cells (T_{reg})—or counteract the inhibition of effector T cells (T_{eff}). Low dose cyclophosphamide is a chemotherapeutic agent with immune modulatory function and has been shown to specifically inhibit T_{reg} but not T_{eff} cells (Motoyoshi et al. 2006). In patients with treatment refractory solid malignancies, compared to administration of the virus alone, administration of intratumoral oncolytic adenovirus and low-dose cyclophosphamide resulted in higher disease control and overall survival (Cerullo et al. 2011). This improved response was associated with a reduction in T_{reg} cells and an increase in cytotoxic T cells. A different chemotherapeutic drug, temozolomide, has also been shown to reduce T_{reg} numbers at low doses (Banissi et al. 2009). The combination of temozolomide with an oncolytic adenovirus is currently under investigation for the treatment of glioblastoma (NCT01956734).

In addition, monoclonal antibodies (mAb) against immune checkpoint proteins have shown encouraging results in cancer immunotherapy and have been combined with oncolytic viruses. In a murine melanoma model, intratumoral injection of Newcastle Disease virus accompanied by systemic treatment with an mAb against CTLA-4 reduced tumor growth, improved survival, and protected mice from tumor rechallenge (Zamarin et al. 2014). However, systemic treatment with checkpoint-blocking antibodies can lead to severe immune-related adverse effects (Voskens et al. 2013; Hodi et al. 2010; Postow et al. 2015; Robert et al. 2011), thus driving investigators to discover more effective local therapies that will have systemic responses. Dias et al. demonstrates that intratumoral treatment with an adenovirus engineered to express a complete human mAb against CTLA-4 leads to 43-fold higher mAb concentration in tumors vs. plasma of mice. The average plasma concentration is below what is reported as tolerated in humans (Dias et al 2012). More recently, attenuated measles virus encoding mAb against CTLA-4 or PD-1 was shown to delay tumor growth and prolong survival in murine melanoma (Engeland et al. 2014). Similarly, Du et al. reveals that in lung cancer and melanoma murine models treatment with adenovirus expressing anti-CTLA-4 significantly delays tumor growth and results in complete regression when combined with a second virus encoding GM-CSF (Du et al. 2014).

In addition to immunosuppressive cells in the tumor microenvironment, components of the extracellular matrix (ECM) such as hyaluronan contribute to tumor immune evasion. Hyaluronan synthase 2 expressed in breast cancer stem-like cells is critical for the interaction of tumor cells with tumor-associated macrophages (TAM) and its deficiency or inhibition reduced metastatic disease (Okuda et al. 2012). VCN-01, a novel adenovirus engineered to avoid tropism for liver and spleen and to express hyaluronidase to degrade ECM accumulates in murine tumors after systemic administration with only transient presence in the liver. Furthermore, anti-tumor efficacy after systemic administration of the virus was comparable to that observed after intratumoral delivery (Rodríguez-García et al. 2015). Two phase I clinical trials with VCN-01 alone or in combination with gemcitabine in patients with pancreatic cancer and advanced solid tumors are currently underway (NCT02045589, NCT02045602).

4 Conclusions

The primary goal of cancer immunotherapy is to induce a durable antitumor immune response while leaving normal host cells unharmed. Personalized vaccines have shown encouraging results, since they can be directed against patient-specific TAAs (Di Nicola et al. 2008; Timmerman et al. 2002; Schuster et al. 2011). A whole tumor cell approach obviates the need to identify TAAs, but manufacturing an ex vivo product is resource intensive, and time consuming limiting opportunity to optimize the vaccine in iterative clinical trials. In contrast, "off-the-shelf" vaccines are easier to manufacture, but mandate the identification of shared TAAs—ideally ones in which tumors are highly dependent—to minimize risk of escape variants. An in situ vaccine combines the best aspects of each strategy. By inducing immunogenic tumor cell death and antigen release at a single tumor site, in situ vaccination is personalized, and thus patient specific. The approach obviates the need for patient-specific TAA identification. Patients can be vaccinated against the tumor's entire TAA repertoire, as opposed to a single TAA. Furthermore, injectable immunomodulators such as cytokines, TLR agonists or viruses can be mass-produced, are not resource intensive and are therefore practical to optimize in iterative patient cohorts.

As the field of cancer therapy continues to incorporate immunotherapy as an integral treatment strategy, the effort to identify therapies that augment the benefit of checkpoint-blocking agents will continue to develop. Intratumoral therapies will be among the most likely to induce this desired effect as they may increase the response rate, while minimizing toxicity (Simmons et al. 2008). Intratumoral therapy effectively converts patients from "low intratumoral T-cell infiltration type" to a "T-cell inflamed phenotype" increasing the likelihood of response to checkpoint blockade therapy (Tumeh et al. 2014; Sharma and Allison 2015). In a field of potential candidates to be combined with checkpoint blockade, in situ vaccination represents one of the promising strategies. Ultimately, the opportunities to expand the armamentarium of tumor-specific immunotherapies with in situ vaccination strategies are continuing to increase with ongoing scrutiny in the laboratory and continued success in our patients.

References

Adams, S., Kozhaya, L., Martiniuk, F., Meng, T.C., Chiriboga, L., Liebes, L., Hochman, T., Shuman, N., Axelrod, D., Speyer, J., Novik, Y., Tiersten, A., Goldberg, J.D., Formenti, S.C., Bhardwaj, N., Unutmaz, D., Demaria, S.: Topical TLR7 agonist imiquimod can induce immune-mediated rejection of skin metastases in patients with breast cancer. Clin. Cancer Res. **18**, 6748–6757 (2012)

Agrawal, N., Bettegowda, C., Cheong, I., Geschwind, J.F., Drake, C.G., Hipkiss, E.L., Tatsumi, M., Dang, L.H., Diaz Jr., L.A., Pomper, M., Abusedera, M., Wahl, R.L., Kinzler, K.W., Zhou, S., Huso, D.L., Vogelstein, B.: Bacteriolytic therapy can generate a potent immune response against experimental tumors. Proc Natl Acad Sci U S A **101**, 15172–15177 (2004)

Alemany, R.: Oncolytic adenoviruses in cancer treatment. Biomedicines **2**, 36–49 (2014)

Amos, S.M., Pegram, H.J., Westwood, J.A., John, L.B., Devaud, C., Clarke, C.J., Restifo, N.P., Smyth, M.J., Darcy, P.K., Kershaw, M.H.: Adoptive immunotherapy combined with intratumoral TLR agonist delivery eradicates established melanoma in mice. Cancer Immunol. Immunother. **60**, 671–683 (2011)

Andtbacka, R.H., Kaufman, H.L., Collichio, F., Amatruda, T., Senzer, N., Chesney, J., Delman, K.A., Spitler, L.E., Puzanov, I., Agarwala, S.S., Milhem, M., Cranmer, L., Curti, B., Lewis, K., Ross, M., Guthrie, T., Linette, G.P., Daniels, G.A., Harrington, K., Middleton, M.R., Miller Jr., W.H., Zager, J.S., Ye, Y., Yao, B., Li, A., Doleman, S., VanderWalde, A., Gansert, J., Coffin, R.S.: Talimogene Laherparepvec improves durable response rate in patients with advanced Melanoma. J Clin Oncol **33**(25), 2780–8 (2015). doi:10.1200/JCO.2014.58.3377

AJ Clin Oncol. 2015 Sep 1;33(25):2780-8. doi: 10.1200/JCO.2014.58.3377. Talimogene Laherparepvec Improves Durable Response Rate in Patients With Advanced Melanoma. Andtbacka RH, Kaufman HL, Collichio F, Amatruda T, Senzer N, Chesney J, Delman KA,

Spitler LE, Puzanov I, Agarwala SS, Milhem M, Cranmer L, Curti B, Lewis K, Ross M, Guthrie T, Linette GP, Daniels GA, Harrington K, Middleton MR, Miller WH Jr, Zager JS, Ye Y, Yao B, Li A, Doleman S,VanderWalde A, Gansert J, Coffin RS. (2015b)

Andtbacka, R.H.I., Curti, B.D., Kaufman, H., Daniels, G.A., Nemunaitis, J.J., Spitler, L.E., Hallmeyer, S., Lutzky, J., Schultz, S.M., Whitman, E.D., Zhou, K., Karpathy, R., Weisberg, J.I., Grose, M., Shafren, D.:. Final data from CALM: a phase II study of Coxsackievirus A21 (CVA21) oncolytic virus immunotherapy in patients with advanced melanoma. J. Clin. Oncol. (Meeting Abstracts) **33**(15_suppl) (May 20 Supplement) 9030 (2015c)

Anwer, K., Barnes, M.N., Fewell, J., Lewis, D.H., Alvarez, R.D.: Phase-I clinical trial of IL-12 plasmid/lipopolymer complexes for the treatment of recurrent ovarian cancer. Gene Ther. **17**, 360–369 (2010)

Appledorn, D.M., Patial, S., McBride, A., Godbehere, S., van Rooijen, N., Parameswaran, N., Amalfitano, A.: Adenovirus vector-induced innate inflammatory mediators, MAPK signaling, as well as adaptive immune responses are dependent upon both TLR2 and TLR9 in vivo. J. Immunol. **181**, 2134–2144 (2008)

Ardigo, M., Cota, C., Berardesca, E.: Unilesional mycosis fungoides successfully treated with imiquimod. Eur. J. Dermatol. **16**, 446 (2006)

Ariffin, N., Khorshid, M.: Treatment of mycosis fungoides with imiquimod 5% cream. Clin. Exp. Dermatol. **31**, 822–823 (2006)

Atkins, M.B., Lotze, M.T., Dutcher, J.P., Fisher, R.I., Weiss, G., Margolin, K., Abrams, J., Sznol, M., Parkinson, D., Hawkins, M., Paradise, C., Kunkel, L., Rosenberg, S.A.: High-dose recombinant interleukin 2 therapy for patients with metastatic melanoma: analysis of 270 patients treated between 1985 and 1993. J. Clin. Oncol. **17**, 2105–2116 (1999)

Atkins, M.B., Robertson, M.J., Gordon, M., Lotze, M.T., Decoste, M., Dubois, J.S., Ritz, J., Sandler, A.B., Edington, H.D., Garzone, P.D., Mier, J.W., Canning, C.M., Battiato, L., Tahara, H., Sherman, M.L.: Phase I evaluation of intravenous recombinant human interleukin 12 in patients with advanced malignancies. Clin. Cancer Res. **3**, 409–417 (1997)

Banchereau, R., Baldwin, N., Cepika, A.M., Athale, S., Xue, Y., Yu, C.I., Metang, P., Cheruku, A., Berthier, I., Gayet, I., Wang, Y., Ohouo, M., Snipes, L., Xu, H., Obermoser, G., Blankenship, D., Oh, S., Ramilo, O., Chaussabel, D., Palucka, K., Pascual, V.: Transcriptional specialization of human dendritic cell subsets in response to microbial vaccines. Nat. Commun. **5**, 5283 (2014)

Banissi, C., Ghiringhelli, F., Chen, L., Carpentier, A.F.: Treg depletion with a low-dose metronomic temozolomide regimen in a rat glioma model. Cancer Immunol. Immunother. **58**, 1627–1634 (2009)

Bartlett, D.L., Liu, Z., Sathaiah, M., Ravindranathan, R., Guo, Z., He, Y., Guo, Z.S.: Oncolytic viruses as therapeutic cancer vaccines. Mol. Cancer **12**, 103 (2013)

Benencia, F., Courreges, M.C., Conejo-Garcia, J.R., Mohamed-Hadley, A., Zhang, L., Buckanovich, R.J., Carroll, R., Fraser, N., Coukos, G.: HSV oncolytic therapy upregulates interferon-inducible chemokines and recruits immune effector cells in ovarian cancer. Mol. Ther. **12**, 789–802 (2005)

Benencia, F., Courreges, M.C., Fraser, N.W., Coukos, G.: Herpes virus oncolytic therapy reverses tumor immune dysfunction and facilitates tumor antigen presentation. Cancer Biol. Ther. **7**, 1194–1205 (2008)

Bennett, J.J., Malhotra, S., Wong, R.J., Delman, K., Zager, J., St-Louis, M., Johnson, P., Fong, Y.: Interleukin 12 secretion enhances antitumor efficacy of oncolytic herpes simplex viral therapy for colorectal cancer. Ann. Surg. **233**, 819–826 (2001)

Berendt, M.J., North, R.J., Kirstein, D.P.: The immunological basis of endotoxin-induced tumor regression. Requirement for T-cell-mediated immunity. J. Exp. Med. **148**, 1550–1559 (1978)

Bhardwaj, N., Merad, M., Kim-Schulze, S., Crowley, B., Davis, T., Salazar, A., Brody, J.: Converting tumors into vaccine manufacturing factories: DC recruitment, activation and clinical responses with a flt3L-primed in situ vaccine for low-grade lymphoma [nct01976585]. J. Immunother. Cancer **2**(Suppl 3), 45 (2014)

Blander, J.M., Medzhitov, R.: Toll-dependent selection of microbial antigens for presentation by dendritic cells. Nature **440**, 808–812 (2006)

Bourke, E., Bosisio, D., Golay, J., Polentarutti, N., Mantovani, A.: The toll-like receptor repertoire of human B lymphocytes: inducible and selective expression of TLR9 and TLR10 in normal and transformed cells. Blood **102**, 956–963 (2003)

Braidwood, L., Dunn, P.D., Hardy, S., Evans, T.R., Brown, S.M.: Antitumor activity of a selectively replication competent herpes simplex virus (HSV) with enzyme prodrug therapy. Anticancer Res **29**, 2159–2166 (2009)

Breitbach, C.J., Arulanandam, R., de Silva, N., Thorne, S.H., Patt, R., Daneshmand, M., Moon, A., Ilkow, C., Burke, J., Hwang, T.H., Heo, J., Cho, M., Chen, H., Angarita, F.A., Addison, C., Mccart, J.A., Bell, J.C., Kirn, D.H.: Oncolytic vaccinia virus disrupts tumor-associated vasculature in humans. Cancer Res. **73**, 1265–1275 (2013)

Breitbach, C.J., Burke, J., Jonker, D., Stephenson, J., Haas, A.R., Chow, L.Q., Nieva, J., Hwang, T.H., Moon, A., Patt, R., Pelusio, A., le Boeuf, F., Burns, J., Evgin, L., de Silva, N., Cvancic, S., Robertson, T., Je, J.E., Lee, Y.S., Parato, K., Diallo, J.S., Fenster, A., Daneshmand, M., Bell, J.C., Kirn, D.H.: Intravenous delivery of a multi-mechanistic cancer-targeted oncolytic poxvirus in humans. Nature **477**, 99–102 (2011)

Breitbach, C.J., Moon, A., Burke, J., Hwang, T.H., Kirn, D.H.: A phase 2, open-label, randomized study of Pexa-Vec (JX-594) administered by intratumoral injection in patients with unresectable primary hepatocellular carcinoma. Methods Mol. Biol. **1317**, 343–357 (2015)

Bridle, B.W., Boudreau, J.E., Lichty, B.D., Brunellière, J., Stephenson, K., Koshy, S., Bramson, J.L., Wan, Y.: Vesicular stomatitis virus as a novel cancer vaccine vector to prime antitumor immunity amenable to rapid boosting with adenovirus. Mol. Ther. **17**, 1814–1821 (2009)

Bridle, B.W., Stephenson, K.B., Boudreau, J.E., Koshy, S., Kazdhan, N., Pullenayegum, E., Brunellière, J., Bramson, J.L., Lichty, B.D., Wan, Y.: Potentiating cancer immunotherapy using an oncolytic virus. Mol. Ther. **18**, 1430–1439 (2010)

Brody, J.D., Ai, W.Z., Czerwinski, D.K., Torchia, J.A., Levy, M., Advani, R.H., Kim, Y.H., Hoppe, R.T., Knox, S.J., Shin, L.K., Wapnir, I., Tibshirani, R.J., Levy, R.: In situ vaccination with a TLR9 agonist induces systemic lymphoma regression: a phase I/II study. J. Clin. Oncol. **28**, 4324–4332 (2010)

Brody, J.D., Goldstein, M.J., Czerwinski, D.K., Levy, R.: Immunotransplantation preferentially expands T-effector cells over T-regulatory cells and cures large lymphoma tumors. Blood **113**, 85–94 (2009)

Broz, M.L., Binnewies, M., Boldajipour, B., Nelson, A.E., Pollack, J.L., Erle, D.J., Barczak, A., Rosenblum, M.D., Daud, A., Barber, D.L., Amigorena, S., Van't Veer, L.J., Sperling, A.I., Wolf, D.M., Krummel, M.F.: Dissecting the tumor myeloid compartment reveals rare activating antigen-presenting cells critical for T cell immunity. Cancer Cell **26**, 638–652 (2014)

Brunda, M.J., Luistro, L., Warrier, R.R., Wright, R.B., Hubbard, B.R., Murphy, M., Wolf, S.F., Gately, M.K.: Antitumor and antimetastatic activity of interleukin 12 against murine tumors. J. Exp. Med. **178**, 1223–1230 (1993)

Calista, D., Riccioni, L., Bagli, L., Valenzano, F.: Long-term remission of primary cutaneous neutrophil-rich CD30+ anaplastic large cell lymphoma treated with topical imiquimod. A case report. J. Eur. Acad. Dermatol. Venereol. (2015). doi:10.1111/jdv.13070

Carpentier, A., Metellus, P., Ursu, R., Zohar, S., Lafitte, F., Barrie, M., Meng, Y., Richard, M., Parizot, C., Laigle-Donadey, F., Gorochov, G., Psimaras, D., Sanson, M., Tibi, A., Chinot, O., Carpentier, A.F.: Intracerebral administration of CpG oligonucleotide for patients with recurrent glioblastoma: a phase II study. Neuro Oncol. **12**, 401–408 (2010)

Cerullo, V., Diaconu, I., Kangasniemi, L., Rajecki, M., Escutenaire, S., Koski, A., Romano, V., Rouvinen, N., Tuuminen, T., Laasonen, L., Partanen, K., Kauppinen, S., Joensuu, T., Oksanen, M., Holm, S.L., Haavisto, E., Karioja-Kallio, A., Kanerva, A., Pesonen, S., Arstila, P.T., Hemminki, A.: Immunological effects of low-dose cyclophosphamide in cancer patients treated with oncolytic adenovirus. Mol. Ther. **19**, 1737–1746 (2011)

Cerullo, V., Diaconu, I., Romano, V., Hirvinen, M., Ugolini, M., Escutenaire, S., Holm, S.L., Kipar, A., Kanerva, A., Hemminki, A.: An oncolytic adenovirus enhanced for toll-like receptor

9 stimulation increases antitumor immune responses and tumor clearance. Mol. Ther. **20**, 2076–2086 (2012)

Cheema, T.A., Wakimoto, H., Fecci, P.E., Ning, J., Kuroda, T., Jeyaretna, D.S., Martuza, R.L., Rabkin, S.D.: Multifaceted oncolytic virus therapy for glioblastoma in an immunocompetent cancer stem cell model. Proc. Natl. Acad. Sci. U. S. A. **110**, 12006–12011 (2013)

Chicoine, M.R., Won, E.K., Zahner, M.C.: Intratumoral injection of lipopolysaccharide causes regression of subcutaneously implanted mouse glioblastoma multiforme. Neurosurgery **48**, 607–614 (2001). discussion 614–615

Choi, K.J., Kim, J.H., Lee, Y.S., Kim, J., Suh, B.S., Kim, H., Cho, S., Sohn, J.H., Kim, G.E., Yun, C.O.: Concurrent delivery of GM-CSF and B7-1 using an oncolytic adenovirus elicits potent antitumor effect. Gene Ther. **13**, 1010–1020 (2006)

Chong, A., Loo, W.J., Banney, L., Grant, J.W., Norris, P.G.: Imiquimod 5% cream in the treatment of mycosis fungoides—a pilot study. J. Dermatolog. Treat. **15**, 118–119 (2004)

Colombo, M.P., Trinchieri, G.: Interleukin-12 in anti-tumor immunity and immunotherapy. Cytokine Growth Factor Rev. **13**, 155–168 (2002)

Conner, J., Braidwood, L.: Expression of inhibitor of growth 4 by HSV1716 improves oncolytic potency and enhances efficacy. Cancer Gene Ther. **19**, 499–507 (2012)

Coors, E.A., Schuler, G., von den Driesch, P.: Topical imiquimod as treatment for different kinds of cutaneous lymphoma. Eur. J. Dermatol. **16**, 391–393 (2006)

Cripe, T.P., Ngo, M.C., Geller, J.I., Louis, C.U., Currier, M.A., Racadio, J.M., Towbin, A.J., Rooney, C.M., Pelusio, A., Moon, A., Hwang, T.H., Burke, J.M., Bell, J.C., Kirn, D.H., Breitbach, C.J.: Phase 1 study of intratumoral Pexa-Vec (JX-594), an oncolytic and immunotherapeutic vaccinia virus, in pediatric cancer patients. Mol. Ther. **23**, 602–608 (2015)

Currie, G.A.: Eighty years of immunotherapy: a review of immunological methods used for the treatment of human cancer. Br. J. Cancer **26**, 141–153 (1972)

D'Andrea, A., Rengaraju, M., Valiante, N.M., Chehimi, J., Kubin, M., Aste, M., Chan, S.H., Kobayashi, M., Young, D., Nickbarg, E., et al.: Production of natural killer cell stimulatory factor (interleukin 12) by peripheral blood mononuclear cells. J. Exp. Med. **176**, 1387–1398 (1992)

Davis, M.B., Vasquez-Dunddel, D., Fu, J., Albesiano, E., Pardoll, D., Kim, Y.J.: Intratumoral administration of TLR4 agonist absorbed into a cellular vector improves antitumor responses. Clin. Cancer Res. **17**, 3984–3992 (2011)

Deeths, M.J., Chapman, J.T., Dellavalle, R.P., Zeng, C., Aeling, J.L.: Treatment of patch and plaque stage mycosis fungoides with imiquimod 5% cream. J. Am. Acad. Dermatol. **52**, 275–280 (2005)

Dewan, M.Z., Vanpouille-Box, C., Kawashima, N., Dinapoli, S., Babb, J.S., Formenti, S.C., Adams, S., Demaria, S.: Synergy of topical toll-like receptor 7 agonist with radiation and low-dose cyclophosphamide in a mouse model of cutaneous breast cancer. Clin. Cancer Res. **18**, 6668–6678 (2012)

di Nicola, M., Zappasodi, R., Carlostella, C., Mortarini, R., Pupa, S.M., Magni, M., Devizzi, L., Matteucci, P., Baldassari, P., Ravagnani, F., Cabras, A., Anichini, A., Gianni, A.M.: Vaccination with autologous tumor-loaded dendritic cells induces clinical and immunological responses in indolent B cell lymphoma patients with relapsed and measurable disease: a pilot study. Blood **113**, 6668–6678 (2008)

Diaconu, I., Cerullo, V., Hirvinen, M.L., Escutenaire, S., Ugolini, M., Pesonen, S.K., Bramante, S., Parviainen, S., Kanerva, A., Loskog, A.S., Eliopoulos, A.G., Pesonen, S., Hemminki, A.: Immune response is an important aspect of the antitumor effect produced by a CD40L-encoding oncolytic adenovirus. Cancer Res. **72**, 2327–2338 (2012)

Dias, J.D., Hemminki, O., Diaconu, I., Hirvinen, M., Bonetti, A., Guse, K., Escutenaire, S., Kanerva, A., Pesonen, S., Löskog, A., Cerullo, V., Hemminki, A.: Targeted cancer immunotherapy with oncolytic adenovirus coding for a fully human monoclonal antibody species for C TLA-4. Gene Ther. **10**, 988–998 (2012)

Didona, B., Benucci, R., Amerio, P., Canzona, F., Rienzo, O., Cavalieri, R.: Primary cutaneous CD30+ T-cell lymphoma responsive to topical imiquimod (Aldara). Br. J. Dermatol. **150**, 1198–1201 (2004)

Dovedi, S.J., Melis, M.H., Wilkinson, R.W., Adlard, A.L., Stratford, I.J., Honeychurch, J., Illidge, T.M.: Systemic delivery of a TLR7 agonist in combination with radiation primes durable antitumor immune responses in mouse models of lymphoma. Blood **121**, 251–259 (2013)

Dranoff, G., Jaffee, E., Lazenby, A., Golumbek, P., Levitsky, H., Brose, K., Jackson, V., Hamada, H., Pardoll, D., Mulligan, R.C.: Vaccination with irradiated tumor cells engineered to secrete murine granulocyte-macrophage colony-stimulating factor stimulates potent, specific, and long-lasting anti-tumor immunity. Proc. Natl. Acad. Sci. U. S. A. **90**, 3539–3543 (1993)

Du, T., Shi, G., Li, Y.M., Zhang, J.F., Tian, H.W., Wei, Y.Q., Deng, H., Yu, D.C.: Tumor-specific oncolytic adenoviruses expressing granulocyte macrophage colony-stimulating factor or anti-CTLA4 antibody for the treatment of cancers. Cancer Gene Ther. **21**, 340–348 (2014)

Dummer, R., Urosevic, M., Kempf, W., Kazakov, D., Burg, G.: Imiquimod induces complete clearance of a PUVA-resistant plaque in mycosis fungoides. Dermatology **207**, 116–118 (2003)

Egilmez, N.K., Jong, Y.S., Sabel, M.S., Jacob, J.S., Mathiowitz, E., Bankert, R.B.: In situ tumor vaccination with interleukin-12-encapsulated biodegradable microspheres: induction of tumor regression and potent antitumor immunity. Cancer Res. **60**, 3832–3837 (2000)

Ehst, B.D., Dreno, B., Vonderheid, E.C.: Primary cutaneous CD30+ anaplastic large cell lymphoma responds to imiquimod cream. Eur. J. Dermatol. **18**, 467–468 (2008)

Elsedawy, N.B., Russell, S.J.: Oncolytic vaccines. Expert Rev. Vaccines **12**, 1155–1172 (2013)

Engeland, C.E., Grossardt, C., Veinalde, R., Bossow, S., Lutz, D., Kaufmann, J.K., Shevchenko, I., Umansky, V., Nettelbeck, D.M., Weichert, W., Jäger, D., von Kalle, C., Ungerechts, G.: CTLA-4 and PD-L1 checkpoint blockade enhances oncolytic measles virus therapy. Mol. Ther. **22**, 1949–1959 (2014)

Engelhardt, R., Mackensen, A., Galanos, C., Andreesen, R.: Biological response to intravenously administered endotoxin in patients with advanced cancer. J. Biol. Response Mod. **9**, 480–491 (1990)

Escors, D.: Tumour immunogenicity, antigen presentation and immunological barriers in cancer immunotherapy. New J. Sci. **2014**, 25 (2014)

Fan, R., Wang, C., Wang, Y., Ren, P., Gan, P., Ji, H., Xia, Z., Hu, S., Zeng, Q., Huang, W., Jiang, Y., Huang, X.: Enhanced antitumoral efficacy and immune response following conditionally replicative adenovirus containing constitutive HSF1 delivery to rodent tumors. J. Transl. Med. **10**, 101 (2012)

Fiszer-Maliszewska, L., den Otter, W., Madej, J.A., Mordarski, M.: Therapeutic potential of biological response modifiers against transplantable mouse tumors of spontaneous origin. II. Local interleukin 2 treatment of tumors of different immunogenic strength. Arch. Immunol. Ther. Exp. (Warsz.) **46**, 293–300 (1998)

Formenti, S.C., Demaria, S.: Systemic effects of local radiotherapy. Lancet Oncol. **10**, 718–726 (2009)

Fransen, M.F., Sluijter, M., Morreau, H., Arens, R., Melief, C.J.: Local activation of CD8 T cells and systemic tumor eradication without toxicity via slow release and local delivery of agonistic CD40 antibody. Clin. Cancer Res. **17**, 2270–2280 (2011)

Fransen, M.F., van der Sluis, T.C., Ossendorp, F., Arens, R., Melief, C.J.: Controlled local delivery of CTLA-4 blocking antibody induces CD8+ T-cell-dependent tumor eradication and decreases risk of toxic side effects. Clin. Cancer Res. **19**, 5381–5389 (2013)

Fujimura, T., Nakagawa, S., Ohtani, T., Ito, Y., Aiba, S.: Inhibitory effect of the polyinosinic-polycytidylic acid/cationic liposome on the progression of murine B16F10 melanoma. Eur. J. Immunol. **36**, 3371–3380 (2006)

Fukuhara, H., Ino, Y., Kuroda, T., Martuza, R.L., Todo, T.: Triple gene-deleted oncolytic herpes simplex virus vector double-armed with interleukin 18 and soluble B7-1 constructed by bacterial artificial chromosome-mediated system. Cancer Res. **65**, 10663–10668 (2005)

Furumoto, K., Soares, L., Engleman, E.G., Merad, M.: Induction of potent antitumor immunity by in situ targeting of intratumoral DCs. J. Clin. Invest. **113**, 774–783 (2004)

Fyfe, G., Fisher, R.I., Rosenberg, S.A., Sznol, M., Parkinson, D.R., Louie, A.C.: Results of treatment of 255 patients with metastatic renal cell carcinoma who received high-dose recombinant interleukin-2 therapy. J. Clin. Oncol. **13**, 688–696 (1995)

Galanis, E., Hersh, E.M., Stopeck, A.T., Gonzalez, R., Burch, P., Spier, C., Akporiaye, E.T., Rinehart, J.J., Edmonson, J., Sobol, R.E., Forscher, C., Sondak, V.K., Lewis, B.D., Unger, E.C., O'Driscoll, M., Selk, L., Rubin, J.: Immunotherapy of advanced malignancy by direct gene transfer of an interleukin-2 DNA/DMRIE/DOPE lipid complex: phase I/II experience. J. Clin. Oncol. **17**, 3313–3323 (1999)

Gitlin, L., Barchet, W., Gilfillan, S., Cella, M., Beutler, B., Flavell, R.A., Diamond, M.S., Colonna, M.: Essential role of mda-5 in type I IFN responses to polyriboinosinic:polyribocytidylic acid and encephalomyocarditis picornavirus. Proc. Natl. Acad. Sci. U. S. A. **103**, 8459–8464 (2006)

Goshima, F., Esaki, S., Luo, C., Kamakura, M., Kimura, H., Nishiyama, Y.: Oncolytic viral therapy with a combination of HF10, a herpes simplex virus type 1 variant and granulocyte-macrophage colony-stimulating factor for murine ovarian cancer. Int. J. Cancer **134**, 2865–2877 (2014)

Goto, S., Sakai, S., Kera, J., Suma, Y., Soma, G.I., Takeuchi, S.: Intradermal administration of lipopolysaccharide in treatment of human cancer. Cancer Immunol. Immunother. **42**, 255–261 (1996)

Grauer, O.M., Molling, J.W., Bennink, E., Toonen, L.W., Sutmuller, R.P., Nierkens, S., Adema, G.J.: TLR ligands in the local treatment of established intracerebral murine gliomas. J. Immunol. **181**, 6720–6729 (2008)

Gudmundsdottir, H., Wells, A.D., Turka, L.A.: Dynamics and requirements of T cell clonal expansion in vivo at the single-cell level: effector function is linked to proliferative capacity. J. Immunol. **162**, 5212–5223 (1999)

Guo, J., Zhu, J., Sheng, X., Wang, X., Qu, L., Han, Y., Liu, Y., Zhang, H., Huo, L., Zhang, S., Lin, B., Yang, Z.: Intratumoral injection of dendritic cells in combination with local hyperthermia induces systemic antitumor effect in patients with advanced melanoma. Int. J. Cancer **120**, 2418–2425 (2007)

Gutwald, J.G., Groth, W., Mahrle, G.: Peritumoral injections of interleukin 2 induce tumour regression in metastatic malignant melanoma. Br. J. Dermatol. **130**, 541–542 (1994)

Harrington, K.J., Hingorani, M., Tanay, M.A., Hickey, J., Bhide, S.A., Clarke, P.M., Renouf, L.C., Thway, K., Sibtain, A., Mcneish, I.A., Newbold, K.L., Goldsweig, H., Coffin, R., Nutting, C.M.: Phase I/II study of oncolytic HSV GM-CSF in combination with radiotherapy and cisplatin in untreated stage III/IV squamous cell cancer of the head and neck. Clin. Cancer Res. **16**, 4005–4015 (2010)

Henriques, L., Palumbo, M., Guay, M.P., Bahoric, B., Basik, M., Kavan, P., Batist, G.: Imiquimod in the treatment of breast cancer skin metastasis. J. Clin. Oncol. **32**, e22–e25 (2014)

Heo, J., Reid, T., Ruo, L., Breitbach, C.J., Rose, S., Bloomston, M., Cho, M., Lim, H.Y., Chung, H.C., Kim, C.W., Burke, J., Lencioni, R., Hickman, T., Moon, A., Lee, Y.S., Kim, M.K., Daneshmand, M., Dubois, K., Longpre, L., Ngo, M., Rooney, C., Bell, J.C., Rhee, B.G., Patt, R., Hwang, T.H., Kirn, D.H.: Randomized dose-finding clinical trial of oncolytic immunotherapeutic vaccinia JX-594 in liver cancer. Nat. Med. **19**, 329–336 (2013)

Hodi, F.S., O'Day, S.J., McDermott, D.F., Weber, R.W., Sosman, J.A., Haanen, J.B., Gonzalez, R., Robert, C., Schadendorf, D., Hassel, J.C., Akerley, W., van den Eertwegh, A.J., Lutzky, J., Lorigan, P., Vaubel, J.M., Linette, G.P., Hogg, D., Ottensmeier, C.H., Lebbé, C., Peschel, C., Quirt, I., Clark, J.I., Wolchok, J.D., Weber, J.S., Tian, J., Yellin, M.J., Nichol, G.M., Hoos, A., Urba, W.J.: Improved survival with ipilimumab in patients with metastatic melanoma. N. Engl. J. Med. **363**, 711–723 (2010)

Hoeller, C., Jansen, B., Heere-Ress, E., Pustelnik, T., Mossbacher, U., Schlagbauer-Wadl, H., Wolff, K., Pehamberger, H.: Perilesional injection of r-GM-CSF in patients with cutaneous melanoma metastases. J. Invest. Dermatol. **117**, 371–374 (2001)

Hoffman, D.M., Figlin, R.A.: Intratumoral interleukin 2 for renal-cell carcinoma by direct gene transfer of a plasmid DNA/DMRIE/DOPE lipid complex. World J. Urol. **18**, 152–156 (2000)

Horton, H.M., Dorigo, O., Hernandez, P., Anderson, D., Berek, J.S., Parker, S.E.: IL-2 plasmid therapy of murine ovarian carcinoma inhibits the growth of tumor ascites and alters its cytokine profile. J. Immunol. **163**, 6378–6385 (1999)

Hou, S., Kou, G., Fan, X., Wang, H., Qian, W., Zhang, D., Li, B., Dai, J., Zhao, J., Ma, J., Li, J., Lin, B., Wu, M., Guo, Y.: Eradication of hepatoma and colon cancer in mice with Flt3L gene therapy in combination with 5-FU. Cancer Immunol. Immunother. **56**, 1605–1613 (2007)

Houot, R., Levy, R.: T-cell modulation combined with intratumoral CpG cures lymphoma in a mouse model without the need for chemotherapy. Blood **113**, 3546–3552 (2009)

Hu, J.C., Coffin, R.S., Davis, C.J., Graham, N.J., Groves, N., Guest, P.J., Harrington, K.J., James, N.D., Love, C.A., Mcneish, I., Medley, L.C., Michael, A., Nutting, C.M., Pandha, H.S., Shorrock, C.A., Simpson, J., Steiner, J., Steven, N.M., Wright, D., Coombes, R.C.: A phase I study of OncoVEXGM-CSF, a second-generation oncolytic herpes simplex virus expressing granulocyte macrophage colony-stimulating factor. Clin. Cancer Res. **12**, 6737–6747 (2006)

Huang, X.F., Ren, W., Rollins, L., Pittman, P., Shah, M., Shen, L., Gu, Q., Strube, R., Hu, F., Chen, S.Y.: A broadly applicable, personalized heat shock protein-mediated oncolytic tumor vaccine. Cancer Res. **63**, 7321–7329 (2003)

Hwang, T.H., Moon, A., Burke, J., Ribas, A., Stephenson, J., Breitbach, C.J., Daneshmand, M., de Silva, N., Parato, K., Diallo, J.S., Lee, Y.S., Liu, T.C., Bell, J.C., Kirn, D.H.: A mechanistic proof-of-concept clinical trial with JX-594, a targeted multi-mechanistic oncolytic poxvirus, in patients with metastatic melanoma. Mol. Ther. **19**, 1913–1922 (2011)

Ino, Y., Saeki, Y., Fukuhara, H., Todo, T.: Triple combination of oncolytic herpes simplex virus-1 vectors armed with interleukin-12, interleukin-18, or soluble B7-1 results in enhanced antitumor efficacy. Clin. Cancer Res. **12**, 643–652 (2006)

Ishihara, M., Seo, N., Mitsui, J., Muraoka, D., Tanaka, M., Mineno, J., Ikeda, H., Shiku, H.: Systemic CD8+ T cell-mediated tumoricidal effects by intratumoral treatment of oncolytic herpes simplex virus with the agonistic monoclonal antibody for murine glucocorticoid-induced tumor necrosis factor receptor. PLoS One **9**, e104669 (2014)

Jackaman, C., Bundell, C.S., Kinnear, B.F., Smith, A.M., Filion, P., van Hagen, D., Robinson, B.W., Nelson, D.J.: IL-2 intratumoral immunotherapy enhances CD8+ T cells that mediate destruction of tumor cells and tumor-associated vasculature: a novel mechanism for IL-2. J. Immunol. **171**, 5051–5063 (2003)

Jahrsdörfer, B., Hartmann, G., Racila, E., Jackson, W., Mühlenhoff, L., Meinhardt, G., Endres, S., Link, B.K., Krieg, A.M., Weiner, G.J.: CpG DNA increases primary malignant B cell expression of costimulatory molecules and target antigens. J. Leukoc. Biol. **69**, 81–88 (2001)

Jahrsdorfer, B., Muhlenhoff, L., Blackwell, S.E., Wagner, M., Poeck, H., Hartmann, E., Jox, R., Giese, T., Emmerich, B., Endres, S., Weiner, G.J., Hartmann, G.: B-cell lymphomas differ in their responsiveness to CpG oligodeoxynucleotides. Clin. Cancer Res. **11**, 1490–1499 (2005)

Kashiwagi, I., Morita, R., Schichita, T., Komai, K., Saeki, K., Matsumoto, M., Takeda, K., Nomura, M., Hayashi, A., Kanai, T., Yoshimura, A.: Smad2 and Smad3 inversely regulate TGF-beta autoinduction in Clostridium butyricum-activated dendritic cells. Immunity **43**, 65–79 (2015)

Kaufman, H.L., Ingemar Andtbacka, R.H., Collichio, F.A., Amatruda, T., Senzer, N.N., Chesney, J., Delman, K.A., Spitler, L.E., Puzanov, I., Ye, Y., Li, A., Gansert, J.L., Coffin, R., Ross, M.I.: Primary overall survival (OS) from OPTiM, a randomized phase III trial of talimogene laherparepvec (T-VEC) versus subcutaneous (SC) granulocyte-macrophage colony-stimulating factor (GM-CSF) for the treatment (tx) of unresected stage IIIB/C and IV melanoma. J. Clin. Oncol. **32**, 5s (2014) (suppl; abstr 9008a)

Kaufman, H.L., Kim, D.W., Deraffele, G., Mitcham, J., Coffin, R.S., Kim-Schulze, S.: Local and distant immunity induced by intralesional vaccination with an oncolytic herpes virus encoding GM-CSF in patients with stage IIIc and IV melanoma. Ann. Surg. Oncol. **17**, 718–730 (2010)

Kerkmann, M., Rothenfusser, S., Hornung, V., Towarowski, A., Wagner, M., Sarris, A., Giese, T., Endres, S., Hartmann, G.: Activation with CpG-A and CpG-B oligonucleotides reveals two distinct regulatory pathways of type I IFN synthesis in human plasmacytoid dendritic cells. J. Immunol. **170**, 4465–4474 (2003)

Kim, J.H., Oh, J.Y., Park, B.H., Lee, D.E., Kim, J.S., Park, H.E., Roh, M.S., Je, J.E., Yoon, J.H., Thorne, S.H., Kirn, D., Hwang, T.H.: Systemic armed oncolytic and immunologic therapy for cancer with JX-594, a targeted poxvirus expressing GM-CSF. Mol. Ther. **14**, 361–730 (2006)

Kim, Y.H., Gratzinger, D., Harrison, C., Brody, J.D., Czerwinski, D.K., Ai, W.Z., Morales, A., Abdulla, F., Xing, L., Navi, D., Tibshirani, R.J., Advani, R.H., Lingala, B., Shah, S., Hoppe, R.T., Levy, R.: In situ vaccination against mycosis fungoides by intratumoral injection of a TLR9 agonist combined with radiation: a phase 1/2 study. Blood **119**, 355–63 (2012)

Kimata, H., Imai, T., Kikumori, T., Teshigahara, O., Nagasaka, T., Goshima, F., Nishiyama, Y., Nakao, A.: Pilot study of oncolytic viral therapy using mutant herpes simplex virus (HF10) against recurrent metastatic breast cancer. Ann. Surg. Oncol. **13**, 1078–1084 (2006)

Kobayashi, T., Walsh, P.T., Walsh, M.C., Speirs, K.M., Chiffoleau, E., King, C.G., Hancock, W.W., Caamano, J.H., Hunter, C.A., Scott, P., Turka, L.A., Choi, Y.: TRAF6 is a critical factor for dendritic cell maturation and development. Immunity **19**, 353–363 (2003)

Kohrt, H.E., Chu, J., Brody, J., Czerwinski, D.K., Chester, C., Sadaram, M., Advani, R., Kim, Y.H., Hoppe, R.T., Knox, S.J., Wapnir, I., Tibshirani, R.J., Levy, R.: Dose-escalated, intratumoral TLR9 agonist and low-dose radiation induce abscopal effects in follicular lymphoma. Blood **124**, 3092 (2014)

Kolstad, A., Kumari, S., Walczak, M., Madsbu, U., Hagtvedt, T., Bogsrud, T.V., Kvalheim, G., Holte, H., Aurlien, E., Delabie, J., Tierens, A., Olweus, J.: Sequential intranodal immunotherapy induces antitumor immunity and correlated regression of disseminated follicular lymphoma. Blood **125**, 82–89 (2015)

Kreiter, S., Diken, M., Selmi, A., Diekmann, J., Attig, S., Hüsemann, Y., Koslowski, M., Huber, C., Türeci, Ö., Sahin, U.: FLT3 ligand enhances the cancer therapeutic potency of naked RNA vaccines. Cancer Res. **71**, 6132–6142 (2011)

Kuang, M., Liu, S.Q., Saijo, K., Uchimura, E., Huang, L., Leong, K.W., Lu, M.D., Huang, J.F., Ohno, T.: Microwave tumour coagulation plus in situ treatment with cytokine-microparticles: induction of potent anti-residual tumour immunity. Int. J. Hyperthermia **21**, 247–257 (2005)

Lang, F.F., Conrad, C., Gomez-Manzano, C., Tufaro, F., Yung, W., Sawaya, R., Weinberg, J., Prabhu, S., Fuller, G., Aldape, K., Fueyo, J.: First-in-human phase I clinical trial of oncolytic Delta-24-RGD (DNX-2401) with biological endpoints: implications for Viro-immunotherapy. Neuro-Oncology **16**, iii39 (2014)

Lee, Y.S., Kim, J.H., Choi, K.J., Choi, I.K., Kim, H., Cho, S., Cho, B.C., Yun, C.O.: Enhanced antitumor effect of oncolytic adenovirus expressing interleukin-12 and B7-1 in an immunocompetent murine model. Clin. Cancer Res. **12**, 5859–5868 (2006)

Leonard, J.P., Sherman, M.L., Fisher, G.L., Buchanan, L.J., Larsen, G., Atkins, M.B., Sosman, J.A., Dutcher, J.P., Vogelzang, N.J., Ryan, J.L.: Effects of single-dose interleukin-12 exposure on interleukin-12-associated toxicity and interferon-gamma production. Blood **90**, 2541–2548 (1997)

Li, J., Song, W., Czerwinski, D.K., Varghese, B., Uematsu, S., Akira, S., Krieg, A.M., Levy, R.: Lymphoma immunotherapy with CpG oligodeoxynucleotides requires TLR9 either in the host or in the tumor itself. J. Immunol. **179**, 2493–500 (2007)

Li, J.L., Liu, H.L., Zhang, X.R., Xu, J.P., Hu, W.K., Liang, M., Chen, S.Y., Hu, F., Chu, D.T.: A phase I trial of intratumoral administration of recombinant oncolytic adenovirus overexpressing HSP70 in advanced solid tumor patients. Gene Ther. **16**, 376–82 (2009)

Liu, B.L., Robinson, M., Han, Z.Q., Branston, R.H., English, C., Reay, P., Mcgrath, Y., Thomas, S.K., Thornton, M., Bullock, P., Love, C.A., Coffin, R.S.: ICP34.5 deleted herpes simplex virus with enhanced oncolytic, immune stimulating, and anti-tumour properties. Gene Ther. **10**, 292–303 (2003)

London, C.A., Lodge, M.P., Abbas, A.K.: Functional responses and costimulator dependence of memory CD4+ T cells. J. Immunol. **164**, 265–272 (2000)

Lu, Y.C., Yeh, W.C., Ohashi, P.S.: LPS/TLR4 signal transduction pathway. Cytokine **42**, 145–151 (2008)

Ma, D.Y., Clarke, E.A.: The role of CD40 and CD154/CD40L in dendritic cells. Semin. Immunol. **21**, 265–272 (2009)

Mach, N., Gillessen, S., Wilson, S.B., Sheehan, C., Mihm, M., Dranoff, G.: Differences in dendritic cells stimulated in vivo by tumors engineered to secrete granulocyte-macrophage colony-stimulating factor or Flt3-ligand. Cancer Res. **60**, 3239–3246 (2000)

Mackie, R.M., Stewart, B., Brown, S.M.: Intralesional injection of herpes simplex virus 1716 in metastatic melanoma. Lancet **357**, 525–526 (2001)

Mahvi, D.M., Henry, M.B., Albertini, M.R., Weber, S., Meredith, K., Schalch, H., Rakhmilevich, A., Hank, J., Sondel, P.: Intratumoral injection of IL-12 plasmid DNA—results of a phase I/IB clinical trial. Cancer Gene Ther. **14**, 717–723 (2007)

Maito, F.L.D.M., Souza, A.P.D.D., Pereira, L., Smithey, M., Hinrichs, D., Bouwer, A., Bonorino, C.: Intratumoral TLR-4 agonist injection is critical for modulation of tumor microenvironment and tumor rejection. ISRN Immunol. **2012**, 926817 (2012)

Maloney, D.G., Liles, T.M., Czerwinski, D.K., Waldichuk, C., Rosenberg, J., Grillo-Lopez, A., Levy, R.: Phase I clinical trial using escalating single-dose infusion of chimeric anti-CD20 monoclonal antibody (IDEC-C2B8) in patients with recurrent B-cell lymphoma. Blood **84**, 2457–2466 (1994)

Mangsbo, S.M., Broos, S., Fletcher, E., Veitonmaki, N., Furebring, C., Dahlen, E., Norlen, P., Lindstedt, M., Totterman, T.H., Ellmark, P.: The human agonistic CD40 antibody ADC-1013 eradicates bladder tumors and generates T-cell-dependent tumor immunity. Clin. Cancer Res. **21**, 1115–1126 (2015)

Marabelle, A., Kohrt, H., Sagiv-Barfi, I., Ajami, B., Axtell, R.C., Zhou, G., Rajapaksa, R., Green, M.R., Torchia, J., Brody, J., Luong, R., Rosenblum, M.D., Steinman, L., Levitsky, H.I., Tse, V., Levy, R.: Depleting tumor-specific Tregs at a single site eradicates disseminated tumors. J. Clin. Invest. **123**, 2447–2463 (2013)

Mariani, C.L., Rajon, D., Bova, F.J., Streit, W.J.: Nonspecific immunotherapy with intratumoral lipopolysaccharide and zymosan A but not GM-CSF leads to an effective anti-tumor response in subcutaneous RG-2 gliomas. J. Neurooncol **85**, 231–240 (2007)

Marron, T., Bhardwaj, N., Crowley, E., Keler, T., Davis, T.A., Brody, J.: Turning a tumor into a vaccine factory: in situ vaccination for low-grade lymphoma. Cancer Immunol. Res. **3**, IA03 (2014)

Marroquin, C.E., Westwood, J.A., Lapointe, R., Mixon, A., Wunderlich, J.R., Caron, D., Rosenberg, S.A., Hwu, P.: Mobilization of dendritic cell precursors in patients with cancer by flt3 ligand allows the generation of higher yields of cultured dendritic cells. J. Immunother. **25**, 278–288 (2002)

Meshii, N., Takahashi, G., Okunaga, S., Hamada, M., Iwai, S., Takasu, A., Ogawa, Y., Yura, Y.: Enhancement of systemic tumor immunity for squamous cell carcinoma cells by an oncolytic herpes simplex virus. Cancer Gene Ther. **20**, 493–498 (2013)

Miller, R.L., Gerster, J.F., Owens, M.L., Slade, H.B., Tomai, M.A.: Imiquimod applied topically: a novel immune response modifier and new class of drug. Int. J. Immunopharmacol. **21**, 1–14 (1999)

Ming Lim, C., Stephenson, R., Salazar, A.M., Ferris, R.L.: TLR3 agonists improve the immunostimulatory potential of cetuximab against EGFR head and neck cancer cells. Oncoimmunology **2**, e24677 (2013)

Morse, M.A., Nair, S., Fernandez-Casal, M., Deng, Y., St Peter, M., Williams, R., Hobeika, A., Mosca, P., Clay, T., Cumming, R.I., Fisher, E., Clavien, P., Proia, A.D., Niedzwiecki, D., Caron, D., Lyerly, H.K.: Preoperative mobilization of circulating dendritic cells by Flt3 ligand administration to patients with metastatic colon cancer. J. Clin. Oncol. **18**, 3883–93 (2000)

Motoyoshi, Y., Kaminoda, K., Saitoh, O., Hamasaki, K., Nakao, K., Ishii, N., Nagayama, Y., Eguchi, K.: Different mechanisms for anti-tumor effects of low- and high-dose cyclophosphamide. Oncol. Rep. **16**, 141–146 (2006)

Nakao, A., Kasuya, H., Sahin, T.T., Nomura, N., Kanzaki, A., Misawa, M., Shirota, T., Yamada, S., Fujii, T., Sugimoto, H., Shikano, T., Nomoto, S., Takeda, S., Kodera, Y., Nishiyama, Y.: A phase I dose-escalation clinical trial of intraoperative direct intratumoral injection of HF10 oncolytic virus in non-resectable patients with advanced pancreatic cancer. Cancer Gene Ther. **18**, 167–175 (2011)

Nasi, M.L., Lieberman, P., Busam, K.J., Prieto, V., Panageas, K.S., Lewis, J.J., Houghton, A.N., Chapman, P.B.: Intradermal injection of granulocyte-macrophage colony-stimulating factor (GM-CSF) in patients with metastatic melanoma recruits dendritic cells. Cytokines Cell. Mol. Ther. **5**, 139–144 (1999)

Nemunaitis, J.: Oncolytic viruses. Invest. New Drugs **17**, 375–386 (1999)

Nemunaitis, J.J., Linette, G.P., Ali, H., Lebel, F., Barrett, J.A., Reed, T., Krishnan, S., Lewis, J.: Ad-RTS-hIL-12+ veledimex regulation of IL-12 expression in advanced breast cancer (BC) and melanoma patients. AACR—Tumor Immunology and Immunotherapy: A New Chapter Poster Session B (meeting abstract) (2014)

Neville, M.E., Robb, R.J., Popescu, M.C.: In situ vaccination against a non-immunogenic tumour using intratumoural injections of liposomal interleukin 2. Cytokine **16**, 239–250 (2001)

Noessner, E., Gastpar, R., Milani, V., Brandl, A., Hutzler, P.J., Kuppner, M.C., Roos, M., Kremmer, E., Asea, A., Calderwood, S.K., Issels, R.D.: Tumor-derived heat shock protein 70 peptide complexes are cross-presented by human dendritic cells. J. Immunol. **169**, 5424–5432 (2002)

Okuda, H., Kobayashi, A., Xia, B., Watabe, M., Pai, S.K., Hirota, S., Xing, F., Liu, W., Pandey, P.R., Fukuda, K., Modur, V., Ghosh, A., Wilber, A., Watabe, K.: Hyaluronan synthase HAS2 promotes tumor progression in bone by stimulating the interaction of breast cancer stem-like cells with macrophages and stromal cells. Cancer Res. **72**, 537–547 (2012)

Otto, F., Schmid, P., Mackensen, A., Wehr, U., Seiz, A., Braun, M., Galanos, C., Mertelsmann, R., Engelhardt, R.: Phase II trial of intravenous endotoxin in patients with colorectal and non-small cell lung cancer. Eur. J. Cancer **32A**, 1712–1718 (1996)

Papanastassiou, V., Rampling, R., Fraser, M., Petty, R., Hadley, D., Nicoll, J., Harland, J., Mabbs, R., Brown, M.: The potential for efficacy of the modified (ICP 34.5(−)) herpes simplex virus HSV1716 following intratumoural injection into human malignant glioma: a proof of principle study. Gene Ther. **9**, 398–406 (2002)

Parato, K.A., Breitbach, C.J., le Boeuf, F., Wang, J., Storbeck, C., Ilkow, C., Diallo, J.S., Falls, T., Burns, J., Garcia, V., Kanji, F., Evgin, L., Hu, K., Paradis, F., Knowes, S., Hwang, T.H., Vanderhyden, B.C., Auer, R., Kirn, D.H., Bell, J.C.: The oncolytic poxvirus JX-594 selectively replicates in and destroys cancer cells driven by genetic pathways commonly activated in cancers. Mol. Ther. **20**, 749–758 (2012)

Park, B.H., Hwang, T., Liu, T.C., Sze, D.Y., Kim, J.S., Kwon, H.C., Oh, S.Y., Han, S.Y., Yoon, J.H., Hong, S.H., Moon, A., Speth, K., Park, C., Ahn, Y.J., Daneshmand, M., Rhee, B.G., Pinedo, H.M., Bell, J.C., Kirn, D.H.: Use of a targeted oncolytic poxvirus, JX-594, in patients with refractory primary or metastatic liver cancer: a phase I trial. Lancet Oncol **9**, 533–542 (2008)

Pawlowska, A.B., Hashino, S., McKenna, H., Weigel, B.J., Taylor, P.A., Blazar, B.R.: In vitro tumor-pulsed or in vivo Flt3 ligand-generated dendritic cells provide protection against acute myelogenous leukemia in nontransplanted or syngeneic bone marrow-transplanted mice. Blood **97**, 1474–1482 (2001)

Pesonen, S., Diaconu, I., Kangasniemi, L., Ranki, T., Kanerva, A., Pesonen, S.K., Gerdemann, U., Leen, A.M., Kairemo, K., Oksanen, M., Haavisto, E., Holm, S.L., Karioja-Kallio, A., Kauppinen, S., Partanen, K.P., Laasonen, L., Joensuu, T., Alanko, T., Cerullo, V., Hemminki, A.: Oncolytic immunotherapy of advanced solid tumors with a CD40L-expressing replicating adenovirus: assessment of safety and immunologic responses in patients. Cancer Res. **72**, 1621–1631 (2012)

Postow, M.A., Chesney, J., Pavlick, A.C., Robert, C., Grossmann, K., McDermott, D., Linette, G.P., Meyer, N., Giguere, J.K., Agarwala, S.S., Shaheen, M., Ernstoff, M.S., Minor, D., Salama, A.K., Taylor, M., Ott, P.A., Rollin, L.M., Horak, C., Gagnier, P., Wolchok, J.D., Hodi, F.S.: Nivolumab and ipilimumab versus ipilimumab in untreated melanoma. N. Engl. J. Med. **372**, 2006–2017 (2015)

Pullen, S.S., Dang, T.T., Crute, J.J., Kehry, M.R.: CD40 signaling through tumor necrosis factor receptor-associated factors (TRAFs). Binding site specificity and activation of downstream pathways by distinct TRAFs. J. Biol. Chem. **274**, 14246–14254 (1999)

Puzanov, I., Milhem, M.M., Ingemar Andtbacka, R.H., Minor, D.R., Hamid, O., Li, A., Chastain, M., Gorski, K., Anderson, A., Vanderwalde, A.M., Chou, J., Kaufman, H.L.: Primary analysis of a phase 1b multicenter trial to evaluate safety and efficacy of talimogene laherparepvec (T-VEC) and ipilimumab (ipi) in previously untreated, unresected stage IIIB-IV melanoma. J. Clin. Oncol. **32**, 5 (2014) (suppl; abstr 9029^)

Radny, P., Caroli, U.M., Bauer, J., Paul, T., Schlegel, C., Eigentler, T.K., Weide, B., Schwarz, M., Garbe, C.: Phase II trial of intralesional therapy with interleukin-2 in soft-tissue melanoma metastases. Br. J. Cancer **89**, 1620–1626 (2003)

Raykov, Z., Grekova, S., Leuchs, B., Aprahamian, M., Rommelaere, J.: Arming parvoviruses with CpG motifs to improve their oncosuppressive capacity. Int. J. Cancer **122**, 2880–2884 (2008)

Reichardt, V.L., Brossart, P., Kanz, L.: Dendritic cells in vaccination therapies of human malignant disease. Blood Rev. **18**, 235–243 (2004)

Richmond, H.M., Lozano, A., Jones, D., Duvic, M.: Primary cutaneous follicle center lymphoma associated with alopecia areata. Clin. Lymphoma Myeloma **8**, 121–124 (2008)

Riediger, C., Wingender, G., Knolle, P., Aulmann, S., Stremmel, W., Encke, J.: Fms-like tyrosine kinase 3 receptor ligand (Flt3L)-based vaccination administered with an adenoviral vector prevents tumor growth of colorectal cancer in a BALB/c mouse model. J. Cancer Res. Clin. Oncol. **139**, 2097–2110 (2013)

Robert, C., Thomas, L., Bondarenko, I., O'Day, S., Weber, J., Garbe, C., Lebbe, C., Baurain, J.F., Testori, A., Grob, J.J., Davidson, N., Richards, J., Maio, M., Hauschild, A., Miller, W.H., Gascon, P., Lotem, M., Harmankaya, K., Ibrahim, R., Francis, S., Chen, T.T., Humphrey, R., Hoos, A., Wolchok, J.D.: Ipilimumab plus dacarbazine for previously untreated metastatic melanoma. N. Engl. J. Med. **364**, 2517–2526 (2011)

Roberts, N.J., Zhang, L., Janku, F., Collins, A., Bai, R.Y., Staedtke, V., Rusk, A.W., Tung, D., Miller, M., Roix, J., Khanna, K.V., Murthy, R., Benjamin, R.S., Helgason, T., Szvalb, A.D., Bird, J.E., Roy-Chowdhuri, S., Zhang, H.H., Qiao, Y., Karim, B., Mcdaniel, J., Elpiner, A., Sahora, A., Lachowicz, J., Phillips, B., Turner, A., Klein, M.K., Post, G., Diaz Jr., L.A., Riggins, G.J., Papadopoulos, N., Kinzler, K.W., Vogelstein, B., Bettegowda, C., Huso, D.L., Varterasian, M., Saha, S., Zhou, S.: Intratumoral injection of Clostridium novyi-NT spores induces antitumor responses. Sci. Transl. Med. **6**, 249ra111 (2014)

Rodríguez-García, A., Giménez-Alejandre, M., Rojas, J.J., Moreno, R., Bazan-Peregrino, M., Cascalló, M., Alemany, R.: Safety and efficacy of VCN-01, an oncolytic adenovirus combining fiber HSG-binding domain replacement with RGD and hyaluronidase expression. Clin. Cancer Res. **21**, 1406–1418 (2015)

Rommelfanger, D.M., Compte, M., Grau, M.C., Diaz, R.M., Ilett, E., Alvarez-Vallina, L., Thompson, J.M., Kottke, T.J., Melcher, A., Vile, R.G.: The efficacy versus toxicity profile of combination virotherapy and TLR immunotherapy highlights the danger of administering TLR agonists to oncolytic virus-treated mice. Mol. Ther. **21**, 348–357 (2013)

Rook, A.H., Wood, G.S., Yoo, E.K., Elenitsas, R., Kao, D.M., Sherman, M.L., Witmer, W.K., Rockwell, K.A., Shane, R.B., Lessin, S.R., Vonderheid, E.C.: Interleukin-12 therapy of cutaneous T-cell lymphoma induces lesion regression and cytotoxic T-cell responses. Blood **94**, 902–908 (1999)

Rosenfeld, M.R., Chamberlain, M.C., Grossman, S.A., Peereboom, D.M., Lesser, G.J., Batchelor, T.T., Desideri, S., Salazar, A.M., Ye, X.: A multi-institution phase II study of poly-ICLC and radiotherapy with concurrent and adjuvant temozolomide in adults with newly diagnosed glioblastoma. Neuro Oncol. **12**, 1071–1077 (2010)

Sahin, T.T., Kasuya, H., Nomura, N., Shikano, T., Yamamura, K., Gewen, T., Kanzaki, A., Fujii, T., Sugae, T., Imai, T., Nomoto, S., Takeda, S., Sugimoto, H., Kikumori, T., Kodera, Y., Nishiyama, Y., Nakao, A.: Impact of novel oncolytic virus HF10 on cellular components of the tumor microenviroment in patients with recurrent breast cancer. Cancer Gene Ther. **19**, 229–237 (2012)

Saji, H., Song, W., Furumoto, K., Kato, H., Engleman, E.G.: Systemic antitumor effect of intratumoral injection of dendritic cells in combination with local photodynamic therapy. Clin. Cancer Res. **12**, 2568–2574 (2006)

Salazar, A.M., Erlich, R.B., Mark, A., Bhardwaj, N., Herberman, R.B.: Therapeutic in situ autovaccination against solid cancers with intratumoral poly-ICLC: case report, hypothesis, and clinical trial. Cancer Immunol. Res. **2**, 720–724 (2014)

Salem, M.L., El-Naggar, S.A., Kadima, A., Gillanders, W.E., Cole, D.J.: The adjuvant effects of the toll-like receptor 3 ligand polyinosinic-cytidylic acid poly (I:C) on antigen-specific CD8+ T cell responses are partially dependent on NK cells with the induction of a beneficial cytokine milieu. Vaccine **24**, 5119–5132 (2006)

Salem, M.L., Kadima, A.N., Cole, D.J., Gillanders, W.E.: Defining the antigen-specific T-cell response to vaccination and poly(I:C)/TLR3 signaling: evidence of enhanced primary and memory CD8 T-cell responses and antitumor immunity. J. Immunother. **28**, 220–228 (2005)

Salmon, H.E.A.: Expansion and activation of CD103+ DC progenitors at the tumor site promote T cell accumulation in melanoma lesions and transform clinical response to BRAF and PD-L1 blockade. Immunity (2016) (in press)

Sangro, B., Mazzolini, G., Ruiz, J., Herraiz, M., Quiroga, J., Herrero, I., Benito, A., Larrache, J., Pueyo, J., Subtil, J.C., Olagüe, C., Sola, J., Sádaba, B., Lacasa, C., Melero, I., Qian, C., Prieto, J.: Phase I trial of intratumoral injection of an adenovirus encoding interleukin-12 for advanced digestive tumors. J. Clin. Oncol. **22**, 1389–1397 (2004)

Schuster, S.J., Neelapu, S.S., Gause, B.L., Janik, J.E., Muggia, F.M., Gockerman, J.P., Winter, J.N., Flowers, C.R., Nikcevich, D.A., Sotomayor, E.M., Mcgaughey, D.S., Jaffe, E.S., Chong, E.A., Reynolds, C.W., Berry, D.A., Santos, C.F., Popa, M.A., McCord, A.M., Kwak, L.W.: Vaccination with patient-specific tumor-derived antigen in first remission improves disease-free survival in follicular lymphoma. J. Clin. Oncol. **29**, 2787–2794 (2011)

Senzer, N.N., Kaufman, H.L., Amatruda, T., Nemunaitis, M., Reid, T., Daniels, G., Gonzalez, R., Glaspy, J., Whitman, E., Harrington, K., Goldsweig, H., Marshall, T., Love, C., Coffin, R., Nemunaitis, J.J.: Phase II clinical trial of a granulocyte-macrophage colony-stimulating factor-encoding, second-generation oncolytic herpesvirus in patients with unresectable metastatic melanoma. J. Clin. Oncol. **27**, 5763–5771 (2009)

Serrone, L., Zeuli, M., Sega, F.M., Cognetti, F.: Dacarbazine-based chemotherapy for metastatic melanoma: thirty-year experience overview. J. Exp. Clin. Cancer Res. **19**, 21–34 (2000)

Shafren, D., Quah, M., Wong, Y., Andtbacka, R.H.I., Kaufman, H.L., Au, G.G.: Combination of a novel oncolytic immunotherapeutic agent, CAVATAK (coxsackievirus A21) and immune-checkpoint blockade significantly reduces tumor growth and improves survival in an immune competent mouse melanoma model. J. Immunother. Cancer **2**, 125–P125 (2014)

Sharma, P., Allison, J.P.: The future of immune checkpoint therapy. Science **348**, 56–61 (2015)

Sharma, S., Dominguez, A.L., Hoelzinger, D.B., Lustgarten, J.: CpG-ODN but not other TLR-ligands restore the antitumor responses in old mice: the implications for vaccinations in the aged. Cancer Immunol. Immunother. **57**, 549–561 (2008)

Shortman, K., Naik, S.H.: Steady-state and inflammatory dendritic-cell development. Nat. Rev. Immunol. **7**, 19–30 (2007)

Si, Z., Hersey, P., Coates, A.S.: Clinical responses and lymphoid infiltrates in metastatic melanoma following treatment with intralesional GM-CSF. Melanoma Res. **6**, 247–255 (1996)

Siders, W.M., Garron, C., Shields, J., Kaplan, J.M.: Induction of antitumor immunity by semi-allogeneic and fully allogeneic electrofusion products of tumor cells and dendritic cells. Clin. Transl. Sci. **2**, 75–79 (2009)

Sidky, Y.A., Borden, E.C., Weeks, C.E., Reiter, M.J., Hatcher, J.F., Bryan, G.T.: Inhibition of murine tumor growth by an interferon-inducing imidazoquinolinamine. Cancer Res. **52**, 3528–3533 (1992)

Simmons, A.D., Moskalenko, M., Creson, J., Fang, J., Yi, S., Vanroey, M.J., Allison, J.P., Jooss, K.: Local secretion of anti-CTLA-4 enhances the therapeutic efficacy of a cancer immunotherapy with reduced evidence of systemic autoimmunity. Cancer Immunol. Immunother. **57**, 1263–1270 (2008)

Singh-Jasuja, H., Toes, R.E., Spee, P., Münz, C., Hilf, N., Schoenberger, S.P., Ricciardi-Castagnoli, P., Neefjes, J., Rammensee, H.G., Arnold-Schild, D., Schild, H.: Cross-presentation of glycoprotein 96-associated antigens on major histocompatibility complex class I molecules requires receptor-mediated endocytosis. J. Exp. Med. **191**, 1965–1974 (2000)

Singh, M., Khong, H., Dai, Z., Huang, X.F., Wargo, J.A., Cooper, Z.A., Vasilakos, J.P., Hwu, P., Overwijk, W.W.: Effective innate and adaptive antimelanoma immunity through localized TLR7/8 activation. J. Immunol. **193**, 4722–4731 (2014)

Slos, P., de Meyer, M., Leroy, P., Rousseau, C., Acres, B.: Immunotherapy of established tumors in mice by intratumoral injection of an adenovirus vector harboring the human IL-2 cDNA: induction of CD8(+) T-cell immunity and NK activity. Cancer Gene Ther. **8**, 321–332 (2001)

Smyth, E.C., Flavin, M., Pulitzer, M.P., Gardner, G.J., Costantino, P.D., Chi, D.S., Bogatch, K., Chapman, P.B., Wolchok, J.D., Schwartz, G.K., Carvajal, R.D.: Treatment of locally recurrent mucosal melanoma with topical imiquimod. J. Clin. Oncol. **29**, e809–e811 (2011)

Soiffer, R., Lynch, T., Mihm, M., Jung, K., Rhuda, C., Schmollinger, J.C., Hodi, F.S., Liebster, L., Lam, P., Mentzer, S., Singer, S., Tanabe, K.K., Cosimi, A.B., Duda, R., Sober, A., Bhan, A., Daley, J., Neuberg, D., Parry, G., Rokovich, J., Richards, L., Drayer, J., Berns, A., Clift, S., Cohen, L.K., Mulligan, R.C., Dranoff, G.: Vaccination with irradiated autologous melanoma cells engineered to secrete human granulocyte-macrophage colony-stimulating factor generates potent antitumor immunity in patients with metastatic melanoma. Proc. Natl. Acad. Sci. U S A **95**(22), 13141–13146 (1998)

Song, W., Levy, R.: Therapeutic vaccination against murine lymphoma by intratumoral injection of naive dendritic cells. Cancer Res. **65**, 5958–5964 (2005)

Spaner, D.E., Miller, R.L., Mena, J., Grossman, L., Sorrenti, V., Shi, Y.: Regression of lymphomatous skin deposits in a chronic lymphocytic leukemia patient treated with the Toll-like receptor-7/8 agonist, imiquimod. Leuk. Lymphoma **46**, 935–939 (2005)

Stavrakoglou, A., Brown, V.L., Coutts, I.: Successful treatment of primary cutaneous follicle centre lymphoma with topical 5 % imiquimod. Br. J. Dermatol. **157**, 620–622 (2007)

Stone, G.W., Barzee, S., Snarsky, V., Santucci, C., Tran, B., Kornbluth, R.S.: Regression of established AB1 murine mesothelioma induced by peritumoral injections of CpG oligodeoxynucleotide either alone or in combination with poly(I:C) and CD40 ligand plasmid DNA. J. Thorac. Oncol. **4**, 802–808 (2009a)

Stone, G.W., Barzee, S., Snarsky, V., Santucci, C., Tran, B., Langer, R., Zugates, G.T., Anderson, D.G., Kornbluth, R.S.: Nanoparticle-delivered multimeric soluble CD40L DNA combined with Toll-Like Receptor agonists as a treatment for melanoma. PLoS One **4**, e7334 (2009b)

Suchin, K.R., Junkins-Hopkins, J.M., Rook, A.H.: Treatment of stage IA cutaneous T-Cell lymphoma with topical application of the immune response modifier imiquimod. Arch. Dermatol. **138**, 1137–1139 (2002)

Suresh, M., Whitmire, J.K., Harrington, L.E., Larsen, C.P., Pearson, T.C., Altman, J.D., Ahmed, R.: Role of CD28-B7 interactions in generation and maintenance of CD8 T cell memory. J. Immunol. **167**, 5565–5573 (2001)

Tan, G., Kasuya, H., Sahin, T.T., Yamamura, K., Wu, Z., Koide, Y., Hotta, Y., Shikano, T., Yamada, S., Kanzaki, A., Fujii, T., Sugimoto, H., Nomoto, S., Nishikawa, Y., Tanaka, M., Tsurumaru, N., Kuwahara, T., Fukuda, S., Ichinose, T., Kikumori, T., Takeda, S., Nakao, A., Kodera, Y.: Combination therapy of oncolytic herpes simplex virus HF10 and bevacizumab against experimental model of human breast carcinoma xenograft. Int. J. Cancer **136**, 1718–30 (2015)

Thaker, P.H., Brady, W.E., Bradley, W.H., Anwer, K., Alvarez, R.D.: Phase I study of intraperitoneal IL-12 plasmid formulated with PEG-PEI-cholesterol lipopolymer administered in combination with pegylated liposomal doxorubicin in recurrent or persistent epithelial ovarian, Fallopian tube, or primary peritoneal cancer patients: an NRG/GOG study. J. Clin. Oncol. (Meeting Abstracts) **33**(Suppl; abstr 5541) (2015)

Timmerman, J.M., Czerwinski, D.K., Davis, T.A., Hsu, F.J., Benike, C., Hao, Z.M., Taidi, B., Rajapaksa, R., Caspar, C.B., Okada, C.Y., van Beckhoven, A., Liles, T.M., Engleman, E.G., Levy, R.: Idiotype-pulsed dendritic cell vaccination for B-cell lymphoma: clinical and immune responses in 35 patients. Blood **99**, 1517–1526 (2002)

Toda, M., Martuza, R.L., Kojima, H., Rabkin, S.D.: In situ cancer vaccination: an IL-12 defective vector/replication-competent herpes simplex virus combination induces local and systemic antitumor activity. J. Immunol. **160**, 4457–4464 (1998)

Todo, T., Martuza, R.L., Dallman, M.J., Rabkin, S.D.: In situ expression of soluble B7-1 in the context of oncolytic herpes simplex virus induces potent antitumor immunity. Cancer Res. **61**, 153–161 (2001)

Tong, Y., Song, W., Crystal, R.G.: Combined intratumoral injection of bone marrow-derived dendritic cells and systemic chemotherapy to treat pre-existing murine tumors. Cancer Res. **61**, 7530–7535 (2001)

Tumeh, P.C., Harview, C.L., Yearley, J.H., Shintaku, I.P., Taylor, E.J., Robert, L., Chmielowski, B., Spasic, M., Henry, G., Ciobanu, V., West, A.N., Carmona, M., Kivork, C., Seja, E., Cherry, G., Gutierrez, A.J., Grogan, T.R., Mateus, C., Tomasic, G., Glaspy, J.A., Emerson, R.O., Robins, H., Pierce, R.H., Elashoff, D.A., Robert, C., Ribas, A.: PD-1 blockade induces responses by inhibiting adaptive immune resistance. Nature **515**, 568–571 (2014)

Tuve, S., Chen, B.M., Liu, Y., Cheng, T.L., Toure, P., Sow, P.S., Feng, Q., Kiviat, N., Strauss, R., Ni, S., Li, Z.Y., Roffler, S.R., Lieber, A.: Combination of tumor site-located CTL-associated antigen-4 blockade and systemic regulatory T-cell depletion induces tumor-destructive immune responses. Cancer Res. **67**, 5929–5939 (2007)

Upadhyay, R., Hammerich, L., Peng, P., Brown, B., Merad, M., Brody, J.D.: Lymphoma: immune evasion strategies. Cancers (Basel) **7**, 736–762 (2015)

Varghese, S., Rabkin, S.D., Liu, R., Nielsen, P.G., Ipe, T., Martuza, R.L.: Enhanced therapeutic efficacy of IL-12, but not GM-CSF, expressing oncolytic herpes simplex virus for transgenic mouse derived prostate cancers. Cancer Gene Ther. **13**, 253–265 (2006)

Vom Berg, J., Vrohlings, M., Haller, S., Haimovici, A., Kulig, P., Sledzinska, A., Weller, M., Becher, B.: Intratumoral IL-12 combined with CTLA-4 blockade elicits T cell-mediated glioma rejection. J. Exp. Med. **210**, 2803–2811 (2013)

Vonderheide, R.H., Glennie, M.J.: Agonistic CD40 antibodies and cancer therapy. Clin. Cancer Res. **19**, 1035–1043 (2013)

Voskens, C.J., Goldinger, S.M., Loquai, C., Robert, C., Kaehler, K.C., Berking, C., Bergmann, T., Bockmeyer, C.L., Eigentler, T., Fluck, M., Garbe, C., Gutzmer, R., Grabbe, S., Hauschild, A., Hein, R., Hundorfean, G., Justich, A., Keller, U., Klein, C., Mateus, C., Mohr, P., Paetzold, S., Satzger, I., Schadendorf, D., Schlaeppi, M., Schuler, G., Schuler-Thurner, B., Trefzer, U., Ulrich, J., Vaubel, J., von Moos, R., Weder, P., Wilhelm, T., Göppner, D., Dummer, R., Heinzerling, L.M.: The price of tumor control: an analysis of rare side effects of anti-CTLA-4 therapy in metastatic melanoma from the ipilimumab network. PLoS One **8**, e53745 (2013)

Wallgren, A.C., Andersson, B., Backer, A., Karlsson-Parra, A.: Direct allorecognition promotes activation of bystander dendritic cells and licenses them for Th1 priming: a functional link between direct and indirect allosensitization. Scand. J. Immunol. **62**, 234–242 (2005)

Wang, C., Dai, Z., Fan, R., Deng, Y., Lv, G., Lu, G.: HSF1 overexpression enhances oncolytic effect of replicative adenovirus. J. Transl. Med. **8**, 44 (2010)

Weide, B., Derhovanessian, E., Pflugfelder, A., Eigentler, T.K., Radny, P., Zelba, H., Pföhler, C., Pawelec, G., Garbe, C.: High response rate after intratumoral treatment with interleukin-2: results from a phase 2 study in 51 patients with metastasized melanoma. Cancer **116**, 4139–4146 (2010)

Won, E.K., Zahner, M.C., Grant, E.A., Gore, P., Chicoine, M.R.: Analysis of the antitumoral mechanisms of lipopolysaccharide against glioblastoma multiforme. Anticancer Drugs **14**, 457–466 (2003)

Wood, C., Srivastava, P., Bukowski, R., Lacombe, L., Gorelov, A.I., Gorelov, S., Mulders, P., Zielinski, H., Hoos, A., Teofilovici, F., Isakov, L., Flanigan, R., Figlin, R., Gupta, R., Escudier, B., C-100-12 RCC Study Group: An adjuvant autologous therapeutic vaccine (HSPPC-96; vitespen) versus observation alone for patients at high risk of recurrence after nephrectomy for renal cell carcinoma: a multicentre, open-label, randomised phase III trial. Lancet **372**, 145–154 (2008)

Wu, C.Y., Monie, A., Pang, X., Hung, C.F., Wu, T.C.: Improving therapeutic HPV peptide-based vaccine potency by enhancing CD4+ T help and dendritic cell activation. J. Biomed. Sci. **17**, 88 (2010)

Yizhi, Y., Xuetao, C., Hong, L., Quanxing, W., Qun, T.: The therapeutic effect of intratumoral injection of GM-CSF gene-modified allogenic macrophages on tumor-bearing mice. Chin. J. Cancer Res. **10**, 1–5 (1998)

Zamarin, D., Holmgaard, R.B., Subudhi, S.K., Park, J.S., Mansour, M., Palese, P., Merghoub, T., Wolchok, J.D., Allison, J.P.: Localized oncolytic virotherapy overcomes systemic tumor resistance to immune checkpoint blockade immunotherapy. Sci. Transl. Med. **6**, 226ra32 (2014)

Zapała, Ł., Wolny, R., Wachowska, M., Jakóbisiak, M., Lasek, W.: Synergistic antitumor effect of JAWSII dendritic cells and interleukin 12 in a melanoma mouse model. Oncol. Rep. **29**, 1208–1214 (2013)

Zhang, H., Liu, L., Yu, D., Kandimalla, E.R., Sun, H.B., Agrawal, S., Guha, C.: An in situ autologous tumor vaccination with combined radiation therapy and TLR9 agonist therapy. PLoS One **7**, e38111 (2012)

Zhang, W., Fulci, G., Wakimoto, H., Cheema, T.A., Buhrman, J.S., Jeyaretna, D.S., Stemmer Rachamimov, A.O., Rabkin, S.D., Martuza, R.L.: Combination of oncolytic herpes simplex viruses armed with angiostatin and IL-12 enhances antitumor efficacy in human glioblastoma models. Neoplasia **15**, 591–599 (2013)

Zhu, J., Huang, X., Yang, Y.: Innate immune response to adenoviral vectors is mediated by both Toll-like receptor-dependent and -independent pathways. J. Virol. **81**, 3170–3180 (2007a)

Zhu, X., Fallert-Junecko, B.A., Fujita, M., Ueda, R., Kohanbash, G., Kastenhuber, E.R., McDonald, H.A., Liu, Y., Kalinski, P., Reinhart, T.A., Salazar, A.M., Okada, H.: Poly-ICLC promotes the infiltration of effector T cells into intracranial gliomas via induction of CXCL10 in IFN-alpha and IFN-gamma dependent manners. Cancer Immunol. Immunother. **59**, 1401–1409 (2010)

Zhu, X., Nishimura, F., Sasaki, K., Fujita, M., Dusak, J.E., Eguchi, J., Fellows-Mayle, W., Storkus, W.J., Walker, P.R., Salazar, A.M., Okada, H.: Toll like receptor-3 ligand poly-ICLC promotes the efficacy of peripheral vaccinations with tumor antigen-derived peptide epitopes in murine CNS tumor models. J. Transl. Med. **5**, 10 (2007b)

Chapter 7
Novel Targets and Their Assessment for Cancer Treatment

Sheila Ranganath and AnhCo Nguyen

1 Drug Discovery in I/O: Can the Promise Become Reality?

There are many excellent scientific reviews on the role of the immune checkpoint (please refer to Dranoff 2013; Topalian et al. 2015; Sharma and Allison 2015) in human disease. Recent clinical results using modulators of two of these immune checkpoint proteins highlight the promise of immune modulation as a means to treat cancer. But the rapid emergence of many novel targets in the immune oncology space is outpacing the ability to validate and test the effects of their modulation, either as monotherapy or in combination, leading to the following question moving forward: Do we understand the biology with sufficient depth to enable meaningful new treatment regimens?

This review intends to address how novel targets from I/O can be evaluated and then describe methods to assess them for cancer drug discovery and development using integrated profiling that is different from current methods used to evaluate either the biology of the targets or the clinical response to existing checkpoint blockade therapeutics.

Recent oncology drug discovery has focused on tumor-specific targets that have been identified by genomics, genetic screens, or overexpression in clinical samples (Stock et al. 2015). Drug candidates that engage the target are then advanced into preclinical models, which may or may not have translational value for predicting efficacy in human patients. Composite preclinical models using immune-deficient host animals and implanted tumors (xenografts), from cell lines or patients, lack the clarity of defined genetic models such as yeast, the fly, or the worm, but do represent the multiclonal nature of adult human cancer (Budhu et al. 2014). However,

S. Ranganath, Ph.D. • A. Nguyen, Ph.D. (✉)
Enumeral Inc., Cambridge, MA, USA
e-mail: cokey@enumeral.com

P.D. Rennert (ed.), *Novel Immunotherapeutic Approaches to the Treatment of Cancer*, DOI 10.1007/978-3-319-29827-6_7

these models were not predictive for any of the multiple mechanisms of tumor resistance which are observed in the clinic. The regulatory pathways of gene expression in normal embryonic growth and abnormal malignant growth in transformed cells have fine distinctions, and the redundant pathways for cell signaling are difficult to effectively and permanently target (Aparicio et al. 2015; Gacche 2015). The industry has struggled in trying to effectively and durably target these oncogenic signaling pathways (Fig. 7.1). With a few notable exceptions, the "magic bullet" to specifically target tumors has failed to deliver cures in most oncology treatment settings.

The recent positive clinical experience with immuno-oncology agents is beginning to redefine the pathway for how drugs are discovered and developed for cancer treatment. One could argue that historically, treatment with drugs that targeted cellular oncogenic mechanisms demonstrated robust initial responsiveness, but the required repeated treatment invoked the inevitable resistance mechanisms (Ercan et al. 2015). These mechanisms that transformed cells employ to assure their survival have been so varied and numerous as to confer resistance to classical DNA-damaging agents, mAbs, and kinase inhibitors. Virtually all treatments, including radiation therapy (XRT), can be thwarted by the ability of malignant cells to ultimately recover and survive. The role of curative or adjuvant therapy has been established only where there is minimal residual disease after debulking.

The immune system has always been of great interest in oncology, mainly because of provocative reports of spontaneous regression of various pediatric cancers, as well as adult melanoma and renal cell tumors (Chan and Wolchok 2015). In melanoma, attempts to elicit long-term durable responses (that may lead eventually to cures) justified allowing riskier assets into drug development pipelines. As opposed to earlier oncology drug discovery assets, programs with less convincing preclinical models were advanced. Anti-CTLA-4 (Yervoy) and anti-PD-1 antibodies (Opdivo and Keytruda) showed relatively modest efficacy in preclinical mouse

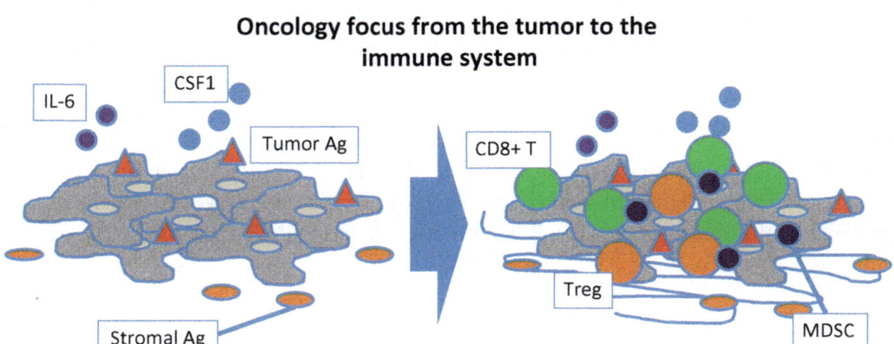

Fig. 7.1 Immune oncology focuses on immuno-modulation and targeting immune cell function (*right*) which is a paradigm shift from tumor-specific targets and tumor-associated growth factors (*left*)

models. However, the clinical trial data shows that these indeed are the first class of antitumor agents which have demonstrated efficacy paired with durable responses. Most importantly, these agents work in late-stage metastatic cancer patients who have become refractory following many rounds of prior treatments (Hodi et al. 2010; Schadendorf et al. 2015; Weber et al. 2015). While these agents appear to work only in subsets of patients, they are and will be the anchor for cancer treatment in the future, likely nucleating combination therapies when paired with other therapeutic modalities such as radiation or chemotherapy.

With the expansion of cancer-focused drug discovery to include immune-oncology, there is even greater need to understand how these targets are different and why immunomodulation might have failed in the past. There are many reasons for why I/O assets had been de-emphasized as early studies with anti-CD3 (OKT3) or exogenous IL-2 and IL-12 were met with very limited clinical benefit yet many serious adverse events (Dhir et al. 2012; Brady et al. 2014; Young et al. 2014).

The potential for safety issues unique to the human population with immune modulation was magnified by the TGN-1412 phase 1 trial of an anti-CD28 monoclonal antibody, where the entire patient cohort in the Phase 1 experienced severe organ damage from cytokine release syndrome causing cardiovascular shock within hours of infusion (Eastwood et al. 2013). Conversely, tumor lysate vaccines, peptide vaccines, and exogenous priming of antigen-presenting cells (APCs), while so far reported as very safe even with long-term administration, also have not demonstrated remarkable survival benefit in clinical phase trials, presumably because they are not eliciting strong enough immune responses (Butterfield 2015). One exception to this is Provenge, (sipuleucel T), a dendritic cell vaccine therapy which was approved for commercial use for advanced prostate cancer in the USA (Strauss et al. 2015).

For novel targets in cancer drug discovery, many now embrace the notion that the immune system "is" the drug. Therapeutic agents which can modulate or augment the immune system may be the new foundation for antitumor therapies whether alone, in sequence, or in combination with cytotoxic drugs and radiation, to debulk tumor mass and expose tumor neoantigens to the immune system, and tumor vaccines which will target the tumor in vivo for the immune response (Binder et al. 2015).

2 Lessons from the Clinic: How I/O Targets Are Different

New clinical studies of drugs that modify epigenetics, tumor metabolism, and immune oncology are demonstrating overall response rates (ORR), progression-free survival (PFS), and overall survival (OS) data that are presenting clinicians with new ways to select subsets of patients, and combat various types of cancers. The clinical data from epigenetics- and tumor metabolism-based therapeutics, while promising, is still early. Concerns about resistance and durability of response will only be answered in larger clinical trials. However, there is enough data from I/O drug trials demonstrating remarkable durable benefit to patients. These studies suggest that our understanding of the biology associated with the immune system requires a subtle shift in how we confirm the relevance of new targets. With the good (re: efficacy), there is also the bad (re: safety): immune-modulatory drugs come with the liability of greatly increased systemic autoimmunity. Cytotoxic and even cytostatic chemotherapy agents are known to affect all rapidly dividing cells, and have toxicity profiles that include all renewable cell populations. Drugs that interfere with constitutive cell pathways, such as TKIs, also have both on-target and off-target effects, such as general gastrointestinal toxicity (Welsh and Corrie 2015). On the other hand, I/O drugs have demonstrated a less predictable and somewhat more widespread pattern of toxicity that has been termed "immune-related serious adverse events (irSAEs)." While on-mechanism, this set of side effects can limit treatment, and in the case of Yervoy (anti-CTLA-4) this has meant treatment discontinuation. As much promise as I/O drugs have for unmet need in cancer, more effort is needed to identify why patients do respond/do not respond as well how to create more selective drugs that may limit as toxic autoimmunity in the intent-to-treat patient (ITT) cohorts.

Next-generation target identification/selection, i.e., novel I/O targets, should seek the same/better efficacy of the first-generation therapeutics. At the same time, it is essential to understand potential irSAEs in humans. In comparison with recent "targeted therapy" development which has been guided by precision medicines aimed at specific oncogenes or specific mutations in oncogenes (Chong and Jänne 2013), I/O drug discovery seeks to (1) increase antigenicity of tumors (e.g., increase cross-presentation), (2) attenuate immunosuppressive factors (e.g., checkpoint blockade), or (3) activate the immune system (e.g., co-receptor agonism) (Table 7.1).

The biggest challenge for novel targets in I/O drug discovery is how to understand immune-checkpoint targets and to be able to predict how these drugs will work in humans—before infusion of drug into a human patient. Current preclinical models for I/O are not yet sufficiently developed to accurately reflect how I/O therapeutics modulate immune effector cell activity in humans (Gould et al. 2015; Budhu et al. 2015). Ideally, a robust preclinical model for immunotherapy would contain appropriately selected human immune cells and allow for prediction of efficacy and adverse events. Recent data suggests that graft-versus-host disease may still

Table 7.1 Targets in immune-oncology drug discovery

Blockade	Agonism
PD-1	OX40
LAG3	CD137
TIM-3	CD40
CTLA-4	ICOS
KIR2DL	GITR
TIGIT	2B4
VISTA	CD27
CEACAM1	CD40L

Chen and Mellman (2013), Topalian et al. (2015), Lesokhin et al. (2015)

dominate preclinical models for immune-checkpoint drug discovery (Fernandez de Sanmamamed et al. 2015). Validation, therefore, should be human focused and needs to integrate the right set of tools to bridge this gap.

3 Target Validation in Immune Oncology

The era of genomics and proteomics has created even more putative targets than ever (Wei and Cleary 2014). There is an even greater imperative to be more "translation efficient": understand drug candidate efficacy with confidence before expensive proof-of-concept studies commence (Guo et al. 2013).

The promise of in silico drug development tools or big data from functional genomics that would replace murine experiments has not been realized, so target validation in small animals continues, cautiously, respectful that findings may not fully translate to disease as it is present in humans. This is particularly true for immunomodulatory drugs, where the human immune system is required to answer the first important questions in the drug discovery program. Typical questions for target validation are the following: What is the evidence for the role of the target in this disease? Is the target a driver of disease or carried along in the process of disease etiology? What would the clinical development plan be and who is in the target patient profile? Before the commitment of resourcing and significant budgeting for the drug discovery program, these questions need to be formally addressed. In-house validation has become a critical issue as clinical drug discovery failures have increased the scrutiny on early discovery efforts. Much has been written about clinical trial failure linking back to incomplete understanding of the drug mechanism of action in preclinical models (Morgan et al. 2012). Many have reported difficulties in reproducing published data (10–25 % success in industrial settings) or in the preclinical modeling of the intent-to-treat human population (Begley and Ellis 2012).

3.1 The Need for Predictive Translational Datasets

Predictive translational datasets are difficult to generate for novel targets in immune oncology. There are very few relevant preclinical models that provide an accurate recapitulation of both the human immune system and human tumors. Thus, many studies use syngeneic mouse models to validate the importance of a particular target: i.e., native mouse immune systems, murine tumor cell lines, and surrogate antibodies which recognize (mouse) checkpoint I/O targets, e.g., CTLA-4, PD-1, and TIM-3, on immune cells (Simpson et al. 2013; Latchman et al. 2001; Butte et al. 2007; Sakuishi et al. 2010). These surrogate preclinical models may miss some of the complexity of both human tumors and the human immune system.

3.2 What's Old Is New Again

For validation of "novel" immune-oncology targets for oncology drug discovery, the good news is that these targets are well characterized in immunology efforts in general. Immune-oncology targets have a long history in immune models of infection and autoimmune disorders. In fact, the term "exhaustion" comes from studies with CD8+ effector T cells in acute versus chronic viral infection (Barber et al. 2006; Odorizzi and Wherry 2012; Penaloza-MacMaster et al. 2014) in preclinical models devised to mimic infection in humans. In these studies, it is observed that regulatory T cells (expressing CTLA-4) and multiple immune checkpoint molecules, e.g., LAG3, 2B4, TIM-3, and PD-1, are involved in dampening the immune response over time. This is driven by sustained exposure to antigen over time (favoring tolerance) as well as evasion mechanisms, e.g., downregulation of MHC molecules, and recruitment of suppressor cells (Schietinger and Greenberg 2014).

3.3 First-Generation Immune Checkpoint Blockade

In clinical trials, there was sufficient durable response observed in patients leading to the rapid approval of Yervoy, a fully human anti-CTLA-4 IgG4 antibody (Hodi et al. 2010). These patients have been longitudinally followed and in some cases show a remarkable duration of response (OS > 10 years). What is not well understood is why the responses with Yervoy were limited to a subset, about 20 %, of patients (Schadendorf et al. 2015). This response differed greatly from the response rate of 80–90 % in preclinical mouse models (Fu et al. 2011; Sharma and Allison 2015). In addition, the synergistic antitumor effect of CTLA-4/PD-1 blockade in preclinical models has not been fully recapitulated in the clinic (Curran et al. 2010; Larkin et al. 2015), but the toxicity observed did translate to humans. These pioneering studies with CTLA4 checkpoint blockade emphasize the importance of translating both efficacy and safety from preclinical drug discovery to patients in the clinic.

3.4 PD-1

In contrast to CTLA-4, preclinical research focused on PD-1 did not predict the significant clinical efficacy that we now observe with PD-1 checkpoint blockade in metastatic melanomas, metastatic lung cancers (Dranoff 2013; Brahmer et al. 2015), and mismatch-repair (MMR)-deficient cancers (Le et al. 2015). Here, the preclinical models grossly underestimated the antitumor efficacy of PD-1 blockade observed in clinical trials (Sakuishi et al. 2010; Hamid et al. 2013; Robert et al. 2015). As has been observed with CTLA-4 blockade, PD-1 blockade only works in a subset of patients (10–40 %). Preclinical studies with PD-1 blockade did not predict the range or severity of irSAEs observed in some patients. Is this because of differential PD-1 expression between mice and humans (Keir et al. 2008) or deeper biological differences between mouse and human immune effector cells at the site of action? Or is the inefficiency in translational findings due to the non-physiologic nature of tumor engraftment in most preclinical models? Understanding these questions is fundamental to target validation for increasing the efficacy of anti-CTLA-4 and anti-PD-1 as well as new targets in I/O.

3.5 The Need to Understand I/O Adverse Events

While we have observed breakthroughs in efficacy and durability of response, there is also the potential liability associated with known and novel targets that can arise from immunomodulation in cancer. The safety profile of a given therapeutic is an under-emphasized aspect of drug discovery in oncology because the regulatory bar for oncology drugs is thought to be lower; that is, in meeting an unmet medical need some safety risk may be acceptable. Effective checkpoint blockade, by definition, means that adverse events may be part of the drug mechanism: these therapeutics can be lethal to patients with so-called immune-related serious adverse events (irSAEs) (Topalian et al. 2012; Kong and Flynn 2014). In clinical trials, 22 % of patients receiving ipilimumab at 10 mg/kg had grade 3/4 irSAEs. In other clinical trials, ~5–10 % of patients receiving anti-PD-1 therapy had grade 3/4 irSAEs. These drug-associated adverse events include complications such as pneumonitis, colitis, and hepatitis with a predictable pattern of kinetics (Weber et al. 2015). Durable responses also imply chronic treatment which suggests that drug-related adverse events will be increased. Safety, therefore, is a key concern in I/O drug discovery (Dranoff 2013). Biologically, this regulatory system has been selected to dampen immune responses and the data suggests that polymorphisms in checkpoint inhibitory receptors correlate with autoimmune disorders such as diabetes, multiple sclerosis, and rheumatoid arthritis (Odorizzi and Wherry 2012). In the best-case scenario, the autoimmune toxicity can be predicted accurately from preclinical models, e.g., CTLA-4 (Tivol et al. 1995; Waterhouse et al. 1995).

4 Current Tools

With the focus now on teasing out meaningful data from human-based samples, it is now worth exploring the current tools used to inform drug discovery. Current target discovery and validation tools can be split into routine tools versus tools still in development. The distinction is important with regard to the ability of a scientist to use something off the shelf versus a platform technology which still requires expert operators.

4.1 The Right Dataset Matters

Recent data examining response and non-response after treatment with checkpoint blockade are excellent training sets for what is possible to glean from human-based sampling and have generated intriguing results (Carthon et al. 2010). These studies, using state-of-the-art tools, hint at how checkpoint blockade works mechanistically in the tumor microenvironment. Simply put, there are no better translational datasets available than ones from current clinical trials. The heterogeneity of human biology is already taken into account, sampling can be done pre- and post-treatment, and patient samples can be annotated by responsiveness and disease staging (Kitano et al. 2013; Sivendran et al. 2014).

Using high-resolution immunohistochemistry (IHC) (Tumeh et al. 2014), next-generation sequencing (NGS) (Rizvi et al. 2015), or high-throughput multi-plex fluorescence-activated cell sorting (FACS) combined with NGS (Kwong et al. 2015; Cooper et al. 2014) investigators are attacking the problem of how to identify biomarkers for response to checkpoint blockade. For PD-1-targeted therapies, in particular, this issue has been problematic because of the inability to rely upon PD-L1 (PD-1 ligand) as a consistent stratifying marker for responsiveness—in some cases PD-L1 expression clearly correlates with response (Topalian et al. 2012; Powles et al. 2014; Carbognin et al. 2015). But there are large studies which also demonstrate clinical benefit in patient cohorts that are PD-L1 negative by IHC (Herbst et al. 2014).

4.2 Response Markers

The unreliability of using PD-L1 as a biomarker for responsiveness means one must turn to deeper biology as the source for answers (Schumacher et al. 2015; Awad and Hammerman 2015). For CTLA-4-based therapy, robust data identified ICOS by gene expression and then confirmed increased ICOS expression by FACS in Yervoy-treated patients (Ng Tang et al. 2013). For PD-1-based therapies, several significant papers in the past year have addressed responsiveness and biomarker utility. CD8 T cell infiltrate, for example, correlates better with response to PD-1 blockade than tumor-based PD-L1 positivity in metastatic melanoma patients (Tumeh et al. 2014). NGS efforts suggest that there is a correlation between tumor mutation burden and potential immunogenicity for checkpoint blockade (Rizvi et al. 2015; Schumacher and Schreiber 2015). This concept has empirical support, based on recently published data, once again using NGS (whole-exome sequencing) that suggests that mismatch-repair-deficient tumors are significantly more responsive to PD1 checkpoint blockade (40 % ORR, 78 % PFS) compared with mismatch-repair-proficient tumors (0 % ORR, 11 % PFS) (Le et al. 2015). This clinical study with mismatch-repair-deficient tumor patients is the validation of an elegant IHC-based evaluation of microsatellite instability (MSI) in primary colorectal cancer. Here the authors demonstrated expression of multiple checkpoint proteins, PD-1, PD-L1, CTLA-4, LAG3, and IDO, in MSI but not microsatellite-stable (MSS) tumors (Llosa et al. 2015). These mismatch-repair status findings lend credence to the notion that tumor genotype can inform clinicians about the TME with regard to checkpoint blockade.

These initial findings build a fundamental understanding as to how checkpoint blockade therapeutics might work. But they also beg for more insights. While tumor-infiltrating lymphocytes (TILs) might correlate with responsiveness, what are these cells doing? Are all the infiltrating T cells tumor antigen specific? Are they all effector cells? Similarly, while tumor mutational burden can correlate with response to checkpoint blockade, there are notable examples of tumor types with "low" mutational burden that are paradoxically responsive to checkpoint blockade, e.g., renal cell carcinoma (RCC) (Brahmer et al. 2012; Topalian et al. 2012; McDermott et al. 2015). Lastly, if mismatch-deficient tumors are ~5–10% of all tumors (Peltomäki 2003), how can we better address the ~90% of mismatch-proficient tumors in patients? Integration of newer tools may aid in answering these questions.

5 Integration: Integrated Profiling at the Single-Cell Level

Because there are still looming questions, e.g., drug mechanism related or target biology related, that need to be answered the drug discovery toolkit needs to evolve to meet the challenge of understanding the human biology of cancer. For many large clinical trials and associated clinical sample studies, simpler and less costly bulk measurements (automated IHC, FACS, bulk NGS) may enable an initial understanding of clinical correlates for response/non-response (Fig. 7.2). However, the knowledge gap from genetically engineered mouse models (GEMMs) to observations from clinical studies is still sufficiently large that we still struggle to obtain a facile understanding of clinical response, let alone clinical non-response to therapeutic drugs (Sharma and Allison 2015).

5.1 FACS as the Standard

One part of the answer may be to augment standard clinical pathology laboratory outputs such as IHC, FACS, or bulk biopsy genomics with single-cell measurements (Chattopadhyay et al. 2014). As these standard analytical platforms report the average response of a heterogeneous population of cell types, these approaches are ill suited for both sensitivity and accuracy (signal to noise) and lost in bulk measurement is the contribution of rare effector cells such as T cells, NK cells, or B cells. Even with polychromatic flow cytometry (Perfetto et al. 2004) which can exceed 17 independent measurements, it is clear that even examining T cells in bulk cannot adequately classify different types of effector T cells, e.g., naïve, central memory, effector cells (Chattopadyay et al. 2006).

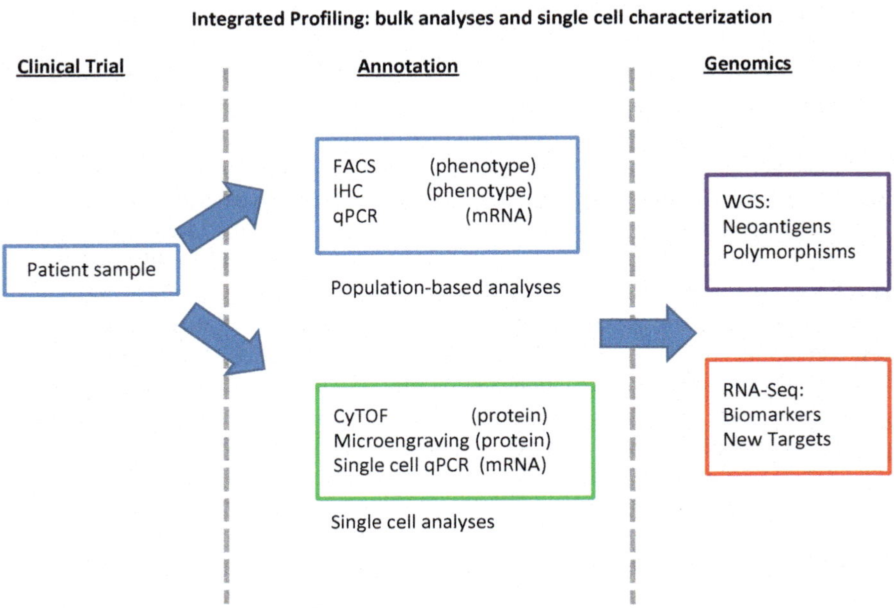

Fig. 7.2 Immune-oncology drug discovery requires a human sample-focused approach with integrated profiling: assessment of rare effector cell types at the single-cell level with functional data to then provide annotation for genomics-based data

5.2 *Mass Spectrometry*

An extension of FACS, which may provide more complete information at the level of the single cell, is to use single cell-based mass spectrometric methods (Bendall et al. 2011). This platform, which is commercially available as the CyTOF platform (Fluidigm), pairs an ability to capture 135 detection channels with more than 40 markers per cell (Bodenmiller et al. 2012). As this platform continues to improve, it may provide tremendous insight into the intracellular-based signaling processes in target cells. One drawback may be loss of genomic information, but pairing a parallel study with a genomics component can potentially augment this.

5.3 *NGS*

The pace at which single-cell genomics has progressed in the past year has been prodigious and a number of approaches have been suggested for leveraging these new methods. While whole-genome sequencing (WGS) of single cells is becoming more commonplace, there are still issues with accuracy and efficiency of genome coverage (Wills and Mead 2015; Zhang et al. 2015). More promising than WGS may be capturing the dynamic RNA-based transcriptome of a single cell isolated from a physiologic patient sample. PCR-based methods to interrogate information for a single cell are widely available (Veldman-Jones et al. 2015). Nanostring-based studies may allow for robust interrogation of RNA following whole-transcriptome-wide sampling. RNA-Seq-based methods have just been published (Macosko et al. 2015; Klein et al. 2015) using droplet-based platform technology, to overcome the limitations of throughput with microfluidics-based or FACS-based single-cell isolation (Moonsamy et al. 2013). These so-called single-cell RNA-Seq (scRNA-Seq) methodologies have uncovered cellular phenotypes that were previously masked by other analytical approaches: new subsets of dendritic cells (Shalek et al. 2013) and novel cell types in retinal development (Macosko et al. 2015). These types of insights could also provide tremendous insight into the dynamics of cells in the TME in response to checkpoint blockade therapy. scRNA-Seq is continually evolving for improved sensitivity (RNA abundance 10–50 transcripts per cell are problematic), but it may be limited by differential expression bias of RNAs in the cell: i.e., the most abundant 1.5 % RNAs account for 43 % of the mapped reads while the least abundant 44 % of RNAs account for 1 % of the reads (Picelli et al. 2014; Grün et al. 2014; Jiang et al. 2011).

5.4 Microengraving

Another platform, which combines proteomics, cell surface marker staining, and genomics, is a platform employing the use of subnanoliter well arrays (Chattopadhyay et al. 2014; Tsioris et al. 2014). This process, called microengraving, isolates single cells in a subnanoliter chamber contained on an ordered array that then enables the capture of secreted cellular products (e.g., cytokines, granzyme B) as well as an ability to assign a cellular surface staining-based phenotype of the respective secreting cell is (e.g., CD3+, CD56+, MHC II+) followed by single-cell recovery for genomics applications (Fig. 7.3). This platform approach not only complements genomics-based studies, but also FACS-based studies. There are few other methods with the ability to link genotype with functionality of rare cells, such as TILs, in paucicellular samples (<50,000 cells) (Zhou et al. 2014). Such a capability forms the basis for potentially bridging the knowledge gap between preclinical and human datasets discussed above.

5.5 Integration and Response Markers

Using the three key examples to date for immune checkpoint responsiveness—(1) increased CD8 T cell infiltrate, (2) upregulation of markers such as ICOS, and (3) mismatch-repair-deficient tumor responsiveness—how could these findings be explored further? Ideally, new efforts should address (1) the precise function of the CD8 T cell infiltrate, (2) the significance of ICOS expression with respect to T cell function, or (3) in the TME from mismatch-repair-deficient tumors what other cell types are present and what are the roles of these cells?

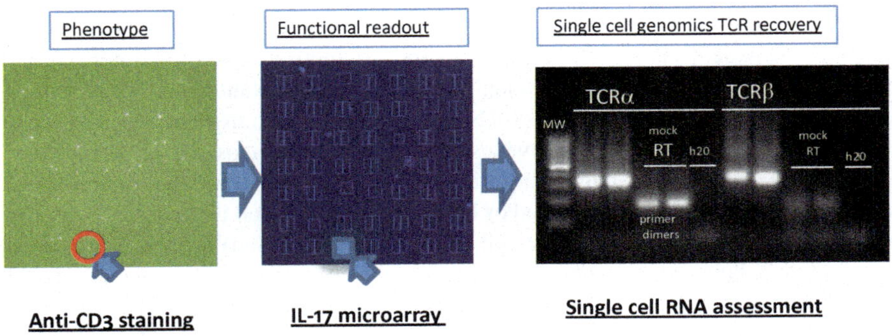

Fig. 7.3 Microengraving is an example of single-cell integrated profiling: cells are loaded at a density that favor single cell per well loading, stained for cell surface markers (*left*), assessed for cytokine secretion (*middle*), and isolated from the subnanoliter well array for single-cell genomics (*right*)

With primary samples from stratified patient cohorts, we can then begin to answer what the aforementioned immune correlates signify for drug discovery and development. Of the TILs present at the margin of a tumor, how many are cytolytic versus exhausted? In ICOS+ T cells, how does this correlate to increased immune cell function in the TME? In mismatch-repair-deficient tumors, what "other" immune cells are present? Are they secreting immunosuppressive cytokines or inflammatory cytokines attracting immunosuppressive cells? These questions can be addressed then, at the single-cell level, when functional analysis can be matched with genomics. A logical extension of this premise is that the understanding of functional cellular interactions in the TME can also begin to unravel the complex and heterogeneous problem of clinical non-response. These studies add impetus to the therapeutic goals of (a) increasing the efficacy and durability elicited by therapeutics in responsive tumors and (b) converting non-responsive tumors (Sharma and Allison 2015). This can be approached therapeutically with the right staging of treatment, such as a regimen of a priming agent such as anti-CTLA4 treatment followed by a checkpoint blockade agent such as anti-PD-1 treatment (as concurrent treatment seems toxic) (Twyman-Saint Victor et al. 2015). But to understand the right therapeutic combination as well as the mechanism of converting refractory patients into responsive patients will require knowledge currently just out of our grasp.

5.6 *Power of Human*

Engaging with clinicians at the frontlines of cancer treatment early and often, combined with the new integrated toolkit of immune oncology, shortens the path to finding efficacy for cancer patients. It is clear that studying the immune system in relation to cancer biology is difficult in preclinical models. The consensus from the literature is that the complexity of human immunology and human tumor biology cannot be modeled adequately.

Combining the right biological samples with an integrated toolkit impacts (in order of importance) clinical efficacy for patients, safety predictions for patients, and next-generation drug discovery efforts. An informed approach could even repurpose approved oncology drugs with limited efficacy, such as PDGFR/VEGFR inhibitors such as sunitinib to predict how they can be used with immune-oncology therapeutics (Amin and Lockhart 2015). These proposed studies could also inform how tumor vaccination or abscopal radiation methods could prime the immune system for checkpoint blockade (Twyman-Saint Victor et al. 2015). Integrated profiling may also be able to in the near future assess nascent autoimmunity, so that combination checkpoint blockade trials can be informed beforehand about potential for irSAEs (Larkin et al. 2015). Toxicity will be an issue for most if not all checkpoint blockade therapeutics in humans, especially as we enter the era of "combinatorial immunotherapy," so this is essential for present and future clinical trials. Lastly, integrated profiling, which incorporates single-cell analysis, has a superior signal-to-noise ratio for genomics-based signatures over historical bulk genomics (Kumar et al. 2014). This is a more promising avenue for target discovery and validation in humans.

While newly approved I/O agents have groundbreaking durable responses in patient subsets (10–40 %), there are still 60–90 % of patients who remain unresponsive. There is work yet to be done on determining the reasons for unresponsiveness before the word "cure" can be used—it should include all patients afflicted with cancer.

References

Aparicio, L.A., Blanco, M., Castosa, R., Concha, A., Valladares, M., Calvo, L., Fiqueroa, A.: Clinical implications of epithelial cell plasticity in cancer progression. Cancer Lett. **336**, 1–10 (2015)

Awad, M.M., Hammerman, P.S.: Durable responses with PD-1 inhibition in lung and kidney cancer and the ongoing search for predictive biomarkers. J. Clin. Oncol. **33**, 1993–1994 (2015)

Amin, M., Lockhart, A.C.: The potential role of immunotherapy to treat colorectal cancer. Expert Opin. Investig. Drugs **24**(3), 329–344 (2015). doi:10.1517/13543784.2015.985376. Epub 2014 Dec 17

Barber, D.L., Wherry, E.J., Masopust, D., Zhu, B., Allison, J.P., Sharpe, A.H., Freeman, G.J., Ahmed, R.: Restoring function in exhausted CD8 T cells during chronic viral infection. Nature **439**, 682–687 (2006)

Begley, C.G., Ellis, L.M.: Drug development: raise standards for preclinical cancer research. Nature **483**, 531–533 (2012)

Bendall, S.C., Simonds, E.F., Qiu, P., Amir el-AD, Krutzik, P.O., Finck, R., Bruggner, R.V., Melamed, R., Trejo, A., Ornatsky, O.I., Balderas, R.S., Plevritis, S.K., Sachs, K., Pe'er, D., Nolan, G.P.: Single-cell mass cytometry of differential immune and drug responses across a human hematopoietic continuum. Science **332**, 687–696 (2011)

Binder, D.C., Fu, Y.X., Weichselbaum, R.R.: Radiotherapy and immune checkpoint blockade: potential interactions and future directions. Trends Mol. Med. **21**, 463–465 (2015)

Bodenmiller, B., Zunder, E.R., Finck, R., Chen, T.J., Savig, E.S., Bruggner, R.V., Simonds, E.F., Bendall, S.C., Sachs, K., Krutzik, P.O., Nolan, G.P.: Multiplexed mass cytometry profiling of cellular states perturbed by small-molecule regulators. Nat. Biotechnol. **30**, 858–867 (2012)

Brahmer, J.R., Tykodi, S.S., Chow, L.Q., Hwu, W.J., Topalian, S.L., Hwu, P., Drake, C.G., Camacho, L.H., Kauh, J., Odunsi, K., Pitot, H.C., Hamid, O., Bhatia, S., Martins, R., Eaton, K., Chen, S., Salay, T.M., Alaparthy, S., Grosso, J.F., Korman, A.J., Parker, S.M., Agrawal, S., Goldberg, S.M., Pardoll, D.M., Gupta, A., Wigginton, J.M.: Safety and activity of anti-PD-L1 antibody in patients with advanced cancer. N. Engl. J. Med. **366**(26), 2455–2465 (2012). doi:10.1056/NEJMoa1200694. Epub 2012 Jun 2

Brady, J.L., Harrison, L.C., Goodman, D.J., Cowan, P.J., Hawthorne, W.J., O'Connell, P.J., Sutherland, R.M., Lew, A.M.: Preclinical screening for acute toxicity of therapeutic monoclonal antibodies in a hu-SCID model. Clin. Transl. Immunol. **3**, e29 (2014)

Brahmer, J., Reckamp, K.L., Baas, P., Crinò, L., Eberhardt, W.E., Poddubskaya, E., Antonia, S., Pluzanski, A., Vokes, E.E., Holgado, E., Waterhouse, D., Ready, N., Gainor, J., Arén Frontera, O., Havel, L., Steins, M., Garassino, M.C., Aerts, J.G., Domine, M., Paz-Ares, L., Reck, M., Baudelet, C., Harbison, C.T., Lestini, B., Spigel, D.R.: N. Engl. J. Med. **373**, 123–135 (2015)

Budhu, S., Wolchok, J., Merghoub, T.: The importance of animal models in tumor immunity and immunotherapy. Curr. Opin. Genet. Dev. **24**, 46–51 (2014). doi:10.1016/j.gde.2013.11.008. Epub 2013 Dec 29

Budhu, S., Wolchok, J., Merghoub, T.: The importance of animal models in tumor immunity and immunotherapy. Curr. Opin. Genet. Dev. **24**, 46–51 (2014)

Butte, M.J., Keir, M.E., Phamduy, T.B., Sharpe, A.H., Freeman, G.J.: Programmed death-1 ligand 1 interacts specifically with the B7-1 costimulatory molecule to inhibit T cell responses. Immunity **27**, 111–122 (2007)

Butterfield, L.H.: Cancer vaccines. Br. Med. J. **350**, h988 (2015)

Carbognin, L., Pilotto, S., Milella, M., Vaccaro, V., Brunelli, M., Caliò, A., Cuppone, F., Sperduti, I., Giannarelli, D., Chilosi, M., Bronte, V., Scarpa, A., Bria, E., Tortora, G.: PLoS One **10**, e0130142 (2015)

Carthon, B.C., Wolchok, J.D., Yuan, J., Kamat, A., Ng Tang, D.S., Sun, J., Ku, G., Troncoso, P., Logothetis, C.J., Allison, J.P., Sharma, P.: Preoperative CTLA-4 blockade: tolerability and immune monitoring in the setting of a presurgical clinical trial. Clin. Cancer Res. **16**, 2861–2871 (2010)

Chattopadhyay, P.K., Price, D.A., Harper, T.F., Betts, M.R., Yu, J., Gostick, E., Perfetto, S.P., Goepfert, P., Koup, R.A., De Rosa, S.C., Bruchez, M.P., Roederer, M.: Quantum dot semiconductor nanocrystals for immunophenotyping by polychromatic flow cytometry. Nat. Med. **12**, 972–977 (2006)

Chattopadhyay, P.K., Gierahn, T.M., Roederer, M., Love, J.C.: Single-cell technologies for monitoring immune systems. Nat. Immunol. **15**, 128–135 (2014)

Chan, T.A., Wolchok, J.D., Snyder, A.: Genetic basis for clinical response to CTLA-4 blockade in melanoma. N. Engl. J. Med. **373**(20), 1984 (2015). doi:10.1056/NEJMc1508163

Chen, D.S., Mellman, I.: Oncology meets immunology: the cancer-immunity cycle. Immunity **39**, 1–10 (2013)

Chong, C.R., Jänne, P.A.: The quest to overcome resistance to EGFR-targeted therapies in cancer. Nat. Med. **19**, 1389–1400 (2013)

Cooper, Z.A., Reuben, A., Amaria, R.N., Wargo, J.A.: Evidence of synergy with combined BRAF-targeted therapy and immune checkpoint blockade for metastatic melanoma. Oncoimmunology **3**, e954956 (2014)

Curran, M.A., Montalvo, W., Yagita, H., Allison, J.P.: PD-1 and CTLA-4 combination blockade expands infiltrating T cells and reduces regulatory T and myeloid cells within B16 melanoma tumors. Proc. Natl. Acad. Sci. U S A **107**, 4275–4280 (2010)

Dhir, V., Fort, M., Mahmood, A., Higbee, R., Warren, W., Narayanan, P., Wittman, V.: A predictive biomimetic model of cytokine release induced by TGN1412 and other therapeutic monoclonal antibodies. J. Immunotoxicol. **9**, 34–42 (2012)

Dranoff, G.: Immunotherapy at large: balancing tumor immunity and inflammatory pathology. Nat. Med. **10**, 1100–1101 (2013)

Eastwood, D., Bird, C., Dilger, P., Hockley, J., Findlay, L., Poole, S., Thorpe, S.J., Wadhwa, M., Thorpe, R., Stebbings, R.: Severity of the TGN1412 trial disaster cytokine storm correlated with IL-2 release. Br. J. Clin. Pharmacol. **76**, 299–315 (2013)

Ercan, D., Choi, H.G., Yun, C.H., Capelletti, M., Xie, T., Eck, M.J., Gray, N.S., Janne, P.A.: EGFR mutations and resistance to Irreversible pyrimidine based EGFR inhibitors. Clin. Cancer Res. **21**, 3913–3923 (2015)

Fernandez de Sanmamamed, M., Lopez Rodriguez, I., Schalper, K.A., Onate, C., Azpilikueta, A., Rodriguez-Ruiz, M.E., Morales-Kastresana, A., Labiano, S., Perez-Gracia, J.L., Martin-Algarra, S., Alfaro, C., Mazzolini, G., Sarno, F., Hidalgo, M., Korman, A.J., Jure-Kunkel, M., Melero, I.: Nivolumab and urelumab enhance antitumor activity of human T lymphocytes engrafted in Rag2–/–IL2Rγnull immunodeficient mice. Cancer Res. **75**, 3466–3478 (2015)

Fu, T., He, Q., Sharma, P.: The ICOS/ICOSL pathway is required for optimal antitumor responses mediated by anti-CTLA-4 therapy. Cancer Res. **71**, 5445–5454 (2011)

Gacche, R.N.: Compensatory angiogenesis and tumor refractoriness. Oncogeneis **4**, e153 (2015)

Gould, S.E., Junttila, M.R., de Sauvage, F.J.: Translational value of mouse models in oncology drug development. Nat. Med. **21**, 431–439 (2015)

Grün, D., Kester, L., van Oudenaarden, A.: Validation of noise models for single-cell transcriptomics. Nat. Methods **11**, 637–640 (2014)

Guo, S., Zou, J., Wang, G.: Advances in the proteomic discovery of novel therapeutic targets in cancer. Drug Des. Devel. Ther. **7**, 1259–1271 (2013)

Hamid, O., Robert, C., Daud, A., Hodi, F.S., Hwu, W.J., Kefford, R., Wolchok, J.D., Hersey, P., Joseph, R.W., Weber, J.S., Dronca, R., Gangadhar, T.C., Patnaik, A., Zarour, H., Joshua, A.M., Gergich, K., Elassaiss-Schaap, J., Algazi, A., Mateus, C., Boasberg, P., Tumeh, P.C., Chmielowski, B., Ebbinghaus, S.W., Li, X.N., Kang, S.P., Ribas, A.: Safety and tumor responses with lambrolizumab (anti-PD-1) in melanoma. Ne. Engl. J. Med. **369**, 134–144 (2013)

Herbst, R.S., Soria, J.C., Kowanetz, M., Fine, G.D., Hamid, O., Gordon, M.S., Sosman, J.A., McDermott, D.F., Powderly, J.D., Gettinger, S.N., Kohrt, H.E., Horn, L., Lawrence, D.P., Rost, S., Leabman, M., Xiao, Y., Mokatrin, A., Koeppen, H., Hegde, P.S., Mellman, I., Chen, D.S., Hodi, F.S.: Predictive correlates of response to the anti-PD-L1 antibody MPDL3280A in cancer patients. Nature **515**, 563–567 (2014)

Hodi, F.S., O'Day, S.J., McDermott, D.F., Weber, R.W., Sosman, J.A., Haanen, J.B., Gonzalez, R., Robert, C., Schadendorf, D., Hassel, J.C., Akerley, W., van den Eertwegh, A.J., Lutzky, J., Lorigan, P., Vaubel, J.M., Linette, G.P., Hogg, D., Ottensmeier, C.H., Lebbé, C., Peschel, C., Quirt, I., Clark, J.I., Wolchok, J.D., Weber, J.S., Tian, J., Yellin, M.J., Nichol, G.M., Hoos, A., Urba, W.J.: Improved survival with ipilimumab in patients with metastatic melanoma. N. Engl. J. Med. **363**, 711–723 (2010)

Jiang, L., Schlesinger, F., Davis, C.A., Zhang, Y., Li, R., Salit, M., Gingeras, T.R., Oliver, B.: Synthetic spike-in standards for RNA-seq experiments. Genome Res. **21**, 1543–1551 (2011)

Keir, M.E., Butte, M.J., Freeman, G.J., Sharpe, A.H.: PD-1 and its ligands in tolerance and immunity. Annu. Rev. Immunol. **26**, 677–704 (2008)

Kitano, S., Tsuji, T., Liu, C., Hirschhorn-Cymerman, D., Kyi, C., Mu, Z., Allison, J.P., Gnjatic, S., Yuan, J.D., Wolchok, J.D.: Enhancement of tumor-reactive cytotoxic CD4+ T cell responses after ipilimumab treatment in four advanced melanoma patients. Cancer Immunol. Res. **1**, 235–244 (2013)

Klein, A.M., Mazutis, L., Akartuna, I., Tallapragada, N., Veres, A., Li, V., Peshkin, L., Weitz, D.A., Kirschner, M.W.: Droplet barcoding for single-cell transcriptomics applied to embryonic stem cells. Cell **161**, 1187–1201 (2015)

Kong, Y.C., Flynn, J.C.: Opportunistic autoimmune disorders potentiated by immune-checkpoint inhibitors anti-CTLA-4 and anti-PD-1. Front. Immunol. **5**, 206 (2014)

Kumar, R.M., Cahan, P., Shalek, A.K., Satija, R., DaleyKeyser, A.J., Li, H., Zhang, J., Pardee, K., Gennert, D., Trombetta, J.J., Ferrante, T.C., Regev, A., Daley, G.Q., Collins, J.J.: Deconstructing transcriptional heterogeneity in pluripotent stem cells. Nature **516**, 56–61 (2014)

Kwong, L.N., Boland, G.M., Frederick, D.T., Helms, T.L., Akid, A.T., Miller, J.P., Jiang, S., Cooper, Z.A., Song, X., Seth, S., Kamara, J., Protopopov, A., Mills, G.B., Flaherty, K.T., Wargo, J.A., Chin, L.: Co-clinical assessment identifies patterns of BRAF inhibitor resistance in melanoma. J. Clin. Invest. **125**, 1459–1470 (2015)

Larkin, J., Chiarion-Sileni, V., Gonzalez, R., Grob, J.J., Cowey, C.L., Lao, C.D., Schadendorf, D., Dummer, R., Smylie, M., Rutkowski, P., Ferrucci, P.F., Hill, A., Wagstaff, J., Carlino, M.S., Haanen, J.B., Maio, M., Marquez-Rodas, I., McArthur, G.A., Ascierto, P.A., Long, G.V., Callahan, M.K., Postow, M.A., Grossmann, K., Sznol, M., Dreno, B., Bastholt, L., Yang, A., Rollin, L.M., Horak, C., Hodi, F.S., Wolchok, J.D.: Combined Nivolumab and Ipilimumab or Monotherapy in Untreated Melanoma. N. Engl. J. Med. **373**, 23–34 (2015)

Latchman, Y.E., Liang, S.C., Wu, Y., Chernova, T., Sobel, R.A., Klemm, M., Kuchroo, V.K., Freeman, G.J., Sharpe, A.H.: PD-L1-deficient mice show that PD-L1 on T cells, antigen-presenting cells, and host tissues negatively regulates T cells. Proc. Natl. Acad. Sci. U. S. A. **101**(29), 10691–10696 (2004). Epub 2004 Jul 12

Le, D.T., Uram, J.N., Wang, H., Bartlett, B.R., Kemberling, H., Eyring, A.D., Skora, A.D., Luber, B.S., Azad, N.S., Laheru, D., Biedrzycki, B., Donehower, R.C., Zaheer, A., Fisher, G.A., Crocenzi, T.S., Lee, J.J., Duffy, S.M., Goldberg, R.M., de la Chapelle, A., Koshiji, M., Bhaijee, F., Huebner, T., Hruban, R.H., Wood, L.D., Cuka, N., Pardoll, D.M., Papadopoulos, N., Kinzler, K.W., Zhou, S., Cornish, T.C., Taube, J.M., Anders, R.A., Eshleman, J.R., Vogelstein, B., Diaz Jr., L.A.: N. Engl. J. Med. **372**, 2509–2520 (2015)

Lesokhin, A.M., Callahan, M.K., Postow, M.A., Wolchok, J.D.: On being less tolerant: enhanced cancer immunosurveillance enabled by targeting checkpoints and agonists of T cell activation. Sci. Transl. Med. **7**, 280sr1 (2015)

Llosa, N.J., Cruise, M., Tam, A., Wicks, E.C., Hechenbleikner, E.M., Taube, J.M., Blosser, R.L., Fan, H., Wang, H., Luber, B.S., Zhang, M., Papadopoulos, N., Kinzler, K.W., Vogelstein, B., Sears, C.L., Anders, R.A., Pardoll, D.M., Housseau, F.: The vigorous immune microenvironment of microsatellite instable colon cancer is balanced by multiple counter-inhibitory checkpoints. Cancer Discov. **5**, 43–51 (2015)

Macosko, E.Z., Basu, A., Satija, R., Nemesh, J., Shekhar, K., Goldman, M., Tirosh, I., Bialas, A.R., Kamitaki, N., Martersteck, E.M., Trombetta, J.J., Weitz, D.A., Sanes, J.R., Shalek, A.K., Regev, A., McCarroll, S.A.: Highly parallel genome-wide expression profiling of individual cells using nanoliter droplets. Cell **161**, 1202–1214 (2015)

McDermott, D.F., Drake, C.G., Sznol, M., Choueiri, T.K., Powderly, J.D., Smith, D.C., Brahmer, J.R., Carvajal, R.D., Hammers, H.J., Puzanov, I., Hodi, F.S., Kluger, H.M., Topalian, S.L., Pardoll, D.M., Wigginton, J.M., Kollia, G.D., Gupta, A., McDonald, D., Sankar, V., Sosman, J.A., Atkins, M.B.: Survival, durable response, and long-term safety in patients with previously treated advanced renal cell carcinoma receiving nivolumab. J. Clin. Oncol. **33**, 2013–2020 (2015)

Moonsamy, P.V., Williams, T., Bonella, P., Holcomb, C.L., Höglund, B.N., Hillman, G., Goodridge, D., Turenchalk, G.S., Blake, L.A., Daigle, D.A., Simen, B.B., Hamilton, A., May, A.P., Erlich, H.A.: High throughput HLA genotyping using 454 sequencing and the Fluidigm Access Array™ System for simplified amplicon library preparation. Tissue Antigens **81**, 141–149 (2013)

Morgan, P., Van Der Graaf, P.H., Arrowsmith, J., Feltner, D.E., Drummond, K.S., Wegner, C.D., Street, S.D.: Can the flow of medicines be improved? Fundamental pharmacokinetic and pharmacological principles toward improving Phase II survival. Drug Discov. Today **17**, 419–424 (2012)

Ng Tang, D., Shen, Y., Sun, J., Wen, S., Wolchok, J.D., Yuan, J., Allison, J.P., Sharma, P.: Increased frequency of ICOS+ CD4 T cells as a pharmacodynamic biomarker for anti-CTLA-4 therapy. Cancer Immunol. Res. **1**, 229–234 (2013)

Odorizzi, P.M., Wherry, E.J.: Inhibitory receptors on lymphocytes: insights from infections. J. Immunol. **188**, 2957–2965 (2012)

Peltomäki, P.: Role of DNA mismatch repair defects in the pathogenesis of human cancer. J. Clin. Oncol. **21**, 1174–1179 (2003)

Penaloza-MacMaster, P., Kamphorst, A.O., Wieland, A., Araki, K., Iyer, S.S., West, E.E., O'Mara, L., Yang, S., Konieczny, B.T., Sharpe, A.H., Freeman, G.J., Rudensky, A.Y., Ahmed, R.: Interplay between regulatory T cells and PD-1 in modulating T cell exhaustion and viral control during chronic LCMV infection. J. Exp. Med. **211**, 1905–1918 (2014)

Perfetto, S.P., Chattopadhyay, P.K., Roederer, M.: Seventeen-colour flow cytometry: unravelling the immune system. Nat. Rev. Immunol. **4**, 648–655 (2004)

Picelli, S., Faridani, O.R., Björklund, A.K., Winberg, G., Sagasser, S., Sandberg, R.: Full-length RNA-seq from single cells using Smart-seq2. Nat. Protoc. **9**, 171–181 (2014)

Powles, T., Eder, J.P., Fine, G.D., Braiteh, F.S., Loriot, Y., Cruz, C., Bellmunt, J., Burris, H.A., Petrylak, D.P., Teng, S.L., Shen, X., Boyd, Z., Hegde, P.S., Chen, D.S., Vogelzang, N.J.: Nature **515**, 558–562 (2014)

Rizvi, N.A., Hellmann, M.D., Snyder, A., Kvistborg, P., Makarov, V., Havel, J.J., Lee, W., Yuan, J., Wong, P., Ho, T.S., Miller, M.L., Rekhtman, N., Moreira, A.L., Ibrahim, F., Bruggeman, C., Gasmi, B., Zappasodi, R., Maeda, Y., Sander, C., Garon, E.B., Merghoub, T., Wolchok, J.D., Schumacher, T.N., Chan, T.A.: Cancer immunology. Mutational landscape determines sensitivity to PD-1 blockade in non-small cell lung cancer. Science **348**, 124–128 (2015)

Robert, C., Schachter, J., Long, G.V., Arance, A., Grob, J.J., Mortier, L., Daud, A., Carlino, M.S., McNeil, C., Lotem, M., Larkin, J., Lorigan, P., Neyns, B., Blank, C.U., Hamid, O., Mateus, C., Shapira-Frommer, R., Kosh, M., Zhou, H., Ibrahim, N., Ebbinghaus, S., Ribas, A., KEYNOTE-006 Investigators: N. Engl. J. Med. **372**, 2521–2532 (2015)

Sakuishi, K., Apetoh, L., Sullivan, J.M., Blazar, B.R., Kuchroo, V.K., Anderson, A.C.: Targeting Tim-3 and PD-1 pathways to reverse T cell exhaustion and restore anti-tumor immunity. J. Exp. Med. **207**, 2187–2194 (2010)

Schadendorf, D., Hodi, F.S., Robert, C., Weber, J.S., Margolin, K., Hamid, O., Patt, D., Chen, T.T., Berman, D.M., Wolchok, J.D.: Pooled analysis of long-term survival data from phase II and phase III trials of ipilimumab in unresectable or metastatic melanoma. J. Clin. Oncol. **33**, 1889–1894 (2015)

Schietinger, A., Greenberg, P.D.: Tolerance and exhaustion: defining mechanisms of T cell dysfunction. Trends Immunol. **35**, 51–60 (2014)

Schumacher, T.N., Schreiber, R.D.: Neoantigens in cancer immunotherapy. Science **348**, 69–74 (2015)

Schumacher, T.N., Kesmir, C., van Buuren, M.M.: Biomarkers in cancer immunotherapy. Cancer Cell **27**, 12–14 (2015)

Shalek, A.K., Satija, R., Adiconis, X., Gertner, R.S., Gaublomme, J.T., Raychowdhury, R., Schwartz, S., Yosef, N., Malboeuf, C., Lu, D., Trombetta, J.J., Gennert, D., Gnirke, A., Goren, A., Hacohen, N., Levin, J.Z., Park, H., Regev, A.: Single-cell transcriptomics reveals bimodality in expression and splicing in immune cells. Nature **498**, 236–240 (2013)

Sharma, P., Allison, J.P.: The future of immune checkpoint therapy. Science **348**, 56–61 (2015)

Simpson, T.R., Li, F., Montalvo-Ortiz, W., Sepulveda, M.A., Bergerhoff, K., Arce, F., Roddie, C., Henry, J.Y., Yagita, H., Wolchok, J.D., Peggs, K.S., Ravetch, J.V., Allison, J.P., Quezada, S.A.: Fc-dependent depletion of tumor-infiltrating regulatory T cells co-defines the efficacy of anti-CTLA-4therapy against melanoma. J. Exp. Med. **210**, 1695–1710 (2013)

Sivendran, S., Chang, R., Pham, L., Phelps, R.G., Harcharik, S.T., Hall, L.D., Bernardo, S.G., Moskalenko, M.M., Sivendran, M., Fu, Y., de Moll, E.H., Pan, M., Moon, J.Y., Arora, S., Cohain, A., DiFeo, A., Ferringer, T.C., Tismenetsky, M., Tsui, C.L., Friedlander, P.A., Parides, M.K., Banchereau, J., Chaussabel, D., Lebwohl, M.G., Wolchok, J.D., Bhardwaj, N., Burakoff, S.J., Oh, W.K., Palucka, K., Merad, M., Schadt, E.E., Saenger, Y.M.: J. Invest. Dermatol. **134**, 2202–2211 (2014)

Stock, J.K., Jones, N.P., Hammonds, T., Roffey, J., Dillon, C.: J. Biomol. Screen. **20**, 305–317 (2015)

Strauss, J., Madan, R.A., Figg, W.D.: Evaluating Immune responses after sipuleucel-T therapy. Cancer Biol. Ther. **16**, 1119–1121 (2015)

Tivol, E.A., Borriello, F., Schweitzer, A.N., Lynch, W.P., Bluestone, J.A., Sharpe, A.H.: Loss of CTLA-4 leads to massive lymphoproliferation and fatal multiorgan tissue destruction, revealing a critical negative regulatory role of CTLA-4. Immunity **3**, 541–547 (1995)

Topalian, S.L., Hodi, F.S., Brahmer, J.R., Gettinger, S.N., Smith, D.C., McDermott, D.F., Powderly, J.D., Carvajal, R.D., Sosman, J.A., Atkins, M.B., Leming, P.D., Spigel, D.R., Antonia, S.J., Horn, L., Drake, C.G., Pardoll, D.M., Chen, L., Sharfman, W.H., Anders, R.A., Taube, J.M., McMiller, T.L., Xu, H., Korman, A.J., Jure-Kunkel, M., Agrawal, S., McDonald, D., Kollia, G.D., Gupta, A., Wigginton, J.M., Sznol, M.: Safety, activity, and immune correlates of anti-PD-1 antibody in cancer. N. Engl. J. Med. **366**, 2443–2454 (2012)

Topalian, S.L., Drake, C.G., Pardoll, D.M.: Immune checkpoint blockade: a common denominator approach to cancer therapy. Cancer Cell **27**, 450–461 (2015)

Tsioris, K., Torres, A.J., Douce, T.B., Love, J.C.: A new toolbox for assessing single cells. Annu. Rev. Chem. Biomol. Eng. **5**, 455–477 (2014)

Tumeh, P.C., Harview, C.L., Yearley, J.H., Shintaku, I.P., Taylor, E.J., Robert, L., Chmielowski, B., Spasic, M., Henry, G., Ciobanu, V., West, A.N., Carmona, M., Kivork, C., Seja, E., Cherry, G., Gutierrez, A.J., Grogan, T.R., Mateus, C., Tomasic, G., Glaspy, J.A., Emerson, R.O., Robins, H., Pierce, R.H., Elashoff, D.A., Robert, C., Ribas, A.: Nature **515**, 568–571 (2014)

Twyman-Saint Victor, C., Rech, A.J., Maity, A., Rengan, R., Pauken, K.E., Stelekati, E., Benci, J.L., Xu, B., Dada, H., Odorizzi, P.M., Herati, R.S., Mansfield, K.D., Patsch, D., Amaravadi, R.K., Schuchter, L.M., Ishwaran, H., Mick, R., Pryma, D.A., Xu, X., Feldman, M.D., Gangadhar, T.C., Hahn, S.M., Wherry, E.J., Vonderheide, R.H., Minn, A.J.: Radiation and dual checkpoint blockade activate non-redundant immune mechanisms in cancer. Nature **520**, 373–377 (2015)

Veldman-Jones, M.H., Brant, R., Rooney, C., Geh, C., Emery, H., Harbron, C.G., Wappett, M., Sharpe, A., Dymond, M., Barrett, J.C., Harrington, E.A., Marshall, G.: Evaluating robustness and sensitivity of the NanoString technologies nCounter platform to enable multiplexed gene expression analysis of clinical samples. Cancer Res. **75**, 2587–2593 (2015)

Waterhouse, P., Penninger, J.M., Timms, E., Wakeham, A., Shahinian, A., Lee, K.P., Thompson, C.B., Griesser, H., Mak, T.W.: Lymphoproliferative disorders with early lethality in mice deficient in Ctla-4. Science **270**, 985–988 (1995)

Weber, J.S., D'Angelo, S.P., Minor, D., Hodi, F.S., Gutzmer, R., Neyns, B., Hoeller, C., Khushalani, N.I., Miller Jr., W.H., Lao, C.D., Linette, G.P., Thomas, L., Lorigan, P., Grossmann, K.F., Hassel, J.C., Maio, M., Sznol, M., Ascierto, P.A., Mohr, P., Chmielowski, B., Bryce, A., Svane, I.M., Grob, J.J., Krackhardt, A.M., Horak, C., Lambert, A., Yang, A.S., Larkin, J.: Nivolumab versus chemotherapy in patients with advanced melanoma who progressed after anti-CTLA-4 treatment (CheckMate 037): a randomised, controlled, open-label, phase 3 trial. Lancet Oncol. **16**, 375–384 (2015a)

Weber, J.S., Yang, J.C., Atkins, M.B., Disis, M.L.: Toxicities of Immunotherapy for the Practitioner. J. Clin. Oncol. **33**, 2092–2099 (2015b)

Wei, M.C., Cleary, M.L.: Novel methods and approaches to acute lymphoblastic leukemia drug discovery. Expert Opin. Drug Discov. **9**, 1435–1446 (2014)

Welsh, S.J., Corrie, P.G.: Management of BRAF and MEK inhibitor toxicities in patients with metastatic melanoma. Ther. Adv. Med. Oncol. **7**, 122–136 (2015)

Wills, Q.F., Mead, A.J.: Application of single cell genomics in cancer: promise and challenges. Hum. Mol. Genet. **24**, R74–R84 (2015)

Young, P.A., Morrison, S.L., Timmerman, J.M.: Antibody-cytokine fusion proteins for treatment of cancer: engineering cytokines for improved efficacy and safety. Semin. Oncol. **41**, 623–636 (2014)

Zhang, C.Z., Adalsteinsson, V.A., Francis, J., Cornils, H., Jung, J., Maire, C., Ligon, K.L., Meyerson, M., Love, J.C.: Calibrating genomic and allelic coverage bias in single-cell sequencing. Nat. Commun. **6**, 6822 (2015)

Zhou, P., Shaffer, D.R., Alvarez Arias, D.A., Nakazaki, Y., Pos, W., Torres, A.J., Cremasco, V., Dougan, S.K., Cowley, G.S., Elpek, K., Brogdon, J., Lamb, J., Turley, S.J., Ploegh, H.L., Root, D.E., Love, J.C., Dranoff, G., Hacohen, N., Cantor, H., Wucherpfennig, K.W.: In vivo discovery of immunotherapy targets in the tumour microenvironment. Nature **506**, 52–57 (2014)

Chapter 8
The New Frontier of Antibody Drug Conjugates: Targets, Biology, Chemistry, Payloads

Christopher D. Thanos and Paul D. Rennert

Abbreviations

ADC	Antibody-drug conjugate
ALL	Acute lymphoblastic leukemia
ASH	American Society of Hematology
BTD	Breakthrough therapy designation
CLL	Chronic lymphocytic leukemia
CR	Complete response
CRi	CR with incomplete hematologic recovery
DLBCL	Diffuse large B cell lymphoma
DLT	Dose-limiting toxicity
DM1	Derivative of maytansine
DOR	Duration of response
FL	Follicular lymphoma
FR	Folate receptor
FTD	Fast track designation
IC	Investigator's choice
IHC	Immunohistochemistry
mAb	Monoclonal antibody
MCC	[N-maleimidomethyl] cyclohexane-1-carboxylate
MMAE	Monomethyl auristatin E
MMAF	Monomethyl auristatin F

C.D. Thanos
Halozyme Therapeutics, Inc., 11388 Sorrento Valley Road, San Diego, CA, USA

P.D. Rennert (✉)
SugarCone Biotech LLC, Holliston, MA 01746, USA

Aleta Biotherapeutics, Natick, MA 01746, USA
e-mail: rennertp@sugarconebiotech.com

P.D. Rennert (ed.), *Novel Immunotherapeutic Approaches to the Treatment of Cancer*, DOI 10.1007/978-3-319-29827-6_8

MTD	Maximum tolerated dose
NHL	Non-Hodgkin lymphoma
ORR	Objective response rate
OS	Overall survival
PFS	Progression-free survival
TNBC	Triple-negative breast cancer

1 Introduction

The ADC field has been rejuvenated by the recent approvals of Adcetris® (brentuximab vedotin) for $CD30^+$ relapsed Hodgkin lymphoma and relapsed anaplastic large-cell lymphoma in 2011 and Kadcyla® (ado-trastuzumab emtansine, T-DM1) for the treatment of $HER2^+$ metastatic breast cancer in 2013. These drugs emerged from the leaders in ADC technology at the time: Adcetris® is from Seattle Genetics (partnered with Takeda) and Kadcyla® was developed by Roche/Genentech using ADC technology licensed from Immunogen. In addition, there are a large number of targets under investigation using diverse ADC chemistries, linkers, and payloads. Many of these early-stage clinical studies will fail, as attrition takes a toll on novel technologies: programs will fail based on efficacy criteria, or toxicity, or both. In some cases the failure will be traced to the underlying technology, and in others to the selection of target antigen. In any case, failures in this field have been common, and our hope is that the percentage of failures begins to decrease going forward. With that in mind, we have selected a number of interesting mid-stage clinical candidates and next-generation ADC technologies, to review in more detail.

2 New Targets for B Cell Leukemias and Lymphomas

The B cell lineage leukemias and lymphomas comprise a diverse group of tumors that represent many stages of abnormal B cell development (Seifert et al. 2013) and the success of Adcetris® has stimulated robust drug development in these hematologic malignancies. These efforts are helped by the fact that the diversity of B cell malignancies has been defined, in part, by the overexpression of specific cell surface proteins; these then serve as antigenic targets for ADCs. As noted in the introduction, Adcetris® targets CD30, a protein found on Hodgkin lymphoma and a variety of B cell leukemias and lymphomas as well as on some T cell malignancies. Other B cell surface-expressed proteins have been targeted with ADCs; these include CD19, CD37, CD79b, BCMA, and others (see Table 8.1).

The attractiveness of this particular class of malignancies is based on several key characteristics. First, the B cell lineage is very distinct, and many targets are specific to B cells or subsets of B cells. As is well known from studies with the B lymphocyte-depleting antibody rituximab, most patients can get along pretty well without B

Table 8.1 Examples of B cell-expressed antigens as targets for ADCs

Target antigen	Indications	ADC	Sponsor
CD19	DLBCL; ALL	Coltuximab ravtansine (SAR-3419)	Immunogen
CD19	NHL, ALL	SGN-CD19A	Seattle Genetics
CD22	Aggressive NHL (stopped) ALL	Inotuzumab ozogamicin	Pfizer
CD22	DLBCL and follicular relapsed or refractory NHL	Pinatuzumab vedotin (RG-7593)	Roche Genentech
CD25	B and T cell leukemias and lymphomas	ADCT-301	ADC Therapeutics
CD30	Relapsed Hodgkin lymphoma and systemic anaplastic large-cell lymphoma	Brentuximab vedotin	Seattle Genetics
CD37	CLL and NHL	IMGN529	Immunogen
CD37	CLL and NHL	ASG67E	Agensys
CD70	Relapsed or refractory NHL	Vorsetuzumab mafodotin	Seattle Genetics
CD79b	Relapsed or refractory NHL	Polatuzumab vedotin	Roche Genentech
CD79b	DLBCL and follicular relapsed or refractory NHL	RG-7596	Roche Genentech
CD138	Multiple myeloma	Indatuximab ravtansine (BT-062)	BioTest
BCMA	Multiple myeloma	GSK2857916	GlaxoSmithKline

cells. This means the risk of on-target toxicity is generally low. Second, many types of B cell leukemias and lymphomas are mitotically active, with cell division a defining feature of disease, making these good cells to target with payloads that interfere with cell division. Third, and quite uniquely, there is dramatic diversity in the class of B cell malignancies, and many niche subtypes remain poorly treated by more traditional therapies. Many subtypes are sufficiently rare that the indications qualify for orphan disease status. Thus there remains unmet need and a tractable landscape from a regulatory perspective, from a commercial perspective, and of course from the clinical perspective.

Currently the most advanced novel ADC targeting B cell lymphomas is denintuzumab mafodotin (formally SGN-CD19a) from Seattle Genetics. Denintuzumab mafodotin is in Phase 1 clinical trials for CD19-positive acute lymphoblastic leukemia (ALL), Burkitt lymphoma, and several of the B-cell non-Hodgkin lymphomas (NHL) (NCT01786135, NCT01786096). A Phase 2 trial of denintuzumab mafodotin in combination with rituximab and chemotherapy in diffuse large B cell lymphoma (DLBCL) has not yet begun recruiting (NCT02592876). The data to date include interim Phase 1 analyses presented at the 2014 American Society of Hematology (ASH) conference that demonstrated that denintuzumab mafodotin was well tolerated in relapsed, refractory NHL and induced objective responses, with an overall objective response rate (ORR) of 35 % in this dose–response setting. In addition 20 % of patients achieved a complete remission (CR) (Abstract #1741,

ASH 2014). While the durability of response is not yet known, these are compelling Phase 1 data. Similar data were reported from an early analysis of a trial enrolling patients with ALL and Burkitt lymphoma (Abstract #963, ASH 2014). The previously mentioned Phase 2 combination trial in DLBCL, a difficult-to-treat subset of NHL, was based on these encouraging Phase 1 data. The focus on DLBCL and other generally difficult-to-treat lymphomas like relapsed/refractory follicular lymphoma (FL) mirrors Seattle Genetics continuing campaign to expand the label for Adcetris®. At the American Society of Clinical Oncology conference (ASCO 2015), Seattle Genetics presented updated results from the Adcetris® studies in DLBCL and FL. In the Phase 2 DLBCL trial, newly diagnosed, high-risk patients (stage III/IV) received Adcetris® plus a rituximab/chemotherapy regimen (R-CHOP) compared to R-CHOP alone as standard of care (Abstract #8506, *ASCO 2015*). The ORR was 80 %, with 67 % achieving CR. The activity of Adcetris® plus R-CHOP was better in CD30-positive DLBCL patients, with a higher CR (76 %) and an estimated progression-free survival (PFS) rate at 12 months of 86 %. To put these numbers in perspective however, R-CHOP alone in a similar patient population produced an ORR of 85 % and a CR of >70 % (Delarue et al. 2013). So the real challenge here will be to monitor relapses and longer term PFS and overall survival (OS). We can also look at results with other therapeutics targeting DLBCL. For example the BTK inhibitor ibrutinib, when added to R-CHOP, produced 100 % ORR and 67 % CR results in a small Phase 1 study (Younes et al. 2014). A very large Phase 3 study in DLBCL is under way. Kite Pharma has treated NHL patients with the CAR T cell therapeutic KTE-C19. In early results, an ORR of 92 % was achieved with a CR of 62 %. Of seven evaluable patients with refractory DLBCL, four achieved complete remission, three of which had reported durations ranging from 9 to 22 months (Kochenderfer et al. 2015). While very preliminary, these results suggest that denintuzumab mafodotin is at least competitive with other modalities, and the differentiation will come as we observe longer term relapse rates, PFS, OS, and other more meaningful readouts. Several updates of the Phase 1 studies were presented at the ASH 2015 meeting. Results from the ALL trial were updated to include 71 patients, showing a complete remission rate of 35 %, and DOR of nearly 7 months (Abstract #1328, ASH 2015). In the relapsed/refractory NHL setting, 60 patients were reported, with an ORR of 50 % in the relapsed cohort and 21 % in the refractory cohort. As noted above, most of these patients presented with DLBCL, a difficult-to-treat population. Of note in the relapsed setting 32 % of patients had complete remission with a median DOR of 10 months (Abstract #182, ASH 2015).

Denintuzumab mafodotin carries an MMAF warhead. Interestingly, Seattle Genetics has announced that it is also developing SGN-CD19b, which possess a next-generation PBD warhead, and also targets CD19, presumably with the same targeting antibody. The differences between these two warheads will be discussed below.

In contrast to the approved drug Adcetris®, most other B cell-targeted ADCs, like denintuzumab mafodotin, are early in their clinical development. An ADC targeting CD79b is undergoing development at Roche/Genentech. CD79b is a component of the B cell receptor and is expressed in nearly all types of B cell malignancies, including NHL. The ADC, called polatuzumab vedotin, is part of the Seattle Genetics/Genentech partnership. Polatuzumab vedotin is linked to the microtubule-disrupting agent monomethyl auristatin E (MMAE). Early studies with the ADC were hampered by toxicity at the highest doses tested; however a more recent clinical trial is using a lower dose of polatuzumab in combination with rituximab (Palanca-Wessels et al. 2015; Pfeifer et al. 2015).

In the dose escalation Phase 1 trial (NCT01290549) the safety and clinical activity of polatuzumab vedotin were assessed across a range of doses (0.1–2.4 mg/kg every 3 weeks) in patients with relapsed or refractory NHL and chronic lymphocytic leukemia (CLL). While these malignancies are expected to express CD79b, confirmation of expression was not required for enrollment. The primary endpoints of the study were to assess drug tolerability and establish the maximum tolerated dose (MTD), and thereby identify a dose for use in Phase 2 monotherapy trials, or in combination trials with rituximab or obinutuzumab (both anti-CD20 mAbs with direct cytotoxic activity) and chemotherapy (NCT1992653; NCT02257567). The MTD was reached in both NHL and CLL, with CLL patients being more sensitive to toxicity. The major severe adverse events (AEs; grade 3 or 4) occurred in over half of patients (58 %) treated at the MTD and included neutropenia, anemia, and peripheral sensory neuropathy. Other serious AEs were reported in 38 % of patients and included diarrhea and lung infection/pathology. The AE numbers were even higher (77 %) in the patients treated with the polatuzumab/rituximab combination. Fortunately, the ORR was just over 50 % in NHL patients given monotherapy and 78 % in NHL patients given the combination therapy. ORR in CLL was 0 % regardless of therapy (Palanca-Wessels et al. 2015). The median follow-up period for patients receiving the MTD dose was 14 months. In an abstract scheduled for presentation at the 2015 ASH meeting (Abstract #2726, ASH 2015), a small relapsed/refractory NHL cohort was analyzed after treatment with polatuzumab vedotin and rituximab plus chemotherapy. CRs were observed in five of seven patients at an early stage of analysis. Toxicities were severe but considered manageable, as was noted above.

In preclinical studies polatuzumab vedotin was analyzed alongside pinatuzumab vedotin, an anti-CD22 ADC, targeting different molecular subtypes of DLBCL. Both ADCs induced cell death in diverse DLBCL cell lines, irrespective of activating mutations in CD79b that induce signaling and support tumor cell proliferation and survival. Of note, target density on cells was not a strong predictor of sensitivity to treatment, suggesting therapeutic value for patients irrespective of the degree of CD79b expression. These preclinical studies have informed the trial design and criteria for a Phase 2 study entitled “A Randomized, Open-Label, Multicenter, Phase II Trial Evaluating the Safety and Activity of Pinatuzumab Vedotin (DCDT2980S) in Combination With Rituximab or Polatuzumab Vedotin (DCDS4501A) in Combination With Rituximab and a Non-Randomized Phase Ib/II Evaluation of Polatuzumab Vedotin in Combination With Obinutuzumab in Patients With Relapsed or Refractory B-cell Non-Hodgkin’s Lymphoma” (NCT01691898).

The interest in CD22 is timely. In October 2015 Pfizer received "Breakthrough Therapy Designation" (BTD) for the anti-CD22 ADC inotuzumab ozogamicin for the treatment of relapsed or refractory ALL. BTD is granted to a drug if it treats a serious or life-threatening condition and preliminary clinical evidence indicates that the drug may demonstrate substantial clinical improvement over available therapies. Inotuzumab ozogamicin is a humanized IgG4 anti-CD22 antibody covalently linked to *N*-acetyl-gamma-calicheamicin dimethyl hydrazide, a toxin that is released once the ADC is internalized, causing double-strand DNA breaks and thereby inducing apoptosis (Ohanian et al. 2015). The BTD was awarded based on results of an open-label Phase 3 active comparator trial in relapsed or refractory ALL, showing the induction of a CR in 80.7 % versus 33.3 % with SOC chemotherapy (Abstract #LB2073, EHA 2015). Most CR patients (78.4 %) were shown to be minimal residual disease (MRD) negative when the cells from the bone marrow were examined by flow cytometry (we'll note in passing here that this is not the same as MRD− by PCR, which is much more sensitive). An important subset of patients were those who were able to proceed to stem cell transplantation—about twice as many patients achieved this important milestone in the inotuzumab ozogamicin cohort as in the chemotherapy cohort. The median DOR was 4.6 months with inotuzumab ozogamicin compared with 3.1 months for chemotherapy. 43 % of patients treated with inotuzumab ozogamicin maintained first complete remission for more than 1 year compared with 35 % in the chemotherapy arm. In addition to the expected toxicities (hematologic cytopenias), 9 % of inotuzumab ozogamicin-treated patients developed hepatobiliary toxicity, particularly veno-occlusive liver disease that most often occurred after SCT, and was fatal in 2 of 15 cases.

In December of 2015 a small trial of inotuzumab ozogamicin in combination with low-intensity chemotherapy and four courses of rituximab as salvage therapy for relapsed/refractory ALL was presented (Abstract #3721, ASH 2015). ORR was 74 % and DOR was limited; however 41 % of patients were able to proceed to allogeneic SCT.

The importance of inotuzumab ozogamicin may be further highlighted as the drug is tested in different treatment classes, including patients who have failed other therapies (e.g., blinatumomab), and as earlier treatment lines are investigated, for example, in elderly patients whose tolerance of chemotherapy is poor. The ability to induce CRs in such a large percentage of treated patients is certainly impressive and ensures that CD22-targeted ADCs will likely find a place in the treatment paradigm for ALL and perhaps other leukemias and lymphomas.

Targets of interest for multiple myeloma (MM) include CD138 and BCMA. The MM field is fascinating, as different targets are being prosecuted via diverse modalities, including bispecific antibodies (e.g., BiTEs, DARTs), CAR-T cell therapies, "naked" antibodies, and ADCs. This will allow us, in time, to assess the efficacy across these therapeutic classes. One interesting ADC being developed for MM is indatuximab ravtansine (BT062, from Biotest Pharmaceuticals). The antibody recognizes CD138, a transmembrane heparin sulfate proteoglycan present on the surface of plasma-type B cells, on epithelial cells, and at a very high level on MM cells.

The antibody is chimeric only the constant domains are human, the rest is of murine origin) and is an IgG4, an isotype which only very weakly induces cytotoxicity through Fc receptors. The IgG4 does not appear to have been mutagenized to prevent "Fab arm exchange" by which IgG4s exchange Fab arms by swapping a heavy chain and attached light chain with a heavy-light chain pair from a different (in this case, endogenous) IgG4, resulting in bispecific antibodies. Whether this phenomena occurs with indatuximab ravtansine is unknown. The payload used on this anti-CD138 mAb is the first-generation microtubule inhibitor maytansinoid (DM4) that requires internalization and lysosomal degradation of the linker to release the DNA-intercalating cytotoxin. DM4 induces apoptosis as a consequence of the inhibition of tubulin polymerization.

Indatuximab ravtansine is in early clinical development. A Phase 1/2a study (NCT01001442) revealed a variety of toxicities, including class effect eye toxicity (corneal damage), and established the dose-limiting toxicity (DLT). Efficacy was limited in the monotherapy setting, with an ORR of only 4 %, although half of patients were recorded as having stable disease. A dose-ranging Phase 1/2 study combining indatuximab ravtansine with lenalidomide/dexamethasone is ongoing (NCT01638936). Early results from the study provided an ORR of 78 % ($n=36$) across all dose levels including CRs, although most patients achieved PR; importantly, nearly all patients had previously failed either lenalidomide with or without bortezomib (Abstract #4763, ASH 2014). Such data will encourage further investigation in these prior treatment failures.

Other ADCs in early clinical development for relapsed or refractory MM include lorvotuzumab mertansine (IMGN901, Immunogen) that targets CD56+ hematologic and other malignancies, currently in Phase 2 trials (see NCT02420873), and GSK2857916, an afucosyl-anti-BCMA mAb conjugated to MMAF using a non-cleavable linker that was in a phase 1 dose escalation trial as of December 2015 (from GlaxoSmithKline and Seattle genetics; NCT02064387).

The MM landscape illustrates the complexity of drug development in the hematologic malignancies, where multiple therapeutic modalities are targeting the same patient population. Relapsed and refractory MM had until recently resisted nearly all forms of treatment, with the most recently approved drugs (carfilzomib and pomalidomide) showing modest efficacy as single agents (i.e., <30 % ORR; <5 months PFS). Such results have been readily bested by standard antibody therapeutics (non-payloaded or "naked" mAbs) targeting CD38 (daratumumab and SAR650982, from Janssen Biotech/Genmab and Sanofi, respectively) and CS1 (elotuzumab, from AbbVie) that routinely have produced >30 % ORR and 7 months of greater PFS in large Phase 2 and Phase 3 clinical trials, and perform even better (as do all MM therapeutics) when given with some combination of lenalidomide, dexamethasone, and/or bortezomib. In addition to these mAb therapies, CAR-T cell therapeutics targeting the relapsed/refractory MM population are under development including CAR-BCMA, CAR-CD38, CAR-CD138, CAR-CS1, and likely other targets. This is a clinical landscape within which ADCs can thrive, if they achieve clinical responses superior to naked mAbs and with less cost and manipulation than CAR T cells.

Another example of an ADC that has demonstrated activity in a difficult indication is SGN-CD33a (Seattle Genetics). This ADC targets CD33, a siglec-family protein expressed on early lineage myeloid precursor cells, on some activated leukocytes including T cells and NK cells, and at higher levels on acute myeloid leukemic (AML) cells (Paul et al. 2000; Hernandez-Caselles et al. 2006; Ehninger et al. 2014). This ADC is composed of an anti-CD33 mAb having genetically engineered cysteines encoded into the amino acid sequence. This allows for uniform site-specific conjugation, an improvement over earlier generation chemistries (see the next section). The linker used is stable in circulation but cleaved in lysosomes, to improve local release of the toxin. The toxin is a pyrrolobenzodiazepine dimer that cross-links DNA and triggers apoptosis.

Interim Phase 1 clinical results were first presented at ASH (Abstract #623, ASH 2014) and then AACR (Abstract #DDT02-04, AACR 2015). This SGN-CD33A dose-escalation study is designed to investigate the safety and efficacy of the ADC in patients with CD33-positive relapsed AML (NCT01902329). The inclusion criteria specified that patients must have either relapsed following an initial CR lasing 3 months or more or alternatively declined intensive induction/consolidation treatment for AML. The drug was given for 3 months (IV q3weeks) and then there was an optional maintenance treatment for patients achieving a CR/CRi. A third cohort received the ADC in combination with azacitidine or decitabine chemotherapy. Data for 52 monotherapy patients was evaluated for antitumor activity. At the dose of 40 mcg/kg, 29 % (5/17) of patients achieved a CR or CRi (CR with incomplete hematologic recovery). Across all dose cohorts, 9/52 patients achieved CR or CRi, and 11/52 patients cleared AML blasts from the bone marrow (morphologic leukemia-free state, MLFS). The remaining 29 patients had residual blasts in the bone marrow.

Additional data was presented in December 2015 (Abstracts #324 and #454, ASH 2015). The abstracts provide the following updates. The dose escalation trial (now $n=87$) successfully identified the DLT dose at 40 mcg/kg. Results from the monotherapy cohort were similar to those reported at AACR. Focusing on the 21 patients treated at the DLT dose of 40 mcg/kg, 33 % achieved a CR/CRi and 20 % achieved morphologic leukemia-free state and median OS was 10 months.

In a second report (Abstract #454, ASH 2015), patients who received hypomethylating treatment for AML were treated with SGN-33A at a single-dose level of 10 mcg/kg (i.e., below the DLT dose). 65 % of patients achieved a CR or CRi, which is similar to historical controls (i.e., those receiving hypomethylating treatment only), but with longer apparent survival.

For an indication notoriously resistant to therapy these numbers are very encouraging. SGN-CD33A was granted orphan drug status by the US FDA. Orphan drug status is granted to drugs being developed to treat indications with significant unmet need and having fewer than 200,000 patients/year and/or no reasonable expectation of recouping R&D and marketing costs. While not an accelerated approval designation, orphan drug status does provide incentives including 7 years of market exclusivity from competitors and exemption from the Affordable Care Act's branded prescription drug fee.

As indicated in Table 8.1 and noted earlier, there are multiple novel ADCs in development for hematologic malignancies. As the comparison with other treatment modalities suggests, some of these therapeutics will become established components of the treatment paradigm for ALL, NHL, MM, and other difficult indications including perhaps the T cell leukemias and acute myeloid leukemia.

3 New Targets for the Treatment of Solid Tumors

Adcetris® stands as the landmark ADC in the field of hematologic malignancies, a position held by Kadcyla® in the treatment of solid tumors. Kadcyla® is the trade name for trastuzumab emtansine, an ADC consisting of the anti-HER2 mAb trastuzumab linked to the cytotoxic agent DM1. The drug was developed for the treatment of HER2+ breast cancer, and is prescribed for patients who have previously failed the combination of naked trastuzumab plus taxane-based chemotherapy.

The number and variety of ADCs targeting solid tumors continue to grow as the field adapts improved linker/payload chemistry to reduce toxicity (see the next section). An abbreviated list of some of the more advanced programs is presented in Table 8.2, and a selection of these will be discussed herein.

Sacituzumab govitecan is one of several novel ADCs being developed for triple-negative breast cancer (TNBC: negative for expression of estrogen receptor, HER2,

Table 8.2 Examples of solid tumor antigens being targeted by ADC therapeutics

Target antigen	Indications	ADC	Sponsor
CAIX	Renal cell carcinoma	BAY-79-4620	Bayer
Ceacam5	Colorectal and other solid tumors	Labetuzumab-SN-3	Immunomedics
CD70	Renal cell carcinoma	AMG-172	Amgen
EGFR	Glioblastoma and other solid tumors	ABT-414	Abbvie
EGFRvIII	Glioblastoma and other solid tumors	AMG-595	Amgen
Folate receptor α	Ovarian cancer	IMGN853	Immunogen
GPNMB	Melanoma, breast cancer	Glembatumumab vedotin	Celldex
Her2	Breast cancer	Trastuzumab emtansine	Immunogen
HuMax-TF	Solid tumors	Tissue factor	Genmab
MUC16	Ovarian and pancreatic cancer	DMUC5754A	Roche Genentech
PSMA	Prostate cancer	RG-7458	Roche Genentech
SLC44A4	Pancreatic cancer	ASG-5ME	Agensys
TROP-2	Pancreatic, gastric, and other cancers	IMMU-132	Immunomedics

and progesterone receptor), a particularly aggressive and difficult-to-treat indication. This therapeutic received the FDA's Fast Track Designation (FTD) in January 2015 for the treatment of TNBC in patients who failed prior lines of therapy. FTD facilitates the development and review of new drugs that are intended to treat serious indications having significant unmet medical need. FTD may also lead to Priority Review status, further accelerating approval. The drug has also garnered both FTD and orphan drug status for the treatment of patients with advanced small-cell lung cancer, and orphan drug status for the treatment of patients with advanced pancreatic cancer. In addition sacituzumab govitecan has been tested in non-small-cell lung, colorectal, esophageal, and urinary bladder cancers. Thus, if successfully developed, sacituzumab govitecan could have important impact in diverse indications. Efficacy data in TNBC is discussed below.

Sacituzumab govitecan (formally IMMU-132, Immunomedics) consists of the anti-trophoblast cell-surface antigen (TROP-2) humanized mAb hRS7 bound to SN-38, an active metabolite of the chemotherapeutic drug irinotecan. TROP-2 is expressed by diverse tumors including breast, colorectal, renal, hepatic, lung, ovarian, and many others. In contrast, expression in normal tissues is limited. Further, sacituzumab govitecan is internalized upon binding to TROP-2, causing selective tumor cell cytotoxicity.

Phase 2 results presented at AACR in April of 2015 included data on treatment of a variety of solid tumors, with sacituzumab govitecan inducing several CRs in TNBC patients who had failed multiple prior lines of therapy. The ORR in TNBC was 26 %. Notably, the therapy performed well in both small-cell lung cancer and NSCLC, with ORR of 32 % and 30 %, respectively, all of which were partial responses. The drug was well tolerated across multiple cycles using a dose regimen developed in Phase 1 (Starodub et al. 2015). At the 2015 AACR-NCI-EORTC International Conference on Molecular Targets and Cancer Therapeutics in November 2015 the Phase 2 trial results were updated to include PFS data (Abstract #LB-C16, AACR Molecular Targets, 2015). At the time of analysis, the interim median PFS was 7 months for the TNBC cohort, compared to a historical PFS of approximately 3.5 months. While median OS data were immature, 87 % of patients were still alive. The ORR had improved to 31.5 %, with all responses partial except the two CRs noted above. A Phase 3 clinical trial in relapsed/refractory TNBC has been registered but was not yet enrolling patients as of December 2015 (NCT02574455).

Another closely watched program is glembatumumab vedotin, one of the three ADCs under development by Celldex in collaboration with Seattle Genetics. Glembatumumab vedotin consists of CR011, a mAb that targets the tumor antigen gpNMB (the NMB glycoprotein) linked to the MMAE toxin. The linked is non-cleavable; thus the ADC must be internalized and processed in late endosomes or lysosomes to release the toxin.

The program is currently in a Phase 2 pivotal clinical trial in advanced or metastatic TNBC (NCT01997333) and in Phase 2 trials of aggressive metastatic melanoma (stage III or IV; NCT02302339, NCT02363283). Indeed expression of gpNMB on diverse tumor types is associated with metastasis and resistance to therapy, and therefore with poor prognosis and reduced OS (Rose et al. 2010). Of note, the use of glembatumumab vedotin is being tested with the premise that higher expression of the target may give better responses. For example in the pivotal Phase 2 study in metastatic breast cancer the inclusion criteria includes positive expression of gpNMB on tumor cells by immunohistochemistry (IHC) staining, based on earlier results from an exploratory study showing benefit in patients in which the target was expressed in >25 % of tumor cells, which are considered high expressors. In these patients the ORR (33 %) was about double that of patients with negative expression (Bendell et al. 2014). The earlier Phase 2 study (EMERGE) reported additional results in 2015 (Yardley et al. 2015) as follows.

Patients ($n=24$) with advanced breast cancer, refractory to prior lines of treatment (minimum of two, and up to seven, as enrolled), were randomized (2:1) to receive glembatumumab vedotin or "Investigator's Choice" (IC) single-agent, approved (i.e., standard of care) chemotherapy. The primary endpoint of the study was ORR and secondary endpoints included safety, DOR, PFS, and OS. Importantly, gpNMB expression levels on biopsied or resected tumor tissue was evaluated by IHC and expression of gpNMB was found on >5 % of tumor cells in essentially all patient samples. Investigators reported that the drug was generally well tolerated. Patient responses were stratified by the intensity of gpNMB staining of tumor cells and this revealed that glembatumumab vedotin-treated patients whose tumor cells expressed higher levels of gpNMB (≥10 % and ≥25 %) had better responses than all other pooled patients. The improved ORR was associated with clinical outcome, as shown by PFS and OS data; specifically OS was 10 months for glembatumumab vedotin-treated patients versus 5.7 months for the IC-treated patients.

In patients with TNBC, gpNMB is frequently expressed and is correlated with metastasis. In subgroup analysis, TNBC patients with >25 % gpNMB expression and treated with glembatumumab vedotin responded well (ORR 40 % versus 0 % in the IC cohort) with a very similar improvement in OS (i.e., about 10 months). These data were sufficient to move the program to a pivotal Phase 2 study, as described above.

In addition to the studies conducted in breast cancer, glembatumumab vedotin is also moving forward in metastatic melanoma, squamous cell lung cancer, osteosarcoma, and uveal melanoma. The early Phase 2 data in advanced metastatic melanoma, while encouraging, have not yet yielded robust responses. Subsetting to patients that express very high levels of gpNMB may improve the therapeutic application of this ADC in advanced melanoma (NCT02302339).

Another example of the potential use of subsetting to identify patients with high expression of the target antigen comes from the early clinical investigation of a novel ADC. Mirvetuximab soravtansine targets cancers that express folate receptor alpha (FR)α, including ovarian cancer, endometrial cancer, a subset of small-cell lung cancer, and several adenocarcinomas. The anti-FRα humanized mAb M9346A is coupled to the maytansinoid toxin DM4 MMAE using an optimized linker. Results from an ongoing Phase 1 clinical trial of mirvetuximab soravtansine were presented at the AACR and ASCO conferences in 2015. This is an interesting program for several reasons. First, the drug is targeting a notoriously difficult-to-treat indication, platinum-based chemotherapy-resistant ovarian cancer. Second, drug dose and administration were varied in an effort to reduce toxicity, notably the various ocular toxicities that are observed with some ADCs (see, e.g., Abstract #5518,

ASCO 2015). Third, as noted, the results in patients expressing very high levels of the target FRα were particularly good.

The Phase 1 results showed that mirvetuximab soravtansine produced notable single-agent activity, particularly for platinum-resistant metastatic ovarian cancer, an indication with a very poor prognosis. Single-agent therapies typically used to treat this indication include non-platinum chemotherapies (e.g., taxanes), having a low ORR (10–15 %) and an OS rate approximately 1 year. Combination chemotherapy for these patients is more toxic but does not improve ORR, PFS, or OS. Against this backdrop the early results obtained with mirvetuximab soravtansine were very good. Of the patients included in the early efficacy analysis ($n=17$) the ORR was 53 %, including one CR. These included patients whose dose regimen was modified to reduce ocular toxicity. Based on these data, the expansion cohort was initiated to enroll additional patients ($n=40$) having FRα-positive platinum-resistant ovarian cancer and orphan drug status was granted in both the US and EU.

Updated results were presented at the AACR-NCI-EORTC conference in November 2015 (Abstract #C47) based on an analysis of 20 patients in Phase I trial who received the Phase 2 selected dose. Patients were categorized as having high (>75 %), medium (50–74 %), or low (25–49 %) tumor cells having strong (3+) or moderate (2+) expression of FRα by IHC. Enrollment criteria for the clinical study required all patients to have at least low expression. For patients with high FRα expression the ORR was 90 % (9/10) including two CRs and seven partial responses. Six of these responders remained on treatment for at least 24 weeks. In contrast patients with medium expression all had tumor regression as a best response and patients with low expression did not respond.

Based on the accumulated results, the Phase 2 study will require patients to have medium or high expression of FRα to qualify for enrollment. A second clinical trial (NCT02606305) will evaluate mirvetuximab soravtansine in earlier lines of therapy of ovarian cancer in combination with other therapies including bevacizumab and platinum-based chemotherapy. Patient enrollment for both trials was scheduled to begin by the end of 2015. Clinical trials in other indications, notably endometrial cancer, are anticipated. Trials of mirvetuximab soravtansine will be supported by a companion diagnostic test to accurately measure expression of FRα in patient tumor tissue samples.

4 Limitations Associated with the Currently Approved ADCs

The two FDA-approved ADCs, Adcetris® and Kadcyla®, are tremendous innovations that have provided a great benefit to patients. However, a body of work has emerged which reveals significant limitations associated with these drugs, offering opportunities for improvement in the design of next-generation ADCs. Adcetris® corresponds to an anti-CD30 targeting mAb carrying multiple cytotoxic warheads conjugated through reduced disulfide bonds. The conjugation chemistry used is maleimide-reactive chemistry, which reacts with reduced thiols. The maleimide group is connected to a

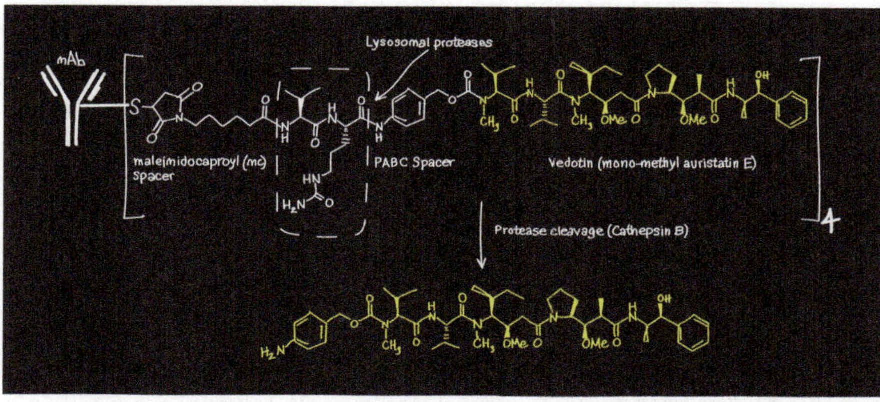

Fig. 8.1 vcPAB-MMAE Conjugation. Reduced thiols are conjugated via a maleimidocaproyl (mc) spacer that are connected to valine-citrulline protease cleavage site that is sensitive to digestion by Cathepsin B. The self-imolating PABC spacer is then released, which frees the active MMAE warhead. Modified from Kitson et al, Chemistry Today, Vol. 31(4) July/August 2013

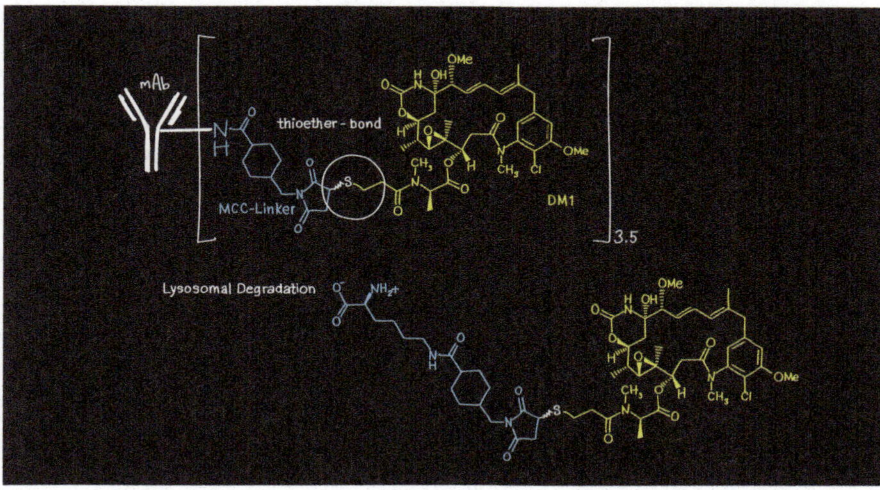

Fig. 8.2 Conjugation of an antibody to random lysine resides via a MCC linker connected to DM1 with a thioether bond. Lysosomcal degradation of the ADC results in the formation of the freed DM1-MCC-lysine adduct. Modified from Kitson et al, Chemistry Today, Vol. 31(4) July/August 2013

valine-citrulline amino acid protease cleavage-site linker, which is attached to a self-immolating PAB moiety that releases the potent cytotoxin MMAE after protease cleavage (Fig. 8.1). Kadcyla® corresponds to the FDA approved, Her-2 targeting antibody, trastuzumab, carrying multiple warheads conjugated through surface lysine residues to an MCC linker attached to DM1, a cytotoxic maytansinoid (Fig. 8.2). The limitations associated with these drugs correspond to (a) plasma-based degradation of the intact ADC in circulation; (b) significant heterogeneity in the drug:mAb ratio (DAR), which is the number of drug molecules conjugated to each mAb, Fig. 8.3; and (c) the type of cytotoxic warhead chosen.

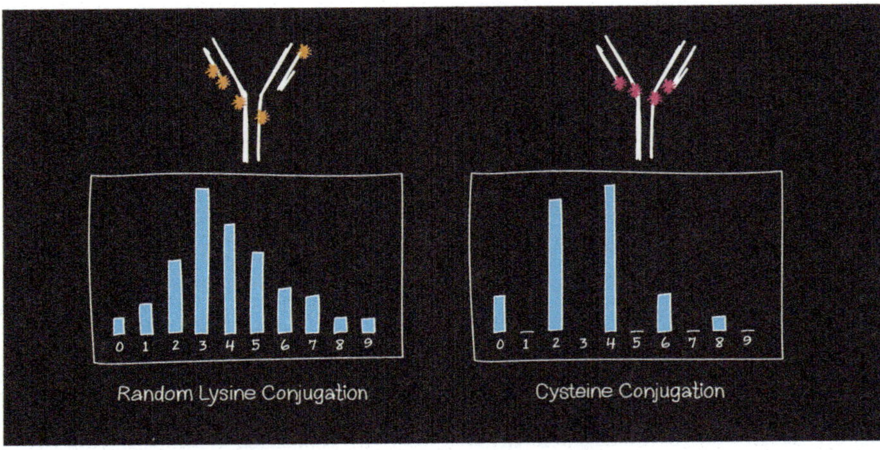

Fig. 8.3 Hypothetical DARs as a result of conjugation to random surface lysines or reduced cysteines

4.1 Conjugation Chemistry Limitations

Both Adcetris® and Kadcyla® use conjugation chemistry that is labile to degradation in plasma. Over time, maleimide exchange between thiol-reactive constituents in plasma results in deterioration of the intact ADC. This raises concerns from efficacy, pharmacokinetics, and toxicity perspectives. Adducts can be formed between plasma albumin and ADC warheads, resulting in the formation of circulating albumin-drug conjugates (Alley et al. 2008; Shen et al. 2012; Pillow et al. 2014). Several new conjugation chemistry formats have emerged to address this limitation and are discussed below.

4.2 Molecular Heterogeneity

ADCs conjugated using the approaches described above generate significantly heterogeneous mixtures of drug product comprised of different levels of drug loaded onto each antibody, which have significantly different properties in vivo. This corresponds to >1E6 species for random lysine-based conjugation chemistry (trastuzumab has over 90 surface lysines) and up to 100 species when conjugated to reduced thiols (Junutula et al. 2008; Wang et al. 2005; Hamblett et al. 2004). Hamblett et al. evaluated the impact of drug load on in vitro activity, in vivo potency, toxicity, and clearance (Hamblett et al. 2004). Using partial antibody reduction and preparative hydrophobic interaction chromatography, they generated defined MMAE-conjugated preparations of the anti-CD30 mAb cAC10—the same mAb used for Adcetris, with DARs of 2, 4, and 8. Interestingly, while the in vitro cell killing potency of ADC increased as more drug was loaded onto the antibody (IC_{50} values DAR8 < DAR4 < DAR2), the in vivo potency was comparable between the DAR 4 and DAR8 ADCs, despite the DAR4 ADC carrying half the amount of MMAE as the DAR 8 ADC. The DAR2 ADC also showed antitumor activity, but required higher doses for an effect to be observed. In addition, the DAR2 ADC had a twofold increased maximum tolerated dose over the DAR 4 ADC, which was twofold higher than that of the DAR 8 ADC. Furthermore, there was a direct correlation between MMAE drug load on the ADC safety and plasma clearance. The DAR 8 ADC cleared three times faster than the DAR 4 ADC and five times faster than the DAR 2 ADC. Higher drug loads per antibody appear to be more toxic; the MTD of the DAR2 ADC was at least two times higher than the MTD of the DAR 4 ADC, which was two times higher than the MTD of the DAR8 ADC. Thus, in the context of mAb of conjugation through reduced disulfides to a maleimide-reactive linker warhead (as is used in Adcetris®), there appears to be an optimal number of conjugations per mAb. Over-conjugation resulted in a more toxic, faster clearing substance that did not provide an enhanced efficacy benefit. Under-conjugation would result in a significant portion of the preparation that remained unconjugated, which could compete with intact for binding to target and negatively impact efficacy. In addition, significant heterogeneity strains the ability to reproducibly manufacture ADC at scale, from a chemistry, manufacturing, and control perspective, which is suboptimal from a production standpoint and introduces risk when working with regulatory agencies.

4.3 Warhead Limitations

While the auristatins and maytansines are the most commonly used warheads, there are several limitations to their use in ADCs, including lack of ability to target quiescent cells, susceptibility to multidrug resistance pathways, and potency. First, both chemotypes are spindle inhibitors that target tubulin, making them most active against rapidly proliferating cells. However, tumor stem cells can exist in a quiescent metabolic state, rendering them more resistant to tubulin inhibition, which could lead to tumor reemergence (Shor et al. 2015). DNA-damaging cytotoxic warheads are distinguished from tubulin inhibitors in that they can promote destruction of both proliferating and non-proliferating tumor cells (Shor et al. 2015). However it should be noted that specificity between proliferating and non-proliferating cells could provide a safety advantage for microtubule inhibitors over other warhead types in the event of off-target ADC activity. Second, drug resistance pathways can become upregulated in response to chemotherapy can impact performance of the ADC. Auristatins (including MMAE), and maytansine, are known substrates for P-glycoprotein, which mediates efflux from cells (Shefet-Carasso and Benhar 2015). A functional genomic approach recently revealed that the ABCC3 drug transporter protein is a mediator of MMAE resistance in $Her2^{+}$ breast cancer (O'Brien et al. 2008). In addition, DM1-based ADCs are susceptible to resistance by tumor cells expressing multidrug transporter protein, MDR1. Third, it is generally recognized that only a small percentage of dosed therapeutic mAbs penetrate deep into solid tumors and recognize their targets (Beckman et al. 2007). For example, a study using radiolabeled antibodies demonstrated that only 0.01 % of the injected dose per gram of tumor was able to penetrate the tumor (Fand et al. 1992). Thus there are efforts in the field to identify novel cytotoxics with improved potency, which will be discussed below.

5 Emerging Next-Generation ADC Technologies

Several interesting new technologies have emerged to address limitations associated with the current FDA-approved ADCs. To address ADC instability in plasma, new chemistries have become available, including a phenyloxadiazole sulfone linker and a bis-alkylating, bridging reagent (Patterson et al. 2014; Badescu et al. 2014). To address molecular heterogeneity, cysteines have been introduced through substitution mutagenesis to achieve site-specific conjugation with a more defined DAR of 2 (Shen et al. 2012; Junutula et al. 2008; Panowksi et al. 2014; Jeffrey et al. 2013). Bifunctional bridging compounds are being developed that re-bridge reduced disulfide bonds between both heavy and light chains and between heavy chains in the hinge region (Badescu et al. 2014), resulting in DAR very close to 4. In addition, nonnatural amino acid-containing mAbs with introduced chemical diversity have emerged, allowing for site-specific, plasma-stable conjugation, and a DAR of 2 (Tian et al. 2014; Zimmerman et al. 2014).

5.1 Improved Conjugation Chemistry

Two recent papers outline interesting new chemistries for conjugation to reduced thiols. First, Patterson et al. performed a head-to-head comparison between a novel phenyloxadiazole sulfone linker and traditional maleimide chemistry, looking for improved conjugate stability in human plasma (Patterson et al. 2014). They tested conjugation to antibodies that were engineered with introduced cysteines for site-specific conjugation (Shen et al. 2012). Interestingly, significantly improved conjugate stability at Fc position S396C was observed for the sulfone linker over the maleimide linker. In addition, conjugation at a second site (light chain position V205C) showed comparable plasma stability between the sulfone and maleimide linker chemistries; however no albumin exchange was observed with sulfone chemistry. In a second paper, Badescu et al. examined the ability of conjugation through a bivalent linker containing two bis-alkylating moieties that react with both sulfur atoms derived from a reduced disulfide bond (Badescu et al. 2014). In doing so, this conjugation effectively re-bridged a reduced disulfide (shown in Fig. 8.4).

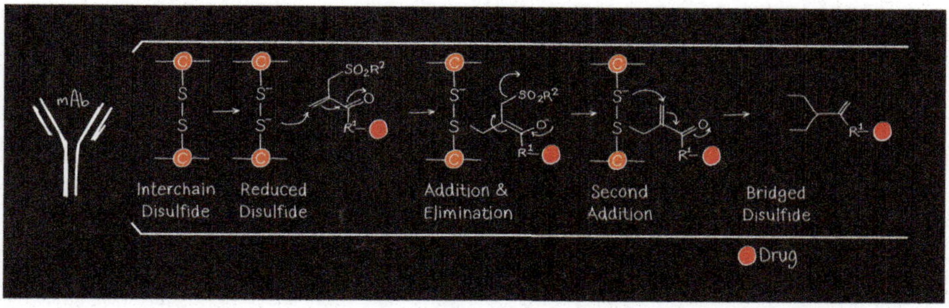

Fig. 8.4 Thiobridge chemistry uses a bis-alkylating reagent to re-bridge reduced disulfide bonds. Modified from Badescu et al, 2014.

Interestingly, use of this chemistry had a twofold effect: (a) the conjugate showed both significant resistance to degradation in human serum and (b) by re-bridging reduced disulfides, significantly less DAR heterogeneity is observed, paving the way for the use of a preparative chromatography step to purify the DAR 4 ADC species only, eliminating unwanted aggregates or unconjugated material. Moreover, use of the re-bridging reagent did not require a mutagenesis step or introduction of a foreign amino acid.

5.2 Addressing Molecular Heterogeneity

Several recent reports outline strategies to generate ADCs with more specific DARs. As mentioned above, engineered cysteines have been introduced at various sites within a mAb, resulting in a more defined DAR after conjugation. Termed THIOMABs substitution of one amino acid with a cysteine residue results in the introduction of two cysteines in the final folded mAb format, and after conjugation this results in a DAR of 2. Junutula et al. assessed the substitution of cysteine at multiple positions on trastuzumab, which differed in solvent accessibility and local physicochemical environment (Junutula et al. 2008). The site with the highest solvent accessibility was most susceptible to loss of the maleimide conjugate. A partially accessible site with a net positive surface charge was more resistant to plasma-mediated degradation, due to hydrolysis of the succinimide ring in the linker, preventing exchange with albumin in plasma. This resulted in a more stable ADC in vivo, as assessed by a rodent pharmacokinetics study, and superior antitumor properties in a human breast cancer xenograft model. In a separate line of experimentation, an anti-MUC16, THIOMAB-based, MMAE-containing ADC showed significantly improved stability, efficacy, and tolerability (in a cynomolgus monkey study), when compared to head-to-head versus the conventionally conjugated ADC, which used endogenous reduced disulfide bonds as the conjugation site.

5.3 *Novel Warheads*

Two interesting new cytotoxins have emerged which address both potency and the ability to target both actively proliferating tumor cells and quiescent stem cells. The first class, pyrrolobenzodiazepine dimers, was pioneered by Spirogen which has since been acquired by Astra Zeneca. PBD family molecules cause cell death through a DNA-cross-linking mechanism (Hartley et al. 2010). Seattle Genetics, working with Spirogen, has published two recent reports testing this warhead in the context of ADCs—first targeting CD33 for hematological malignancies, and second targeting CD70 for solid tumors (Jeffrey et al. 2013; Kung Sutherland et al. 2013). Both papers demonstrated that ADCs carrying this warhead showed profound antitumor responses at low doses, and in both cases the PBD dimer was conjugated through site-specific conjugation to an engineered cysteine residue in the antibody Fc domain at position 239. Interestingly, this position overlaps with a known binding site for Fc receptors that mediate effector function. It is possible that introduction of a solvent-exposed cysteine and conjugation with a PBD warhead generate steric blockade between the ADC and Fc receptors, which would attenuate effector function, but also possibly prevent Fc receptor-mediated cellular internalization.

The second emerging cytotoxin class is based on α-amanitin, a mushroom toxin, which kills cells by inhibiting RNA polymerase II (Pol II) (Moldenhauer et al. 2012). A recent study found that low doses of an anti-EpCAM α-amanitin-based ADC led to strong antitumor activity in human colorectal tumor xenografts (Liu et al. 2015). The authors found that genomic deletion of the p53 gene frequently encompasses essential neighboring genes, the gene for RNA polymerase II (Pol II), which was identified as a gene that is almost always co-deleted with P53 in human cancers. Tumors with hemizygous deletion of RNA polymerase II (Pol II) were highly sensitive to low-dose inhibition by the α-amanitin-based ADC.

6 Summary

The ADC field is entering a golden age of discovery and promise for patients. Multiple investigational drug candidates have pending clinical trial readouts that will serve to validate a new generation of targets across a range of tumor types. Tremendous knowledge has been gained in the study of existing ADC therapeutics and the limitations associated with the technology used; significant investment is under way in next-generation technologies to address those limitations. The combination of new ADC targets and technologies that address conjugate stability, heterogeneity, and warhead potency will deliver breakthrough therapies for years to come, and in many cases become the standard of care. It will be fascinating to follow performance of this class of agents vs. other emerging modalities, such as immune checkpoint inhibitors, cell-based immunotherapies, and oncolytic vaccine strategies.

Moreover, it's tempting to speculate that combination regimens which exploit synergistic benefit between ADCs and other therapeutic modalities may further serve to shift the paradigm from cancer treatment to cure.

References

Alley, S.C., Benjamin, D.R., Jeffrey, S.C., Okeley, N.M., Meyer, D.L., Sanderson, R.J., Senter, P.D.: Contribution of linker stability to the activities of anticancer immunoconjugates. Bioconjug. Chem. **19**, 759–765 (2008)

Badescu, G., Bryant, P., Bird, M., Henseleit, K., Swierkosz, J., Parekh, V., Tommasi, R., Pawlisz, E., Jurlewicz, K., Farys, M., Camper, N., Sheng, X., Fisher, M., Grygorash, R., Kyle, A., Abhilash, A., Frigerio, M., Edwards, J., Godwin, A.: Bridging disulfides for stable and defined antibody drug conjugates. Bioconjug. Chem. **25**, 1124–36 (2014)

Beckman, R.A., Weiner, L.M., Davis, H.M.: Antibody constructs in cancer therapy: protein engineering strategies to improve exposure in solid tumors. Cancer **109**, 170–179 (2007)

Bendell, J., Saleh, M., Rose, A.A., Siegel, P.M., Hart, L., Sirpal, S., Jones, S., Green, J., Crowley, E., Simantov, R., Keler, T., Davis, T., Vahdat, L.: Phase I/II study of the antibody-drug conjugate glembatumumab vedotin in patients with locally advanced or metastatic breast cancer. J. Clin. Oncol. **32**, 3619–3625 (2014)

Delarue, R., Tilly, H., Mounier, N., Petrella, T., Salles, G., Thieblemont, C., Bologna, S., Ghesquieres, H., Hacini, M., Fruchart, C., Ysebaert, L., Ferme, C., Casasnovas, O., van Hoof, A., Thyss, A., Delmer, A., Fitoussi, O., Molina, T.J., Haioun, C., Bosly, A.: Dose-dense rituximab-CHOP compared with standard rituximab-CHOP in elderly patients with diffuse large B-cell lymphoma (the LNH03-6B study): a randomised phase 3 trial. Lancet Oncol. **14**, 525–533 (2013)

Ehninger, A., Kramer, M., Rollig, C., Thiede, C., Bornhauser, M., von Bonin, M., Wermke, M., Feldmann, A., Bachmann, M., Ehninger, G., Oelschlagel, U.: Distribution and levels of cell surface expression of CD33 and CD123 in acute myeloid leukemia. Blood Cancer J. **4**, e218 (2014)

Fand, I., Sharkey, R.M., Grundy, J.P., Goldenberg, D.M.: Localization by whole-body autoradiography of intact and fragmented radiolabeled antibodies in a metastatic human colonic cancer model. Int. J. Rad. Appl. Instrum. B **19**, 87–99 (1992)

Hamblett, K.J., Senter, P.D., Chace, D.F., Sun, M.M., Lenox, J., Cerveny, C.G., Kissler, K.M., Bernhardt, S.X., Kopcha, A.K., Zabinski, R.F., Meyer, D.L., Francisco, J.A.: Effects of drug loading on the antitumor activity of a monoclonal antibody drug conjugate. Clin. Cancer Res. **10**, 7063–7070 (2004)

Hartley, J.A., Hamaguchi, A., Coffils, M., Martin, C.R., Suggitt, M., Chen, Z., Gregson, S.J., Masterson, L.A., Tiberghien, A.C., Hartley, J.M., Pepper, C., Lin, T.T., Fegan, C., Thurston, D.E., Howard, P.W.: SG2285, a novel C2-aryl-substituted pyrrolobenzodiazepine dimer prodrug that cross-links DNA and exerts highly potent antitumor activity. Cancer Res. **70**, 6849–6858 (2010)

Hernandez-Caselles, T., Martinez-Esparza, M., Perez-Oliva, A.B., Quintanilla-Cecconi, A.M., Garcia-Alonso, A., Alvarez-Lopez, D.M., Garcia-Penarrubia, P.: A study of CD33 (SIGLEC-3) antigen expression and function on activated human T and NK cells: two isoforms of CD33 are generated by alternative splicing. J. Leukoc. Biol. **79**, 46–58 (2006)

Jeffrey, S.C., Burke, P.J., Lyon, R.P., Meyer, D.W., Sussman, D., Anderson, M., Hunter, J.H., Leiske, C.I., Miyamoto, J.B., Nicholas, N.D., Okeley, N.M., Sanderson, R.J., Stone, I.J., Zeng, W., Gregson, S.J., Masterson, L., Tiberghien, A.C., Howard, P.W., Thurston, D.E., Law, C.L., Senter, P.D.: A potent anti-CD70 antibody-drug conjugate combining a dimeric pyrrolobenzodiazepine drug with site-specific conjugation technology. Bioconjug. Chem. **24**, 1256–1263 (2013)

Junutula, J.R., Raab, H., Clark, S., Bhakta, S., Leipold, D.D., Weir, S., Chen, Y., Simpson, M., Tsai, S.P., Dennis, M.S., Lu, Y., Meng, Y.G., Ng, C., Yang, J., Lee, C.C., Duenas, E., Gorrell, J., Katta, V., Kim, A., Mcdorman, K., Flagella, K., Venook, R., Ross, S., Spencer, S.D., Lee Wong, W., Lowman, H.B., Vandlen, R., Mx, S.L.I.W.K.O.W.S.K.I., Scheller, R.H., Polakis, P., Mallet, W.: Site-specific conjugation of a cytotoxic drug to an antibody improves the therapeutic index. Nat. Biotechnol. **26**, 925–932 (2008)

Kochenderfer, J.N., Dudley, M.E., Kassim, S.H., Somerville, R.P., Carpenter, R.O., Stetler-Stevenson, M., Yang, J.C., Phan, G.Q., Hughes, M.S., Sherry, R.M., Raffeld, M., Feldman, S., Lu, L., Li, Y.F., Ngo, L.T., Goy, A., Feldman, T., Spaner, D.E., Wang, M.L., Chen, C.C., Kranick, S.M., Nath, A., Nathan, D.A., Morton, K.E., Toomey, M.A., Rosenberg, S.A.: Chemotherapy-refractory diffuse large B-cell lymphoma and indolent B-cell malignancies can be effectively treated with autologous T cells expressing an anti-CD19 chimeric antigen receptor. J. Clin. Oncol. **33**, 540–549 (2015)

Kung Sutherland, M.S., Walter, R.B., Jeffrey, S.C., Burke, P.J., Yu, C., Kostner, H., Stone, I., Ryan, M.C., Sussman, D., Lyon, R.P., Zeng, W., Harrington, K.H., Klussman, K., Westendorf, L., Meyer, D., Bernstein, I.D., Senter, P.D., Benjamin, D.R., Drachman, J.G., Mcearchern, J.A.: SGN-CD33A: a novel CD33-targeting antibody-drug conjugate using a pyrrolobenzodiazepine dimer is active in models of drug-resistant AML. Blood **122**, 1455–1463 (2013)

Liu, Y., Zhang, X., Han, C., Wan, G., Huang, X., Ivan, C., Jiang, D., Rodriguez-Aguayo, C., Lopez-Berestein, G., Rao, P.H., Maru, D.M., Pahl, A., He, X., Sood, A.K., Ellis, L.M., Anderl, J., Lu, X.: TP53 loss creates therapeutic vulnerability in colorectal cancer. Nature **520**, 697–701 (2015)

Moldenhauer, G., Salnikov, A.V., Luttgau, S., Herr, I., Anderl, J., Faulstich, H.: Therapeutic potential of amanitin-conjugated anti-epithelial cell adhesion molecule monoclonal antibody against pancreatic carcinoma. J. Natl. Cancer Inst. **104**, 622–634 (2012)

O'Brien, C., Cavet, G., Pandita, A., Hu, X., Haydu, L., Mohan, S., Toy, K., Rivers, C.S., Modrusan, Z., Amler, L.C., Lackner, M.R.: Functional genomics identifies ABCC3 as a mediator of taxane resistance in HER2-amplified breast cancer. Cancer Res. **68**, 5380–5389 (2008)

Ohanian, M., Kantarjian, H., Guy, D., Thomas, D., Jabbour, E., O'Brien, S.: Inotuzumab ozogamicin in B-cell acute lymphoblastic leukemias and non-Hodgkin's lymphomas. Expert Opin. Biol. Ther. **15**, 601–611 (2015)

Palanca-Wessels, M.C., Czuczman, M., Salles, G., Assouline, S., Sehn, L.H., Flinn, I., Patel, M.R., Sangha, R., Hagenbeek, A., Advani, R., Tilly, H., Casasnovas, O., Press, O.W., Yalamanchili, S., Kahn, R., Dere, R.C., Lu, D., Jones, S., Jones, C., Chu, Y.W., Morschhauser, F.: Safety and activity of the anti-CD79B antibody-drug conjugate polatuzumab vedotin in relapsed or refractory B-cell non-Hodgkin lymphoma and chronic lymphocytic leukaemia: a phase 1 study. Lancet Oncol. **16**, 704–715 (2015)

Panowksi, S., Bhakta, S., Raab, H., Polakis, P., Junutula, J.R.: Site-specific antibody drug conjugates for cancer therapy. MAbs **6**, 34–45 (2014)

Patterson, J.T., Asano, S., Li, X., Rader, C., Barbas III, C.F.: Improving the serum stability of site-specific antibody conjugates with sulfone linkers. Bioconjug. Chem. **25**, 1402–1407 (2014)

Paul, S.P., Taylor, L.S., Stansbury, E.K., Mcvicar, D.W.: Myeloid specific human CD33 is an inhibitory receptor with differential ITIM function in recruiting the phosphatases SHP-1 and SHP-2. Blood **96**, 483–490 (2000)

Pfeifer, M., Zheng, B., Erdmann, T., Koeppen, H., McCord, R., Grau, M., Staiger, A., Chai, A., Sandmann, T., Madle, H., Dorken, B., Chu, Y.W., Chen, A.I., Lebovic, D., Salles, G.A., Czuczman, M.S., Palanca-Wessels, M.C., Press, O.W., Advani, R., Morschhauser, F., Cheson, B.D., Lenz, P., Ott, G., Polson, A.G., Mundt, K.E., Lenz, G.: Anti-CD22 and anti-CD79B antibody drug conjugates are active in different molecular diffuse large B-cell lymphoma subtypes. Leukemia **29**, 1578–1586 (2015)

Pillow, T.H., Tien, J., Parsons-Reponte, K.L., Bhakta, S., Li, H., Staben, L.R., Li, G., Chuh, J., Fourie-O'Donohue, A., Darwish, M., Yip, V., Liu, L., Leipold, D.D., Su, D., Wu, E., Spencer, S.D., Shen, B.Q., Xu, K., Kozak, K.R., Raab, H., Vandlen, R., Lewis Phillips, G.D., Scheller, R.H., Polakis, P., Sliwkowski, M.X., Flygare, J.A., Junutula, J.R.: Site-specific trastuzumab maytansinoid antibody-drug conjugates with improved therapeutic activity through linker and antibody engineering. J. Med. Chem. **57**, 7890–7899 (2014)

Rose, A.A., Grosset, A.A., Dong, Z., Russo, C., MacDonald, P.A., Bertos, N.R., St-Pierre, Y., Simantov, R., Hallett, M., Park, M., Gaboury, L., Siegel, P.M.: Glycoprotein nonmetastatic B is an independent prognostic indicator of recurrence and a novel therapeutic target in breast cancer. Clin. Cancer Res. **16**, 2147–2156 (2010)

Seifert, M., Scholtysik, R., Kuppers, R.: Origin and pathogenesis of B cell lymphomas. Methods Mol. Biol. **971**, 1–25 (2013)

Shefet-Carasso, L., Benhar, I.: Antibody-targeted drugs and drug resistance—challenges and solutions. Drug Resist. Updat. **18**, 36–46 (2015)

Shen, B.Q., Xu, K., Liu, L., Raab, H., Bhakta, S., Kenrick, M., Parsons-Reponte, K.L., Tien, J., Yu, S.F., Mai, E., Li, D., Tibbitts, J., Baudys, J., Saad, O.M., Scales, S.J., McDonald, P.J., Hass, P.E., Eigenbrot, C., Nguyen, T., Solis, W.A., Fuji, R.N., Flagella, K.M., Patel, D., Spencer, S.D., Khawli, L.A., Ebens, A., Wong, W.L., Vandlen, R., Kaur, S., Sliwkowski, M.X., Scheller, R.H., Polakis, P., Junutula, J.R.: Conjugation site modulates the in vivo stability and therapeutic activity of antibody-drug conjugates. Nat. Biotechnol. **30**, 184–189 (2012)

Shor, B., Gerber, H.P., Sapra, P.: Preclinical and clinical development of inotuzumab-ozogamicin in hematological malignancies. Mol. Immunol. **67**, 107–116 (2015)

Starodub, A.N., Ocean, A.J., Shah, M.A., Guarino, M.J., Picozzi Jr., V.J., Vahdat, L.T., Thomas, S.S., Govindan, S.V., Maliakal, P.P., Wegener, W.A., Hamburger, S.A., Sharkey, R.M., Goldenberg, D.M.: First-in-human trial of a novel anti-trop-2 antibody-SN-38 conjugate, sacituzumab govitecan, for the treatment of diverse metastatic solid tumors. Clin. Cancer Res. **21**, 3870–3878 (2015)

Tian, F., Lu, Y., Manibusan, A., Sellers, A., Tran, H., Sun, Y., Phuong, T., Barnett, R., Hehli, B., Song, F., Deguzman, M.J., Ensari, S., Pinkstaff, J.K., Sullivan, L.M., Biroc, S.L., Cho, H., Schultz, P.G., Dijoseph, J., Dougher, M., Ma, D., Dushin, R., Leal, M., Tchistiakova, L., Feyfant, E., Gerber, H.P., Sapra, P.: A general approach to site-specific antibody drug conjugates. Proc. Natl. Acad. Sci. U S A **111**, 1766–1771 (2014)

Wang, L., Amphlett, G., Blattler, W.A., Lambert, J.M., Zhang, W.: Structural characterization of the maytansinoid-monoclonal antibody immunoconjugate, huN901-DM1, by mass spectrometry. Protein Sci. **14**, 2436–2446 (2005)

Yardley, D.A., Weaver, R., Melisko, M.E., Saleh, M.N., Arena, F.P., Forero, A., Cigler, T., Stopeck, A., Citrin, D., Oliff, I., Bechhold, R., Loutfi, R., Garcia, A.A., Cruickshank, S., Crowley, E., Green, J., Hawthorne, T., Yellin, M.J., Davis, T.A., Vahdat, L.T.: EMERGE: a randomized phase II study of the antibody-drug conjugate glembatumumab vedotin in advanced glycoprotein NMB-expressing breast cancer. J. Clin. Oncol. **33**, 1609–1619 (2015)

Younes, A., Thieblemont, C., Morschhauser, F., Flinn, I., Friedberg, J.W., Amorim, S., Hivert, B., Westin, J., Vermeulen, J., Bandyopadhyay, N., de Vries, R., Balasubramanian, S., Hellemans, P., Smit, J.W., Fourneau, N., Oki, Y.: Combination of ibrutinib with rituximab, cyclophosphamide, doxorubicin, vincristine, and prednisone (R-CHOP) for treatment-naive patients with CD20-positive B-cell non-Hodgkin lymphoma: a non-randomised, phase 1b study. Lancet Oncol. **15**, 1019–1026 (2014)

Zimmerman, E.S., Heibeck, T.H., Gill, A., Li, X., Murray, C.J., Madlansacay, M.R., Tran, C., Uter, N.T., Yin, G., Rivers, P.J., Yam, A.Y., Wang, W.D., Steiner, A.R., Bajad, S.U., Penta, K., Yang, W., Hallam, T.J., Thanos, C.D., Sato, A.K.: Production of site-specific antibody-drug conjugates using optimized non-natural amino acids in a cell-free expression system. Bioconjug. Chem. **25**, 351–361 (2014)

Chapter 9
Cellular Therapies: Gene Editing and Next-Gen CAR T Cells

Thomas J. Cradick

1 Introduction

Gene editing has many applications important for cancer research, including identifying and validating targets, screening drug candidates, and making models. Gene editing may grow in importance for therapy redirecting immune cells, advancing adoptive cell therapy (ACT), and correcting mutations. Chimeric antigen receptor (CAR) therapy includes editing the genome of T cells and transferring the edited cells to patients where the edited cells provide an immunologic defense against cancer cells. CAR T therapy therefore links gene therapy, cell therapy, and immunotherapy. This review centers on the developments and promise of gene editing, and possible future developments in cancer treatment. Research continues on each section of modular CAR-T design, while these and other variables are being tested in labs and in clinical trials. These trials have demonstrated the potential of this approach for pediatric and adult cancer patients with the hope of clearing tumors without the toxicity of conventional treatments (Kowolik et al. 2006; Pule et al. 2008; Lipowska-Bhalla et al. 2012; Brentjens et al. 2013; Grupp et al. 2013; Zhu et al. 2015).

Gene therapy has emerged as a promising method to improve patient care and ideally cure genetic diseases. Gene therapy can include any modification of the genetic material of living cells for therapeutic purposes, including gene addition (knockins), knockouts, correction mutations, or other editing (Amado and Chen 1999). Gene editing can use delivery by virus, transposon, mRNA, single or double-stranded DNA, and/or plasmids. The editing is directed by sequence-specific DNA breaks using engineered nucleases, including zinc finger nucleases (ZFNs), transcription activator-like effector nucleases (TALENs), and the clustered regularly

T.J. Cradick (✉)
CRISPR Therapeutics, Cambridge, MA 02139, USA
e-mail: tj@alum.mit.edu

P.D. Rennert (ed.), *Novel Immunotherapeutic Approaches to the Treatment of Cancer*, DOI 10.1007/978-3-319-29827-6_9

interspaced short palindromic repeats (CRISPR) and the CRISPR-associated protein (Cas) systems (CRISPR/Cas) (Gaj et al. 2013). Editing occurs as the DNA breaks are repaired by the cellular repair machinery, which can result in the introduction of insertions, deletions, and/or mutations from repair using the cellular nonhomologous end joining (NHEJ) pathway, or precise homology directed repair (HDR) that uses a supplied donor DNA for the correction template (reviewed in Gaj et al. 2013).

Gene editing, including a growing use of CRISPR/Cas systems, has been used extensively for rapid generation of model cell lines and animals for basic research, drug discovery, testing of anticancer agents, and studies on the mechanisms of drug resistance (Sander and Joung 2014; Sánchez-Rivera and Jacks 2015; Mou et al. 2015; Shuvalov and Barlev 2015). CRISPR/Cas systems are directed to target sites for using new guide RNAs (gRNAs) that are supplied and combine with the Cas9 protein, unlike ZFNs and TALENs, which require different proteins be designed and cloned for each new target. Single guide RNAs (sgRNAs) are approximately 100 nt in length and therefore easier to clone, express, or chemically synthesize (Jinek et al. 2012), allow the creation of large libraries of nucleases when co-expressed with the same protein. Large lentiviral libraries of gRNAs can be used for genome-wide screens to identify oncogenes or mutations that confer drug resistance (see Sect. 3.1) (Chen et al. 2015; Shalem et al. 2014). The speed and efficiency of CRISPR targeting facilitates drug resistance experiments, which remain the gold standard of drug-target validation, and can elucidate drugs' mechanisms of action (Liu et al. 2014a).

Nucleases, including CRISPR/Cas systems, have been used to edit cells ex vivo for introduction back to the patients as adoptive cell therapy (ACT, see Sect. 4). Nucleases also appear promising for editing cells within the patient to correct disease-causing mutations. Gene editing may additionally be used in the future to eliminate susceptibility mutations or variations. T cells are attractive targets for gene editing because the edited T cells can then be used in ACT for a range of functions, including targeting and killing cells displaying tumor associated antigens (TAAs). CAR therapy, therefore combines cell therapy, gene therapy, and immunotherapy. Cells expressing a given TCR or CAR can target a range of antigens, but an especially exciting use is in cancer therapy.

Edited T cells (as well as non-edited T cells with certain specificities) play important roles in antitumor immune responses against TAAs, overcoming immunosuppressive factors and the need for activation and expansion. The resulting clonal T cell expansions lead to tumor killing through immunostimulatory signals. There have been a number of advancements in cancer-directed immunotherapy that have translated to T cell engineering, including enhanced signaling pathways that have dramatically increased the amplification of immune response (Kowolik et al. 2006). In addition to knocking in larger constructs with additional domains fused to the CAR, some second and third generation CAR T methods requires a series gene of editing steps that require higher efficiency editing at each individual step (see Sect. 4.1).

Conventional cancer treatments generally include surgical resection, chemotherapy, and/or radiation, each of which can damage healthy tissues. The use of gene edited T cells similarly have the potential for effects that must be monitored. Research on modified T cells has primarily tracked their antitumor activity and cytotoxicity associated with incorrect or overactivation, but there are additional concerns that may need further study due to the potential of T cells to persist long term and to expand (Scholler et al. 2012). Significant safety concerns include the possible toxic effects of expression of the targeting protein from healthy tissue, which leads to CAR-T killing of healthy tissue, similar to graft-versus-host disease (GVHD). A recent solution to this problem is engineering a suicide gene into the modified T cells, such that drug administration during GVHD can result in apoptosis of the CAR T cells (Springer and Niculescu-Duvaz 2000). The addition of suicide genes to CAR gene editing of T cells for adoptive cell transfer has the potential to alleviate GVHD and improve antitumor efficacy (see Sect. 4.2) (Casucci and Bondanza 2011).

Treatment with CAR T or TCR-modified T cells has resulted in cytokine storm or other toxicity. Possible remedies include improving the binding domain's affinity or specificity, and targeting TAA that are truly only expressed on tumor cells. Other options include adding suicide switches, particularly those that can be controlled pharmacologically (Budde et al. 2013). Similarly, specific inhibitors that react to nontumor cells can be engineered into the cells to prevent activation if an off-target cell that express the target antigen also express an antigen associated with nontumor cells (Fedorov et al. 2013). Much needs to be determined in terms of specificity and cellular expression, but the hope is that the shutdown is transitory, thereby enable future targeting of the desired antigen. Conversely, a low-affinity CAR or TCR can be expressed with a costimulatory receptor that enables activation if both tumor-specific antigens are bound (Srivastava and Riddell 2015). The addition of these features to the cells also involve further gene editing prior to ACT. These additional modifications to CAR T cells require multiple cloning steps (see Sect. 6.1).

2 Engineered Nucleases

Multiple platforms have been developed and used to drive gene editing using engineering nucleases, including ZFNs, TALENs and bacterial CRISPR/Cas systems. These nucleases creates DNA breaks at a specific sequence (Gaj et al. 2013). The breaks may be repaired using the cell's inherent nonhomologous end joining (NHEJ) repair pathway, which can repair correctly or result in insertions, deletions (frameshifts), and/or mutations. The correctly repaired DNA can be recut by the nuclease, resulting in the accumulation of these types of errors, which can be useful when intending to knock out a gene or allele. DNA breaks can also lead to HDR that edits the cut site and surrounding sequence using a supplied donor DNA template (Urnov et al. 2005; Porteus and Baltimore 2003). As NHEJ is the more common repair pathway, research continues on means to increase the rate of repairs by HDR in relevant cell types.

Zinc Finger Nucleases (*ZFNs*) are fusions of Zinc Finger Protein (ZFP) DNA-binding domains to a FokI endonuclease catalytic domain (Kim et al. 1994). ZFPs, and therefore ZFNs, can be selected or engineered to bind to new sequences with novel specificity (reviewed in Urnov et al. 2010; Carroll et al. 2006). The DNA binding domains of ZFNs are smaller than in TALENs and smaller than the Cas9 protein required by CRISPR. This smaller size allows easier packaging of ZFNs for viral delivery. When two ZFNs bind to DNA with correct orientation and spacing, the FokI dimer forms and cleaves the intervening DNA (Porteus and Baltimore 2003). The mis-repair of DNA breaks caused by ZFNs targeting CCR5 result in insertions and deletions that knock out the protein's expression, resulting in T cells resistant to HIV that requires this co-receptor (Perez et al. 2008). Clinical trials demonstrated that CD4 T cells treated with these ZFNs were refractory to HIV infection (Tebas et al. 2014). In the small scale phase 1 clinical trial, ZFN treatment appeared generally safe and well tolerated. All subjects had increase CD4+ T-cell levels, and increased HIV resistance was observed during interruption of antiretroviral drug treatment (Tebas et al. 2014). The specificity of the CCR5-directed ZFNs were studied using different methods (Pattanayak et al. 2011; Gabriel et al. 2011; Fine et al. 2014; Frock et al. 2015), including SELEX (Sander et al. 2013), which was then used to drive the genome search and sequencing of the 20 highest ranked putative off-target sites. Two of the identified sites were in exons and one had a 1.75 % frequency of insertions, deletions, and/or mutations (indels), which was significantly below the on-target percentage (75 %). Intronic or intergenic sites also had indel percentages above background, though their significance would require further work to determine the number of reads in nuclease-treated and mock samples. There are limited means of determining if gene editing may cause proliferative abnormalities or tumor formation, such as transferring the edited cells into NSG mice. Nuclease specificity is increasingly studied; a number of groups have published new off-target analysis methods (Frock et al. 2015; Lindsay and Roth 2014; Tsai et al. 2014a; Kim et al. 2015; Wang et al. 2015a), which are relevant as off-target mutations and chromosomal rearrangements occur as a result of off-target cleavage events.

The effects of using ZFNs targeting exon 1 of PDCD-1 were tested in melanoma tumor infiltrating lymphocytes (TILs). The average allele modification frequency after high flow-through electroporation of the ZFN mRNA was 75 %, with 40–48 % of cells having biallelic PD-1 modification (Beane et al. 2015). This editing rate resulted in a 76 % reduction in cell surface PD-1. In two of three donors tested, the TILs with edited PDCD-1 showed improved in vitro effector function and increased cytokine profile (TNFα, GM-CSF, and IFNγ) when cultured with antigen-specific tumor targets. The treated cells retained an effector memory phenotype and similar proliferative capacity as controls.

Transcription activator-like effector nucleases (*TALENs*) are artificial restriction enzymes generated by fusing a TAL effector DNA-binding domain to a FokI endonuclease catalytic domain. As with ZFNs, two TALENs binding to DNA with correct orientation and spacing allows the FokI dimer to form and cleave the intervening sequence. The TAL DNA-binding domain contains repeats of a highly conserved 33–35 amino acid domain with two amino acids that are highly variable, the Repeat Variable Diresidues (RVDs), which primarily determine the single DNA nucleotide bound by that repeat. TALEN target sites are readily found and TALENs are easier to design than ZFNs due the straightforward pairing of DNA sequence and RVDs (Cermak et al. 2011). Guanines are the exception as they are commonly targeted using either using the RVDs NN or using NK, which provides more specificity, though may lead to less activity (Streubel et al. 2012; Lin et al. 2014a). A number of solutions of different scale were presented that alleviated the difficulty of cloning the large, highly repetitive TAL domains (Cermak et al. 2011; Zhang et al. 2011; Weber et al. 2011; Reyon et al. 2012). As TALENs are large proteins, effective delivery is more challenging. TALENs have been reported with high specificity, though off-target cleavage has also been observed with some TALENs (Mussolino et al. 2011). Although there is significant variety between different TALENs and ZFNs, TALENs have been reported that had higher specificity (less off-target cleavage) than ZFNs targeting overlapping sites (Hendel et al. 2014; Mussolino et al. 2014).

MegaTAL nuclease contain a single TALE domain fused to an additional DNA-binding domain (Boissel et al. 2014). Unlike ZFNs or TALENs, megaTALs cleave as single molecules and are therefore easier to deliver to cells, and compatible with all current viral and nonviral cell delivery methods. MegaTAL specificity has been less studied than other classes of nucleases (Osborn et al. 2015). MegaTALs have been used in CAR T cells, as described in Sect. 5.1.

Clustered, regularly interspaced, short palindromic repeats (*CRISPR*) (Bolotin et al. 2005; Hale et al. 2009; Horvath and Barrangou 2010; Marraffini and Sontheimer 2010; Garneau et al. 2010; Deltcheva et al. 2011) are part of a bacterial defense system for cleaving foreign DNA and provide an exciting new class of nucleases that have the advantage of being RNA-guided, allowing the use of the same CRISPR-associated (Cas) protein for each target in contrast to the need to design and clone new proteins pairs for each target for ZFNs and TALENs (Cong et al. 2013). A short guide RNA strand (gRNA) directs the nuclease to a ~20 bp nucleotide sequence adjacent to protospacer adjacent motif (PAM), such as NGG, which is required by the *Streptococcus pyogenes* (Sp) Cas9 protein (Jinek et al. 2012; Ran et al. 2013a). Cas proteins binding alternative PAMs have been characterized from other species (Esvelt et al. 2013). Having multiple Cas proteins with alternative PAMs increases the sites that can be targeted by CIRSPR/Cas systems. As guide RNA (gRNA) strands typically target a ~20 bp DNA sequence, and non-Watson–Crick base pairing is known to occur (Jiang et al. 2013), it was likely there was the possibility for off-target beyond the level suggested by early work. Studies in tissue culture suggested that CRISPR/Cas systems have the potential for off-target activity, particularly at genomic sites with mismatches to genomic sequences further from the PAM (Cong et al. 2013; Jiang et al. 2013; Gasiunas et al. 2012; Jinek et al. 2013). These examples of off-target cleavage raised awareness about vetting gRNA using bioinformatics to choose unique target sites with few similar sites in the target genome (Fu et al. 2013; Hsu et al. 2013; Cradick et al. 2013).

The high efficiency of CRISPR/Cas cleavage has allowed multiplexing, the simultaneous use of multiple gRNA that enable multiple edits. As CRISPR systems uses alternative RNA to redirect the same protein, multiple guide RNAs can be supplied to direct the nuclease to multiple loci (Cong et al. 2013). Examples of multiplex editing include targeting five genes simultaneously in mouse embryonic stem cells, or two loci targeted in zygotes for simultaneous editing with HDR donors (Wang et al. 2013). This feature, for example, may allow multiple edits within CAR T cells or targeting multiple oncogenic mutations simultaneously (Poirot et al. 2015; Derniame et al. 2014). Multiple concurrent cleavage events increase the need for specific nucleases.

Over the last few years the applications of CRISPR are have grown at a remarkable pace. Methods are rapidly developing for research and therapeutic use. A tremendous number of CRISPR gRNA have been successfully used in a wide range of species and cell types (Gaj et al. 2013; Sander and Joung 2014).

3 Gene Editing with Cancer Therapeutic Applications

3.1 *CRISPR for Identifying and Validating Drug Targets*

An increasingly important step in the drug discovery process is identifying novel, validated targets whose pharmacological modulation may be important therapeutically. It is important to validate the wide landscape of mutations that are identified by sequencing cancer cells or through other means. Validated targets are further studied to identify the subset that may be addressed with small molecule, biological treatments, and/or gene editing.

Inhibiting the function of a single cancer-driving mutation remains a major strategy in anticancer drug development. This step often helps in the development of small molecule inhibitors of the target protein. Only a fraction of the genome has been explored, providing a great opportunity to identify new protein targets. Experiments of this scale are much easier with CRISPR/Cas than with previous technologies. CRISPR/Cas has proven highly effective compared to siRNA gene inactivation, which is often incomplete, and not a true loss-of-function.

Large lentivirus libraries enable high-throughput loss-of-function screens that rapidly identify genes whose activity is important for the specific endpoint being measured. For example, gRNA delivered by lentivirus to cells with Cas9 can be selected using any knockout phenotype that can be assessed by cell sorting. Tracking the viability of gRNA knockouts can be used as an indication of the potential effects of pharmacological inhibition (Shalem et al. 2014; Koike-Yusa et al. 2014; Kasap et al. 2014). The efficiency and specificity of CRISPR genomic screens have allowed identification of novel therapeutic targets, including the genes required for the development of drug resistance in cancer (Shalem et al. 2015; Wang et al. 2014). The cutting efficiencies of ZFNs and TALENs may be sufficient to generate double allelic knockouts, which is an important criterion for knockout screens. The costs to construct a genome-wide ZFN library would be significantly more expensive (suggested to be $15–50 million (Moore 2015)), particularly at the scale used with CRISPR. The GeCKO v2 library consists of 122,417 gRNAs, targeting 19,052 human genes, plus 1000 control gRNAs (Shalem et al. 2014). Lentivirus expressing Cas9 and a large gRNA library designed to target every mouse gene were used to mutate genes in a mouse model of non-small cell lung cancer (NSCLC) (Chen et al. 2015). The cells were transplanted into a mouse and created highly metastatic tumors. The mutations in the primary tumors and in the metastases included known tumor suppressors, and identified some new genes and microRNAs. Cas9-based screening has proven to be a comparatively easy genome-wide method to systematically assay gene phenotypes in tissue culture and in vivo, and is proving invaluable for cancer research.

Current screening strategies have successfully selected known factors and some novel hits by targeting CRISPR/Cas-induced mutations in the first exons of candidate genes (Shalem et al. 2014; Koike-Yusa et al. 2014; Wang et al. 2014; Zhou et al. 2014). To avoid alternative start codons and missing changes that keep the gene in-frame and functional, an alternative approach targeted the key protein domains in hopes of generating a higher proportion of null mutations and increased negative selection. The authors suggest this approach may be used to determine protein domains that sustain cancer cells and are suitable for drug targeting, as they selected previously identified therapeutic targets and new putative targets (Shi et al. 2015). It is possible that future libraries will contain a combination of guides designed using these two or other methods to ensure a higher rate of knockout.

Because of the capacity for genome-wide knockout libraries, CRISPR/Cas became an important tool within a few years. In addition to using Cas9 to cleave target sequences and screen for knockouts, the protein can be modified to exert many other functions. When both the RuvC and HNH nuclease domains are mutated, Cas9 is catalytically "dead." Dead Cas9 (dCas9) functions as a DNA-binding domain that can be fused to the FokI nuclease domain (Guilinger et al. 2014; Tsai et al. 2014b; Aouida et al. 2015), or can be fused to activators, repressors, or other effector domains. Large CRISPR libraries can also be made with dCas9 fused to other effector domains, including activation and repression domains (Zhao et al. 2014). Attaching an activation domain to dCas9 and supplying a gRNA that specifies a promoter region, it is possible to stimulate the expression of that endogenous gene. Libraries can therefore be used to activate (CRISPRa) or inhibit (CRISPRi) gene transcription in human cells (Perez-Pinera et al. 2013; Larson et al. 2013; Qi et al. 2013; Maeder et al. 2013; Gilbert et al. 2014). CRISPR/Cas libraries demonstrate much higher levels of effectiveness and reliability with respect to both loss-of-function and gain-of-function screenings, than other methods such as RNAi (La Russa and Qi 2015). One CRISPR library structure used tethered engineered transcriptional activating complexes for improved function. The Synergistic Activation Mediator (SAM) libraries targeted each human RefSeq coding isoform with 70,290 gRNAs and enabled robust, specific transcriptional activation and screenings (Konermann et al. 2015).

The high output of NGS has provided massive amounts of cancer genomic data, including the mutational landscape in both common and rare cancers. The next challenging step is determining the *functional relevance* of the identified mutations and combinations of mutations, and separate the driver and actionable mutations from other somatic mutations. CRISPR/Cas is also having a major impact in functional genomics to determine the consequences of mutations and a major impact on target validation by allowing genome editing to *ver*ify that it would be effective to target a gene product will have an effect. It is advantageous to validate in cells that have been edited to more closely resemble the human disease. Knockout cell lines can be quickly generated with monoallelic or biallelic edits that allow evaluation of the loss of the target protein and allow comparison to cells that are identical outside this change. These isogenically paired cell lines allow testing and comparison of the observed effects of both the gene edit and the tested molecules. In addition to generating edited tissue culture cells, a growing number of species have been edited using CRISPR both in vitro and in vivo (Sander and Joung 2014).

3.2 Cancer Model Cell Lines and Animals

ZFNs, TALENs and CRISPR have greatly expedited the creation of model cell lines and animals (Geurts et al. 2009). Due to its greater ease of use, CRISPR/Cas can more quickly create model cells or animals by inducing a diverse range of cancer-associated mutations in vitro, including point mutations and chromosomal rearrangements, such as translocations or inversions (Chen et al. 2015; Choi and Meyerson 2014). CRISPR/Cas can use multiple gRNAs ("multiplexing," see Sect. 2) to edit several suspected genes to model cooperating mutations (Heckl et al. 2014). CRISPR/Cas has transformed the ability to make complex mouse models, which are usually generated by modifying embryonic stem (ES) cells. Genetic modification in adult mice can also be achieved to create cancer models using hydrodynamic tail vein injection and CRISPR/Cas systems to target individual or combinations of genes (Liu et al. 2014a). In addition to mutating or correcting endogenous genes, gene editing allows the addition of fusion tags to an endogenous protein, such as antibody epitope tags or green fluorescent protein (GFP). Fluorescent tagging allows visualization of the gene's expression in an antibody-independent manner and testing or screening for molecules altering expression. The speed of generating CRISPR gene edits is promising when facing emerging clinical data. CRISPR/Cas coupled with rapid sequencing, and genetic characterization allows rapid generation of recapitulating cellular and in vivo models. CRISPR has also been used to validate hypotheses generated by high-throughput-sequencing analysis of drug-resistant tumors (Kasap et al. 2014).

3.3 Gene Editing for Direct Cancer Therapy

The same types of nucleases that are capable of creating oncogenic genetic changes for model creation also hold tremendous therapeutic potential; site-specific nucleases enable genetic editing in both forward and reverse directions. In addition to creating cancer models and helping with drug discovery, nucleases can be used to explore therapeutic paths and therapeutically correct individual or multiple mutations (Gaj et al. 2013). In addition, susceptibility genes and oncogenic virus can also be targeted. In some cases, the same nucleases capable of creating oncogenic genetic changes for model creation can be used therapeutically, as the same DNA cleavage can be repaired using supplied donor templates containing the intended sequence.

Advances in sequencing have identified a wide landscape of mutations in cancer cells, which helped to identify targets that may be addressed with small molecule or other treatments, or may be targets for gene editing. A recent study sequencing the coding exons of 623 candidate cancer genes in 188 lung adenocarcinomas revealed more than 1000 somatic mutations and 26 genes that are mutated at significantly high frequencies (Ding et al. 2008). The ease and speed of cloning CRISPR nucleases allows more readily testing to this scale to determine the importance of these mutations, define the key driver mutations, and map the interactions between multiple mutations in cancerous and healthy cells. CRISPR/Cas and other engineered nucleases can also target the identified mutations for therapeutic editing.

There has been an incredible acceleration of CRISPR/Cas research in recent years, including the correction of single-gene mutations and use for multiplex gene modifications (see Sect. 4.1), as may be needed to cure the genetic cause of complex diseases, such as cancer. Hurdles remain for effective in vivo use, including optimizing delivery to the target cells for gene correction and cancer treatment in vivo. Alternative delivery means, including Cas9 mRNA and protein have been demonstrated (Kim et al. 2014), as has the use of smaller Cas and split Cas viral vectors (Ran et al. 2015; Wright et al. 2015). As the large human genome provides many similar sequences and opportunities for off-target cleavage (Fu et al. 2013; Hsu et al. 2013; Cradick et al. 2013), a number of methods have been demonstrated to improve CRISPR specificity, at least with some targets (Kim et al. 2015; Guilinger et al. 2014; Fu et al. 2014; Kleinstiver et al. 2015). New mutation detection methods have increased awareness about the importance of careful choice of unique gRNAs. With the high number of academic and industrial labs using and studying CRISPR/Cas it is likely that significant improvements will continue (see below).

In addition to many examples of editing cells ex vivo, editing adult cells in vivo was demonstrated in several mouse models. CRISPR was used to correct a mutation in the *Fah* gene in mouse hepatocytes, a model for typrosinemia.(Yin et al. 2014) Hydrodynamic injection was used, resulting in Fah expression in ~1/250 liver cells. Upon expansion, the Fah-positive hepatocytes restored the weight loss seen in untreated mutant mice. This proof-of-principle experiment demonstrated the potential to use CIRSPR-cas9 to correct disease genes in vivo in adult mouse liver and other cells.

Gene editing of tumor suppressor genes *PTen* and *p53* was similarly demonstrated in mouse models (Xue et al. 2014). Deletion of each gene, and a combination of both, gave results comparable to Cre-loxP-mediated deletion. Similar to the *Fah* experiment, this work demonstrates the ability of CRISPR/Cs9 to target tumor suppressor genes and generate point mutations in oncogenes in adult mouse liver. The experiments targeting *PTen* and *p53* created mutations in these genes, more useful for creating cancer models, and drug discovery tools, but inclusion of donor DNAs would allow editing or correction of mutations. Another study demonstrated the use of adenovirus delivery of CRISPR/Cas to target *Pte* (Wang et al. 2015b).

Viral insertion studies, sequencing of tumor cells, and a range of other methods have identified many genes that may be suggested as potential therapeutic gene editing targets (Stratton 2011; Weber et al. 2015). To demonstrate editing in a manner that may be used to correct mutations, as with the *Fah* gen above, CRISPR/Cas was used to target the *Ctnnb1* gene, which encodes β-catenin, a transcription factor in the WNT pathway that is frequently mutated in liver cancer (Moon et al. 2004). Single-stranded oligonucleotides were included in the injection with the CRISPR/Cas plasmids to serve as repair donors, leading to low levels of editing that likely can be optimized and improved with sufficient delivery.

Delivery remains a hurdle to effectively target cancer cells with the nuclease and, if needed, the donor DNA that is required as the template for correction of the oncogenic mutations. Means of exclusively delivering the CRISPR systems to cancerous cells would likely increase efficiency and decrease the chance for introduction of mutations throughout the genome. It is especially important to avoid mutating the targeted oncogene in normal cells. It is possible to avoid cleavage in other cell types by limiting expression of the nuclease to the relevant cells. For example, modular logic circuits were designed based on CRISPR/Cas to allow expression only in bladder cancer cells (Liu et al. 2014a). Delivery of Cas9 DNA, mRNA or protein so that delivery is targeting only the intended cell type also limits editing in irrelevant cells. Once safety, specificity and ethical considerations are established, it might also be reasonable to correct cancer susceptibility mutations in individuals with high probability of developing cancer.

It is estimated that in 2013, about 10% of cancer incidence was attributable to viral infections, generally after years of virus persistence (Schiller and Lowy 2014). Hepatitis B virus (HBV) and Hepatitis C virus (HCV) are predominant causes of hepatocellular carcinoma. Targeting oncogenic viruses may be therapeutic in decreasing both viral loads and cancer rates. Nuclease targeting of HBV has been demonstrated in culture and in mouse models, with the hope that cleavage of persistent viral DNA will help prevent and/or treat HBV-associated liver cancer (Cradick et al. 2010; Lin et al. 2014b).

Another therapeutic approach is synthetic lethality, when alteration of a gene results in cell death only in the presence of alterations in another gene, such as a cancer-associated mutation. Neither alteration is lethal by itself; synthetic lethality requires that two defects be present for cell death to occur (Thompson et al. 2015). Synthetic lethality screens can identify genes that are essential only in the context of specific cancer-causing mutations. In hopes of developing therapeutics targeting cancer cells dependent on mutant KRAS, which had previously been thought to be "undruggable," high-throughput RNA interference (RNAi) was used with a mutant KRAS cell line to identify a serine/threonine protein kinase, STK33 that is selectively required for the survival and proliferation of a range of KRAS-dependent cancer cells (Scholl et al. 2009). Cancer cells that are dependent on mutant KRAS exhibit selective sensitivity to suppression of STK33, which has been identified as target for treatment of mutant KRAS-driven cancers. CRISPR/Cas provides an even more promising means of synthetic lethal screening, which can improve on many of the methods that targeted genes using short RNAs (Platt et al. 2014; Scrace et al. 2015).

4 T Cell Genome Editing for Cell Therapy

Gene editing advances increased the ability to stably express transgenes, such as engineered TCR or CARs (Fig. 9.1), in T cells and have greatly advanced adoptive cell therapy and immunotherapy. High avidity T-cell receptors specific for TAAs can

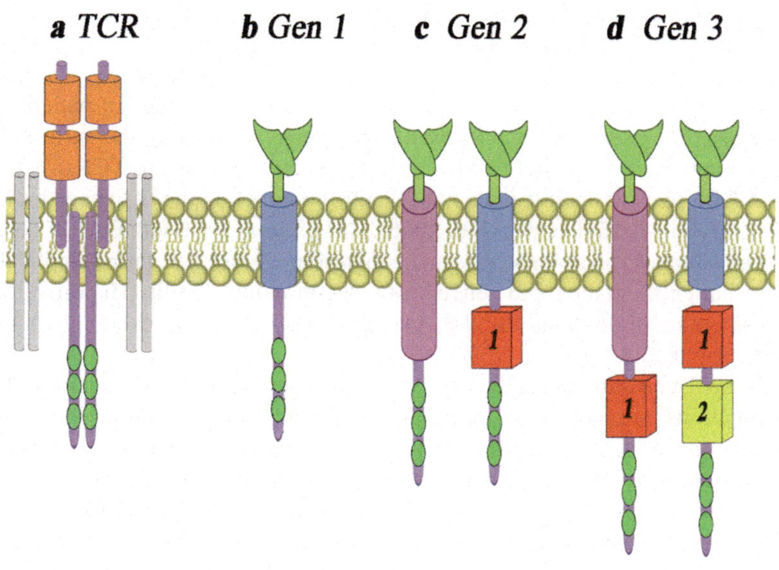

Fig. 9.1 TCR and CAR generations 1, 2 and 3. (From *left* to *right*) (**a**) T cell receptor (TCR) complex containing TCR-α and TCR-β chains, (center), CDζ with three ITAMs (*green ovals*), and two pairs of dimeric signaling modules CD3δ/ε, CD3γ/ε (in *grey*). (**b**, *Gen 1*) The first generation CAR is drawn with the transmembrane domain (*blue cylinder*) and intracellular CDζ. (**c**, *Gen 2*) Two second generation CARs are drawn, (*left*) Single-chain antibody variable fragment (ScFv) domain (*light green*) connected to CD28 (*pink cylinder*) and CDζ, and (*right*) ScFv fused to an additional signaling domain and CDζ. (**d**, *Gen 3*) Two third generation CARs are drawn, (*left*) Single-chain antibody variable fragment (ScFv) domain (*light green*) connected to CD28 (*pink cylinder*), an additional signaling domain and CDζ, and (*right*) ScFv fused to a transmembrane domain, two additional signaling domains and CDζ

be cloned and transduced into T cells that will be reinfused into the patient to direct cytotoxic T-cell activity (Restifo et al. 2012). The receptors' binding domains can be derived from naturally occurring or manmade T-cell receptor (TCR) alpha and beta single-chains (Fig. 9.1a) with the hope of improving the binding affinity, as the binding affinities of endogenous TCRs for TAAs are generally low. TCRs generally recognize protein epitopes presented on the cell surface by the major histocompatibility complex-1 (MHC-1). Ideal TAAs are only expressed on tumor cells, thereby minimizing the risk of toxicity to nontumorous cells (Lipowska-Bhalla et al. 2012; Curran et al. 2012). As normal cells can express low levels of TAAs, alternative strategies are employed (see Sect. 4.1) to avoid targeting these healthy cells.

Chimeric antigen receptors (CARs) are surface receptors engineered to provide a desired specificity to an immune effector cell. Typical CARs have higher affinity than TCRs. The effects of TCR binding, including T cell activation and cytotoxicity, can correlate with the binding affinity up to a threshold amount. A range of binding domains have been used, indicating that the main requirements are high affinity and specificity, though the spatial location of epitope binding and the hinge domain are also important. The binding domains of the TCR are replaced by alternatives, such as single chain antibodies or the single-chain variable fragments (scFv), which are linked binding domains of an immunoglobulin heavy and light chain. The scFv are expressed fused to the transmembrane and intracytoplasmic/endodomains as a single chimeric protein. These linked domains vary through the generations (described below) and are applicable to a broad range of patients, irrespective of HLA phenotype. CARs bind to markers expressed at the surface of the target cell and are not limited to MHC presented epitopes, as are TCRs. A widely used CAR is effective against malignant B cells by targeting the B-lineage molecule CD19 (Zhu et al. 2015; Cooper et al. 2006). Cancer treatment with CAR T cells has several advantages: HLA-independent recognition of antigen, broad applicability for many patients and the rapid delivery of CAR-modified T cells. The use of different transmembrane domains fused to the CAR has led to improved signaling and stability (see Sect. 4.1).

Different T cell subsets can be used in adoptive cell therapy, as they provide different functions and have a direct role in treatment efficacy. In addition to the differences between the major classes of T cells, differences have been found between differentiation states. In a mouse model, more-differentiated effector T cells were less effective for in vivo tumor treatment than naïve and early effector T cells (Gattinoni et al. 2005). Therefore, efficacy may depend on picking the optimal T cell subset, differentiation state, processing methods and other features.

4.1 CAR T Cell Generations

"Generations" of CAR T cells typically refer to the type of fused intracellular signaling domains, which are one of the elements of CAR design that have undergone changes over time. First-generation CARs expressed binding domains on the surface of the T cells linked to the intracellular CD3zeta signaling domain (Fig. 9.1b) (Eshhar et al. 2001). Binding of the scFv to its target results in the transmission of a zeta signal similar to CD3 binding. CD3zeta contains three ITAMs that signal the activation, which is the primary signal from endogenous TCRs (Irving and Weiss 1991). In clinical trials, first generation CARs showed only modest efficacy, due to a combination of insufficient activation, expansion, and persistence of the modified T cells (Lipowska-Bhalla et al. 2012).

Later generations CAR Ts contain multiple added domains or proteins to retarget and reprogram for further amplification of T-cell activation, or to dampen the activation, in the case of adverse reactions. To compensate for the insufficient number of costimulatory molecules on the surface of cancer cells, second-generation CARs were developed with costimulatory domains, such as CD28 or 4-1BB, linked by a spacer region which is typically based on a constant region of either IgG1 or IgG4 (Curran et al. 2012). Second-generation CARs signal through these fusions using these intracellular domains to provide additional signals that compensates for the lack of costimulatory ligands (Fig. 9.1c). CD28 or 4-1BB signaling domains are often added to CD19-directed CARs, which results in remarkable rates of complete remission in patients with refractory B cell malignancies (Jena et al. 2014). Additional costimulatory signaling was added through revising the constructs, adding CD28 and OX40 signaling (Kowolik et al. 2006). The types of genome editing have coevolved with the advancement through different CAR T signaling generations (Fig. 9.2c–e). The combined activating and costimulatory domains included in second generation CAR T cells further program their function and T cell persistence. These types of modification have resulted in varied properties and treatment options that may better match the specific needs of the patient.

Third-generation CARs often combined multiple signaling domains, such as linking CD3-zeta and CD28 and 41BB or OX40, plus additional signaling domains to enhance T cell function (Fig. 9.1d). The second and third generation CAR-T cells have improved activation signals, increased cytokine production, effector function and proliferation. These domains provide the appropriate costimulation, which has proven essential for potent CAR T response. The move to second and third generation systems may help explain why, in addition to cell type differences, viral-mediated transduction of T cells for adoptive immunotherapy has not resulted in adverse outcomes, in contrast to early treatments of HSC. The use of different cell types, though, may affect the integration site preference or availability.

4.2 Other Gene Editing Targets

In addition to adding the CAR, T cells can be further edited to add receptors, switches, and circuits that direct their location, activity, duration, and strength. The number of individual gene editing steps increases as CAR T cells are improved with additional features in addition to the CAR fusion knockin. T cell response and survival can be improved by modulating the expression regulatory molecules, such as

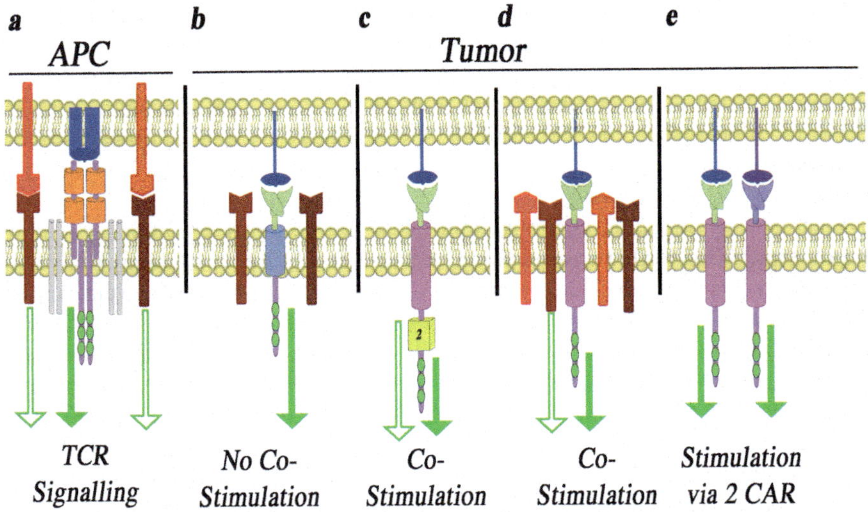

Fig. 9.2 Strategies to provide costimulation in CAR-modified T cells. (**a**) Antigen presenting cell (APC) with antigen in MHC (*blue*) and costimulatory proteins (*red*) interacts with TCR (*center*), CDζ with three ITAMs (*green ovals*), and two pairs of dimeric signaling modules CD3δ/ε, CD3γ/ε (in *grey*) results in activation (*solid arrow*) with costimulation (*outline arrow*). (**b**) A tumor associated antigen (TAA, *blue*) is bound by chimeric antigen receptor (CAR), though signaling is prevented by the lack of costimulation. (**c**) TAA (*blue*) is bound by CAR, signaling is enabled by the secondary signaling domain. (**d**) TAA (*blue*) is bound by CAR, signaling is enabled by pairs of interacting secondary signaling domains expressed on the CAR T cell. (**e**) TAA (*blue*) is bound by one CAR, while a TAA (*purple*) is bound by an additional CAR increasing specificity and allowing signaling

those that control immune responses (reviewed in Mahoney et al. 2015). It has proven important to modulate immune checkpoints—the genes coding for the immune cell's inhibitory receptors. Ligand binding results in inhibition of key effector functions (including activation, proliferation, cytokine release, and cytotoxicity), helping to verify certain genes as key gene editing targets. Excessive T cell activation can result in systemic inflammatory response and cytokine release syndrome (CRS). High levels have been described as a "cytokine storm." One possible solution to CRS is the use of suicide switches (Springer and Niculescu-Duvaz 2000; Casucci and Bondanza 2011).

The number and type of added or edited molecules will depend on effector and target cell types (Devaud et al. 2013). One example of a costimulatory retargeting molecule is expressing the extracellular checkpoint receptor PD-1 fused to intracellular CD28, so that the presence of the tumor-associated checkpoint ligand programmed cell death 1 ligand 1 (PD-L1) results in enhanced, rather than suppressed T cell function (Ankri and Cohen 2014). More editing targets are listed in Box 9.1, including suicide switches and inhibitory CARs (iCARs).

Box 9.1. Additional Editing Targets

In addition to the targets discussed in the main text, a number of genes may been edited in hopes of increasing or modifying therapeutic outcome.

One of the first discovered checkpoint proteins, *CTLA-4* (cytotoxic T-lymphocyte-associated protein 4), plays an important inhibitory role during T cell priming[1], therefore earlier than the PD-1/PD-L1 checkpoint. CTLA4 is a protein receptor that binds CD80 or CD86, the two ligands for CD28, and therefore prevents the costimulatory signals necessary for T cell activation. CTLA4 on the surface of T cells binds to CD80 or CD86 on the surface of antigen presenting cells (APC). This functions as on "off switch," downregulating the immune response and functions as an immune checkpoint. Anti-CTLA4 antibodies were the first approved immune checkpoint blockade therapy[2]. Ipilimumab targets CTLA-4 to down regulate the immune system, and therefore can be used to turn off the inhibitory signal blocking cytotoxic T lymphocytes (CTL) targeting of cancer cells. The higher binding affinity of CTLA-4 compared to CD28 makes it an exciting potential therapy for autoimmune diseases, an immunotherapy strategy for patients with cancer, and a gene editing target. One construct added the gene for a chimeric protein to cells containing an extracellular CTLA4 fused to the intracellular domain of CD28, which allowed binding of CD80 and CD86 and conversion of an immunosuppressive signal to one that stimulates T cells[3].

Programmed cell death-1 (*PD-1*), another key regulator, is expressed on B-cells and activated T cells[4]. PD-1 down modulates effector functions and limits the generation of immune memory. Murine knockout models and studies with blocking antibodies have indicated that these functions are attractive targets, if they can be effectively harnessed though gene editing[2,5,6]. Antigen-specific antigen receptors (iCARs) were developed to constrain T cell responses, limiting cytokine secretion, cytotoxicity or proliferation induced through endogenous TCR. CAR T or TCR activation with one antigen can be countered through binding of another antigen to the iCAR. Constructs were made linking iCARS with the intracellular domains of PD-1 or CTLA4[7].

In addition to the iCARs and other inhibitory signals, other constructs have been added that function as "*suicide genes*" or "suicide switches" to protect from unwanted consequences by specifically eliminating the cells responsible for the unwanted toxicity. Suicide genes allows selective destruction of adoptively transferred cells. These safety switches are important because of the potentially long half-lives of cell therapies. The co-expressed "suicide gene" may limit CAR T cells' immune response time and may irreversibly abrogate such toxicities and adverse events, including cytokine storms. There are a number of different suicide gene technologies, including metabolic, dimerization inducing, and monoclonal mediated. GDEPTs, such as HSV-TK, converts a drug that is nontoxic into a compound that is toxic to the activated

(continued)

Box 9.1. (continued)

gene-modified cells[8]. Small molecules can be added that conditionally dimerize apoptotic molecules, such as caspases. Monoclonal antibodies can be used to eliminate populations of cells that express a cell surface molecule. One example is the RQR8 gene, which depletes the expressing cells when the monoclonal antibody rituximab is administered[9]. These methods that required adding drugs or antibodies once toxicity has been detected, though, may be too late to avoid some adverse events.

There is a wide range of interactions that can be combined with a CAR or TCR to improve tissue associated antigen (TAA) recognition and avoid targeting unintended cells. Examples include adding secondary binding domains, adding negative or inhibitory signals, and expression of other signaling molecules. These combinatorial strategies will require optimization to balance the signals. It is likely that new CAR molecules will be developed with new specificities and it is likely that different costimulatory domains are effective in different T cell subsets, and different costimulatory or signaling pathways are important to effectively target different types of tumor cells. In addition to the molecules above, a number of different molecules have already been tested in CARs. ICOS is a member of the B7 family that is upregulated upon TCR-CD28 signaling. ICOS deficiency leads to impaired effector T cells, memory T cells and Treg cells[10,11]. CARs with ICOS targeting CD33 have been tested[12].

A number of TNFR/TNF superfamily members control aspects of immune function, including the prominent interactions between OX40 and OX40L. These molecules strongly regulate conventional CD4 and CD8 T cells, such that blocking OX40L has resulted in strong therapeutic effect in animal models. Activated T cells express OX40 after TCR and CD28 stimulation. CARs with OX40 targeting CD33 have tested favorably[13].

Box References

1. Freeman, G.J., et al.: Murine B7-2, an alternative CTLA4 counter-receptor that costimulates T cell proliferation and interleukin 2 production. J. Exp. Med. **178**, 2185–2192 (1993)
2. Pardoll, D.M.: The blockade of immune checkpoints in cancer immunotherapy. Nat. Rev. Cancer **12**, 252–264 (2012)
3. Shin, J.H., et al.: Positive conversion of negative signaling of CTLA4 potentiates antitumor efficacy of adoptive T-cell therapy in murine tumor models. Blood **119**, 5678–5687 (2012)
4. Shinohara, T., Taniwaki, M., Ishida, Y., Kawaichi, M., Honjo, T.: Structure and chromosomal localization of the human PD-1 gene (PDCD1). Genomics **23**, 704–706 (1994)

(continued)

Box 9.1. (continued)

5. Topalian, S.L., et al.: Survival, durable tumor remission, and long-term safety in patients with advanced melanoma receiving nivolumab. J. Clin. Oncol. **32**, 1020–1030 (2014)
6. Luke, J.J., Ott, P.A.: PD-1 pathway inhibitors: the next generation of immunotherapy for advanced melanoma. Oncotarget **6**, 3479–3492 (2015)
7. Fedorov, V.D., Themeli, M., Sadelain, M.: PD-1- and CTLA-4-based inhibitory chimeric antigen receptors (iCARs) divert off-target immunotherapy responses. Sci. Transl. Med. **5**, 215ra172 (2013)
8. Springer, C.J., Niculescu-Duvaz, I.: Prodrug-activating systems in suicide gene therapy. J. Clin. Invest. **105**, 1161–1167 (2000)
9. Philip, B., et al.: A highly compact epitope-based marker/suicide gene for easier and safer T-cell therapy. Blood **124**, 1277–1287 (2014)
10. Dong, C., et al.: ICOS co-stimulatory receptor is essential for T-cell activation and function. Nature **409**, 97–101 (2001)
11. Tafuri, A., et al.: ICOS is essential for effective T-helper-cell responses. Nature **409**, 105–109 (2001)
12. Guedan, S., et al.: ICOS-based chimeric antigen receptors program bipolar TH17/TH1 cells. Blood **124**, 1070–1080 (2014)
13. Finney, H.M., Akbar, A.N., Lawson, A.D.: Activation of resting human primary T cells with chimeric receptors: costimulation from CD28, inducible costimulator, CD134, and CD137 in series with signals from the TCR zeta chain. J. Immunol. **172**, 104–113 (2004)

Adding a novel TCR or CAR, plus costimulatory molecules, and modifying regulatory genes, are importance advancements, as is editing to remove the T cell's ability to express an endogenous TCR. Inactivating or editing out a gene segment, such as the TCR alpha region, prevents the rearrangement and expression of alloreactive TCRs that can lead to graft versus host disease (GvHD). These edits, which help create nonautologous CAR T-cells for use "off the shelf" for any individual, is exciting because it allows scaling production, though it requires additional gene editing to prevent expression of the cells' TCR (Poirot et al. 2015). Nonautologous CAR T-cell production can be more readily optimized, and produced in Good Manufacturing Practice (GMP)-compliant facilities without the delays inherent in isolating and modifying each patient's own cells. This is particularly important for critically ill patients and those with low T cell counts that may not be amenable to having cells withdrawn, then waiting for editing of the cells.

5 Delivery Methods and Vectors

In addition to the changes in CAR T components described above, researchers are working on a range of methods to deliver the nucleases and/or donor DNA to the patients' cells. A variety of viral and nonviral methods have been used to integrate the CAR and other constructs into T cells. Viruses have evolved specific mechanisms to evade host responses and deliver their genetic material to the target cell nuclei. Study of natural virus helped lead to the concept of using viruses for gene transfer. Most early gene editing in T cells used either gamma-retrovirus (γ-RV) or lentivirus (LV) to enable stable expression of the CAR (Singh et al. 2008; Kohn et al. 2011; Kay 2011). Viral vectors provide high levels of transduction as this step evolved as part of natural gene delivery of the virus. Virus also provide the ability to stably integrate the target genes into the host genome, thereby ensuring long term gene expression. Viral transduction with γ-RV or LV vectors continue to be the most frequently used methods, though adverse insertional events, including mutagenesis and oncogene activation, are a major worries. Other methods are under development that vary in efficiency, level of expression, cost, and safety. Examples below (Sect. 5.1), employ both viral and then nonviral editing steps.

5.1 Nonviral Delivery

Gene therapy requires delivery into cells, which can be accomplished by a number of methods. The major classes of methods can be divided between those that use recombinant viruses, including LV and γ-RV, and nonviral methods that do not, including transposons. Nonviral vectors are generally used to transfer RNA, small DNA (oligonucleotides) and large DNA (including plasmids). Nonviral methods avoid the chance of immunogenicity and cytotoxicity found with viral vectors, but have technical limitations including efficiency and difficulty with in vivo delivery. Nonviral methods include electroporation, physical methods, chemical carriers, and polymer based vectors. Transposons and donor DNA can be delivered for gene editing. Nucleases can be supplied as plasmid DNA, RNA and/or proteins. As described in Sect. 6.1, the same cells can be edited using both viral and nonviral methods.

5.1.1 Plasmid DNA Delivery

Plasmid delivery is an attractive alternative to virus, as clinical grade plasmids can be quickly produced at approximately 10 % of the cost of GMP-grade virus (Huls et al. 2013). A major limitation of using naked plasmid DNA is the low efficiency of stable integration. The efficiency of integration can be greatly increased using nucleases or transposon/transposase systems (Jasin 1996). Stable expression using plasmids can be generated using Sleeping Beauty (SB) transposon and transposase systems (Aronovich et al. 2011; Hackett et al. 2010). Two DNA plasmids can be introduced to the cells: one plasmid with a transposon coding for a CAR- or TCR-fusion sequence between the terminal inverted repeats that contain binding sites for the transposase and a second plasmid expressing a transposase to insert the transgene into TA dinucleotide repeats (de Jong et al. 2014; Li et al. 2013a). The efficiency of the SB system, therefore combines the low cost and simplicity of naked DNA with gene transfer rates associated with recombinant retroviruses.

Plasmids may also allow transient expression of an engineered nuclease and provide donor DNA as needed for HDR-directed gene editing (Gaj et al. 2013; Durai et al. 2005). A range of donor DNAs have been effectively used that vary in size from 60 to 200 nt oligonucleotides, to plasmids with 400–1500 bp homology arms, to AAV constructs (Gaj et al. 2013). The donor DNA can be supplied with nucleases that are delivered as RNA, DNA or protein.

5.1.2 mRNA Delivery

Delivery of mRNA to cells has allowed effective expression of a number of proteins, including nucleases for genome editing, such as the ZFN mRNAs targeting PD-1 (Beane et al. 2015). Transient CAR-T expression was achieved by ex vivo electroporating T cells with mRNA coding for CARs or TCRs(Yoon et al. 2009; Rabinovich et al. 2009). High-throughput mRNA electroporation can resulting in 80% or more of the cells expressing the construct (Choi et al. 2010). Multiple mRNA can be co-delivered and expressed, as can one or more gRNA and Cas9 mRNA. Expression from mRNA can be a safer alternative than transient vectors or integration, as there is no DNA that may become inserted into the chromosome. The natural metabolism of the mRNA ensures transient expression with a relatively short half-life that limits off-target cleavage. In addition to use for gene correction and editing, transient expression by mRNA electroporation may be especially suited for clinical testing of novel receptors, and/or as a temporary treatment.

Transient expression was tested using a series of anti-CD19 CAR T constructs in a xenograph mouse model and in vitro (Almåsbak et al. 2015). T cells were effectively electroporated with mRNA encoding a CD19-directed CAR. T cells expressing this CAR efficiently killed primary leukemia and lymphoma cells in vitro with minimal toxicity. The mRNA was capped with anti-reverse cap analogue (ARCA), one of many RNA modifications that may further optimize mRNA efficiency. TALEN pairs targeting TCR-α and TCR-β effectively knocked out these genes in both Jurkat and primary T cells when delivered as mRNA. After these genes were knocked out, the cells were transduced with the chains of an influenza virus-specific TCRs leading to functional reprogramming (Poirot et al. 2015; Berdien et al. 2014).

5.1.3 Protein Delivery

For nuclease-directed gene editing, delivery options include DNA, mRNA and nuclease proteins, or combinations thereof. A number of methods have been developed for direct delivery of nuclease proteins, including the use of cell-penetrating peptides to deliver ZFNs, TALENs or Cas9 (Gaj et al. 2012; Liu et al. 2015; Liu et al. 2014b; Ru et al. 2013; Ramakrishna et al. 2014). Transferrin receptor-mediated endocytosis has been demonstrated for ZFNs (Chen et al. 2013). The use of transferrin receptors for tumor targeting has shown promise due to their high expression on the surface of tumor cells (Daniels et al. 2012).

Protein and mRNA delivery, unlike viral or plasmid delivery, prevent integration of the nuclease gene into the chromosome. Protein delivery allows a burst of activity that dissipates as the protein is degraded, thereby limiting the chance for off-target cleavage (after the target site is cleaved). The amount of protein entering the cell therefore becomes the limiting step, and is beginning to be more widely used (Kim et al. 2014; Hendel et al. 2015). For gene editing by HDR, a donor oligonucleotide or plasmid DNA may be co-delivered by electroporation or nanoparticles or delivered using a separate method, such as AAV.

6 Future Generation T Cells

There has been great success through administration of T cells that were genetically edited to express chimeric antigen receptors (CARs) (Lipowska-Bhalla et al. 2012; Zhu et al. 2015; Jena et al. 2014). Recent advances in gene editing, initially using retroviral and lentiviral vectors, have allowed combining gene therapy and cell therapy when engineered CARs or tumor-specific T-cell receptor genes are expressed in immune effector cells (Kay 2011).

CD19 is an attractive therapeutic target as it is expressed during all stages of B-cell differentiation with the important exceptions of hematopoietic stem cells and plasma cells (Kowolik et al. 2006; Singh et al. 2008). Sustained complete response was observed in patients with acute lymphoblastic leukemia and chronic lymphocytic leukemia after treatment with anti-CD19 CAR T cells (reviewed in Zhu et al. 2015). Lentiviruses were used to engineer T cells to express a CAR targeting CD19 and stimulating T cells for activation and proliferation. Since then, CD19 remains the most investigated target for CAR T-cell therapy (Levine 2015). Several institutions have developed and tested alternative next generation CAR T against CD19. These CAR T cells contain different anti-CD19 domains, and different costimulatory domains (see Sect. 4.1), including CD28 or 4-1BB (CD137), which were delivered by lentivirus, retrovirus or Sleeping Beauty. CAR T constructs were recently generated using CCR5-directed megaTAL nucleases (a single TALE-meganuclease chimera) and AAV donor templates containing anti-HIV CAR, or an MND promoter-CD19CAR-T2A-BFP expression cassettes between CCR5 homology arms. Rates of biallelic HDR were not provided in the abstract, though activity was listed as indistinguishable from LV transduced T cells using the identical CD19-CAR construct (Hale et al. 2015).

Comparison of the effects of alternative costimulatory molecules and gene delivery mechanisms are being compiled from the high number of clinical trials and ongoing investigations. Complications with CD19-directed therapy have been reported and their treatment described (Grupp et al. 2013; Teachey et al. 2013). For example, the off-tumor toxicity with CD19 directed T cells can be managed with intravenous immunoglobulin replacement. Cytokine release syndrome (CRS), is treated using tocilizumab, a humanized monoclonal antibody against the interleukin-6 receptor (IL-6R).

6.1 CAR T Cells with Multiple Editing Steps

The improvements in CAR design with the additional costimulatory domains led to dramatic improvements, but were all part of knocking in one, albeit larger gene fusion. An extra editing step was evaluated that allowed testing the feasibility of using allogeneic CAR T cells. In addition to transposon introduction of the CAR construct, ZFNs were used to target the endogenous TCR to limit graft-versus-host disease (Torikai et al. 2012). The efficiency of this procedure was greatly above previous attempts at naked DNA electrotransfer that resulted in low efficiency of chromosomal integration and active selection (Jensen et al. 2010).

An example of next generation CAR T cells that include additional features, and therefore required multiple editing steps, are anti-CD19 CAR+, TCR−, CD52− RQR8+ T cells (Springer and Niculescu-Duvaz 2000; Derniame et al. 2014). These were generated by editing third-party healthy donor cells to generate allogeneic "off-the-shelf" engineered CD19-CAR+ T cells by knocking out the TCR, again to prevent graft-versus-host. The cells are then transduced with the CAR construct. In addition, the T-cells are engineered to co-express the RQR8 gene, which contains target epitopes from both CD34 and CD20 antigens (Philip et al. 2014). This safety feature allows the cells to be depleted using the monoclonal antibody rituximab. Subsequently, the TCR and the CD52 genes are targeted with TALENs, using mRNA electroporation. Knocking out the CD52 gene makes the cells resistant to the lymphodepleting agent alemtuzumab. The final yield of correctly modified cells in a process like this is a product of the efficiency at each step.

Another next generation platform for generating CAR T cells using multiple editing steps is anti-CD19 CAR+ TRAC− dCK− (Valton et al. 2015). These cells are transduced with lentivirus for CAR expression followed by mRNA electroporation of two sets of TALEN pairs targeting the TCR constant region (TRAC) and targeting deoxycytidine kinase (dCK), which is responsible for PNA toxicity. The edited cells are resistant to three different purine nucleotide analogues (PNA) currently used in clinical preconditioning regiments, so that the cells function in lymphodepleting doses of PNAs.

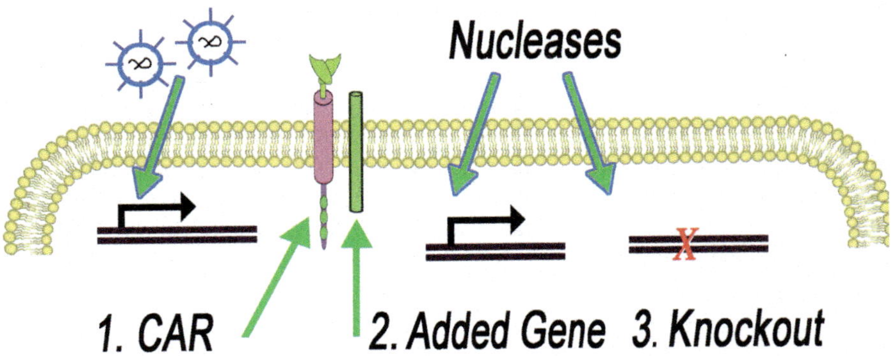

Fig. 9.3 CAR T cell constructed using multiple gene editing steps. Viral transduction can introduce the fusion gene that allows CAR expression. Engineered nucleases can enable multiple editing steps (depicted by two *green arrow*). Gene editing steps can include gene knockout (*red X*), correction or mutational edits or introduce other genes (shown expressing a membrane signaling molecule in *green*)

The two methods described above edit different sets of genes and demonstrate that one can target a range of additional targets, such as those listed in Box 9.1 (Fig. 9.3). The optimal engineered T cells will vary depending on the target cells, patient and therapeutic goal. Possible features include generating "armored CAR" T cells that secrete an inflammatory cytokine (Pegram et al. 2014). Additional options include adding dual CARs or chemokine receptors that may improve targeting of tumor cells (Fig. 9.2e), though adding or editing genes requires the co-transfection of a donor DNA for HDR-directed repair (Pegram et al. 2014). The ability of CRISPR/Cas and multiple gRNAs to effectively target multiple genes ("multiplexing," see Sect. 2) greatly expands our ability to make series of changes (Jiangtao et al. 2015). These examples using multiple editing steps also increases the opportunities for off-target events and emphasize the importance of safe and efficient editing. Final yield is also dependent on the editing activity at each step. This is most evident when multiple sites are cleaved simultaneously, when there is the possibility of translocation between cleavage sites. These examples included data following the edited cells in culture and did not find translocations leading to cellular proliferation (Derniame et al. 2014; Valton et al. 2015). The increased awareness of the importance of specificity and the development of newer testing methods will allow continued improvements and increased usage of editing with TALENs and CRISPR/Cas.

Different nuclease families were used to make allogenic CAR-T cells for a comparison of activity and specificity (Osborn et al. 2015). TALENs, megaTAL and CRISPR/Cas9 nucleases were used to target the first exon of the TCR alpha chain (*TRAC*) that had previously been targeted by ZFNs. Disruption of *TRAC* function prevents TCR expression and undesired endogenous TCR effects, a required step for generating allogenic cells from healthy donors (Torikai et al. 2012). Each of the nucleases successively targets the same region. The nearby and overlapping target sites varied and may account for some of the differences observed, as may differences in delivery. Knockout rates and cell viability were measured and IDLV insertions determined as a genome-wide screen for off-target cleavage. IDLV insertion had previously been demonstrated to detect cleavage for ZFNs, TALENs and CRISPR/Cas9 (Gabriel et al. 2011; Wang et al. 2015a). It is often followed up by NGS to increase sensitivity. The TALEN pair had high activity, though some toxicity in this study, even though the IDLV insertion study failed to locate sequence-confirmed off-target cleavage events. The megaTALs were highly activity at a low dose, though the IDLV insertion assay located validated megaTAL off-target cleavage sites. The authors mention the hopes of improved specifically in newer generations of megaTALs. The CRISPR/Cas9 nuclease displayed low levels of toxicity and low off-target activity, but required chemically modified guide RNAs for highest activity. This gRNA appears to be a unique guide strand without significantly similar sites in the genome when analyzed by COSMID (Cradick et al. 2014). Further studies with improved off-target sensitivity and series of nucleases with overlapping targets will allow better comparison to determine how generalizable these results may be. As ACT may require a series of editing steps, it is exciting that there are multiple nuclease platforms that may serve complementary functions.

7 Improving Specificity

7.1 Improving Transposon Specificity

To circumvent the insertional bias of virus or transposons, their integration preferences can be modified in hopes of redirecting the integration to gene-poor genomic regions, or ideally to specific, safe target sites. The chance of avoiding insertional mutagenesis or proto-oncogenes cannot be completely alleviated unless integration is very specifically directed. A range of methods have been attempted to redirect insertional specificity, including protein engineering through rational design and directed molecular evolution. Adding a known DNA-binding domain has proven a direct route to changing the previous insertional specificity to favor the DNA-binding domain's known specificity. Transposase targeting was altered when fused to either the adeno-associated virus Rep protein (Ammar et al. 2012), ZFPs (Kettlun et al. 2011; Voigt et al. 2012), or custom TALE DNA-binding domains (Voigt et al. 2012). This work will likely continue after the early, limited success, in hopes of more efficient targeting. Similarly, a ZFP fused to Hyperactive SB enzymes has activity, but failed to show integration at the specified genomic-site (Yant et al. 2007). A chimeric ZFP-piggyBac transposase fusion led to higher integration, targeting the ZFP target site, and site-directed transposon integration into an episomal plasmid with the ZFP site. Integration occurred at a chromosomal target with a TTAA-site, but not chromosomal target without at TTAA-site (Kettlun et al. 2011). An excision competent/integration defective (Exc+Int−) version of the piggyBac transposase was developed that was then coupled to ZFPs that directed the transposase and allowed integration (Li et al. 2013b). Tethering to DNA-binding domains may allow efficient integration with specific targeting and improved safety, while, a deeper understanding of the molecular determinants and cellular mechanisms determining insertion site selection may provide alternative methods. It is likely these efforts will lead to more specific targeting.

7.2 *Altering Recombinases*

Although engineer nuclease can cleave novel targets with high specificity, this editing is reliant on cellular DNA repair pathways. Site-specific recombinases, in contrast, function without the need for cellular machinery and are sufficient to direct DNA excision and integration, though they have proven harder to engineer to new specificities. Hybrid recombinases containing activated catalytic domains derived from the resolvase/invertase family of serine recombinases hold promise for genome editing. Directed molecular evolution of site-specific recombinases has provided novel specificities (Eroshenko and Church 2013). The formation of unintended recombinase homodimers can lead to off-target modifications analogous to the off-target mutations caused by ZFNs and TALENs, which were decreased by modifications of the FokI endonuclease dimerization domain (see Sect. 7.5) (Bitinaite et al. 1998; Miller et al. 2007; Szczepek et al. 2007; Miller et al. 2011). Similarly, bacterial selections identified mutations in the Cre recombinase dimerization interface that improve the accuracy of recombination (Eroshenko and Church 2013). To avoid formation of unintended recombinase homodimers that can lead to off-target modifications, rational design and directed evolution were used to reengineer the serine recombinase dimerization interface which reduced homodimer formation >500-fold (Gaj et al. 2014).

7.3 *Changing Viral Integration*

Viral integration into a specified target site may avoid the problems seen with uncontrolled, but nonrandom genomic integration seen with each virus family (Box 9.2). The sites of viral integration may be changed by protein engineering of transposases or through fusions with ZFPs, TAL domains or dCas9 (Jinek et al. 2012; Horvath and Barrangou 2010), or other natural or artificial DNA-binding domain systems. These types of fusions are hoped to lessen targeting to genomic sites, through redirection of viral integration to the binding sites preferred by the DNA-binding proteins. A previously characterized ZFP was fused to viral integrase and the C-terminus of the Vpr that resulted in targeting near the ZFP target site at a 10× higher rate in HeLa cells (Tan et al. 2006). ZFPs were similarly used to target RVs through fusion to the Gag-Pol polyprotein (Lim et al. 2010). Three variants had shifted integration patterns—two variants preferentially targeted four sites, though

Box 9.2. Viral and Transposon Delivery

The virus family *Retroviridae*, including retroviruses and lentiviruses, is among the most widely used viral vectors due to their well understood replication cycle, their ability to integrate into the target genome and high expression levels of foreign genes. Retrovirus evolved as effective gene delivery vectors, as productive infection requires stable integration of their reverse-transcribed RNA into a host cell's chromosome. Covalent integration of viral genomes into the host cell chromatin provides a template for viral gene expression and allows viral replication. As the integrated form of the virus persists for the life of the infected cell and daughter cells, they are effective gene therapy vehicles.

Retroviral vectors have nonrandom integration patterns resulting in highly clustered, cell-specific patterns that correlate with transcriptional patterns and the epigenetic landscape of each cell type[14,15]. Retroviral-based vectors *differ in their preference* for chromatin-associated features and insertion site nucleotide sequence, which lead to differences in insertion site use and in their genotoxic potential[16]. Viral genera-specific patterns appear to exist that describe viral insertion site preference. Early work with retroviral vectors took advantage of the efficient, though mostly random, chromosomal DNA integration capacity of gamma-retrovirus (*g-RV*). Insertions have clustered near genes controlling cell growth and proliferation[17,18]. The insertion sites of *g-RV* favor regulatory regions, including promoters and 5′ regions of genes. The preference of *g-RV* to predominantly target regulatory regions can deregulate gene expression at the transcriptional level. *gRVs* tend to cause disruption of genes more than lentivirus[19,20].

Lentivirus (*LV*) favors integration in *active transcription units* and gene-rich regions of the genome, avoiding regulatory 5′ regions. LV result in clustered integration sites without a bias toward growth-associated genes[7,18]. *LV* tend to insert into transcriptional areas, particularly *actively transcribed genes*. The preference of *LV* for the transcription units of expressed genes can deregulate gene expression post-transcriptionally and may also alter expression by interfering with splicing and/or polyadenylation[21]. LV that preferentially insert into actively transcribed genes include HIV-1[17], simian immunodeficiency virus (SIV)[22], and feline immunodeficiency virus (FIV)[23]. Integrations are highly clustered in the genome, with patterns varying with cell type, transcriptional activity and epigenetic landscape. HIV prefers *actively transcribed genes* within gene dense regions of chromosomes. Murine leukemia virus (MLV) tends to insert near transcription start sites (TSSs) or near CpG islands[24]. Differences in cell types were observed, but a strong link was observed between MLV integration sites and STAT1 binding sites in IFN-γ stimulated HeLa cells, though detecting a protein–protein interaction between STAT1 and MLV integrase was unsuccessful[25].

(continued)

Box 9.2. (continued)

Despite efforts to identify important retroviral or chromosome features that influence integration, the precise determinants are not known. The integration of viral vectors and their genetic cargo into the host cells genome is mediated by pre-integration complexes (PICs), which include the viral integrase and other viral and cellular proteins[26]. Retrvirus-based vectors have been successfully used in research studies and in human gene therapy to correct primary immunodeficiency and genetic deficiency[27], allowing the calculation of the insertion sites. Retroviral integration studies have revealed that the integrase and cognate cellular binding partners are key determinants[28,29].

Adverse insertional events, including mutagenesis and oncogene activation, have raised awareness of the safety implications of retroviral-based vectors used in clinical gene therapy. Integration near a proto-oncogene or disrupting a tumor suppressor gene can lead to the development of tumors. Mapping these locations has been used to identify cancer-related genes[30]. The need to limit insertional mutagenesis in gene therapy is a major force driving mechanistic studies and mapping retroviral integration sites. High-throughput technologies have aided these studies and driven efforts to improve vector safety[18].

Sleeping Beauty (SB) is a typical (class II) transposon system consists of a transposase gene flanked by two inverted terminal repeats, which are the specific binding sites for the transposase protein. Two transposase subunits binding each of the terminal repeats leading excision from a donor sequence and insertion into an acceptor sequence allowing the movement of these genetic elements, which is sometimes described as a hop/jump due to cut and paste.

SB results in precise integration of one copy of the payload genetic sequence flanked by the inverted repeat. Transposon-based delivery vehicles include co-delivery donor plasmids carrying the DNA transposon vector including the gene to be inserted and a plasmid or RNA encoding the transposase. Co-delivering the transposase decreased the size of the delivery plasmid and increases transposition efficiency, but may be more expensive to produce[31]. Viral vector, including LV, Adeno and AAV, have been used to deliver the transposase expression cassette[32–34]. One advantage, though, for use of nonviral vectors is the clinical grade SB transposon production is more reliable and less expensive than virus[31]. SB transposons have few known preferences for integration sites, unlike virus which often target near or in transcribed genes[35,36]. Of the published integrating vectors, SB has less preference for integration either into or proximal to transcriptional units[37]. Insertional site mapping identified 2×10^8 thymine and adenine stacked base pair sites in mammalian cells where insertion randomly occurs without a discernable preference for actively transcribed genes[31].

(continued)

Box 9.2. (continued)

Box References

14. Moiani, A., et al.: Genome-wide analysis of alpharetroviral integration in human hematopoietic stem/progenitor cells. Genes (Basel) **5**, 415–429 (2014)
15. Akhtar, W., et al.: Chromatin position effects assayed by thousands of reporters integrated in parallel. Cell **154**, 914–927 (2013)
16. Mitchell, R.S., et al.: Retroviral DNA integration: ASLV, HIV, and MLV show distinct target site preferences. PLoS Biol. **2**, E234 (2004)
17. Schröder, A.R., et al.: HIV-1 integration in the human genome favors active genes and local hotspots. Cell **110**, 521–529 (2002)
18. Wang, G.P., Ciuffi, A., Leipzig, J., Berry, C.C., Bushman, F.D.: HIV integration site selection: analysis by massively parallel pyrosequencing reveals association with epigenetic modifications. Genome Res. **17**, 1186–1194 (2007)
19. Hacein-Bey-Abina, S., et al.: Insertional oncogenesis in 4 patients after retrovirus-mediated gene therapy of SCID-X1. J. Clin. Invest. **118**, 3132–3142 (2008)
20. Ciuffi, A.: Mechanisms governing lentivirus integration site selection. Curr. Gene Ther. **8**, 419–429 (2008)
21. Moiani, A., et al.: Lentiviral vector integration in the human genome induces alternative splicing and generates aberrant transcripts. J. Clin. Invest. **122**, 1653–1666 (2012)
22. Crise, B., et al.: Simian immunodeficiency virus integration preference is similar to that of human immunodeficiency virus type 1. J. Virol. **79**, 12199–12204 (2005)
23. Kang, Y., et al.: Integration site choice of a feline immunodeficiency virus vector. J. Virol. **80**, 8820–8823 (2006)
24. Derse, D., et al.: Human T-cell leukemia virus type 1 integration target sites in the human genome: comparison with those of other retroviruses. J. Virol. **81**, 6731–6741 (2007)
25. Santoni, F.A., Hartley, O., Luban, J.: Deciphering the code for retroviral integration target site selection. PLoS Comput. Biol. **6**, e1001008 (2010)
26. Levin, A., Rosenbluh, J., Hayouka, Z., Friedler, A., Loyter, A.: Integration of HIV-1 DNA is regulated by interplay between viral rev and cellular LEDGF/p75 proteins. Mol. Med. **16**, 34–44 (2010)
27. Biasco, L., Baricordi, C., Aiuti, A.: Retroviral integrations in gene therapy trials. Mol. Ther. **20**, 709–716 (2012)
28. Demeulemeester, J., De Rijck, J., Gijsbers, R., Debyser, Z.: Retroviral integration: Site matters: Mechanisms and consequences of retroviral integration site selection. Bioessays **37**, 1202–1214 (2015)

(continued)

Box 9.2. (continued)

29. Kvaratskhelia, M., Sharma, A., Larue, R.C., Serrao, E., Engelman, A.: Molecular mechanisms of retroviral integration site selection. Nucleic Acids Res. **42**, 10209–10225 (2014)
30. Nusse, R., Varmus, H.E.: Many tumors induced by the mouse mammary tumor virus contain a provirus integrated in the same region of the host genome. Cell **31**, 99–109 (1982)
31. Hackett, P.B., Largaespada, D.A., Switzer, K.C., Cooper, L.J.: Evaluating risks of insertional mutagenesis by DNA transposons in gene therapy. Transl. Res. **161**, 265–283 (2013)
32. Moldt, B., et al.: Comparative genomic integration profiling of Sleeping Beauty transposons mobilized with high efficacy from integrase-defective lentiviral vectors in primary human cells. Mol. Ther. **19**, 1499–1510 (2011)
33. Ammar, I., et al.: Retargeting transposon insertions by the adeno-associated virus Rep protein. Nucleic Acids Res. **40**, 6693–6712 (2012)
34. Singh, H., Moyes, J.S., Huls, M.H., Cooper, L.J.: Manufacture of T cells using the Sleeping Beauty system to enforce expression of a CD19-specific chimeric antigen receptor. Cancer Gene Ther. **22**, 95–100 (2015)
35. Geurts, A.M., et al.: Structure-based prediction of insertion-site preferences of transposons into chromosomes. Nucleic Acids Res. **34**, 2803–2811 (2006)
36. Hackett, C.S., Geurts, A.M., Hackett, P.B.: Predicting preferential DNA vector insertion sites: implications for functional genomics and gene therapy. Genome Biol. **8**(Suppl 1), S12 (2007)
37. Berry, C., Hannenhalli, S., Leipzig, J., Bushman, F.D.: Selection of target sites for mobile DNA integration in the human genome. PLoS Comput. Biol. **2**, e157 (2006)

without preferred insertions at their ZFP target site. It was suggested that the high affinity and multivalent presentation of the ZFP may have led to the off-target binding at preferred sites, but this type of fusion may allow the use of high efficiency viral systems with specific targeting.

7.4 Improving Nuclease Delivery

There have been great advances in gene editing in a range of cell and animal types (reviewed in Gaj et al. 2013). Cells have been transfected by nuclease RNA, DNA or proteins through a number of methods including transfection or electroporation of nucleic acids (Urnov et al. 2005; Porteus and Carroll 2005), integrase-deficient lentiviral vectors (IDLVs) (Lombardo et al. 2007), adeno-associated virus (AAV) (Ellis et al. 2013), adenovirus and lentiviral vectors (Holkers et al. 2013). Viral methods provide efficient delivery and nuclease expression, raising fears that over and/or prolonged expression may lead to off-target cleavage and DNA insertion. In hopes of fine tuning delivery to each cell, LVP protein delivery was used (Joglekar et al. 2013), though blocking viral insertion was a chief concern. HDR was achieved by co-delivering two different ZFN proteins as part of the lentiviral Gag polypeptide, plus an included donor DNA (Cai et al. 2014). The level of the protein delivery could be tuned by adjusting the ratio of nuclease-Gag fusions to Gag. The rates of gene editing may permit therapeutic use, and it is hoped that future experimental use of CRISPR/Cas systems may lead to higher rates.

To improve the shortcomings of viral vectors, including limited payload, long-term expression, immunogenicity, and genotoxicity, hybrid vectors are under study that have added positive abilities and removed some of these undesired features. Hybrid forms of gene delivery can include combinations of virally derived and synthetic materials, and appear to be a promising approach for developing safe and efficient gene therapy vectors. Noninfectious murine leukemia virus-like particles (M-VLPs) that contained chitosan that functionally replaced the viral envelope protein resulted in transfection efficiencies similar to traditional MLV vectors and had sustained transgene expression (Keswani et al. 2014). An adenoviral vector was constructed that expressed hyperactive insect piggyBac transposase (iPB7) resulting in efficient and persistent expression of a therapeutic transgene (Cooney et al. 2015). DNA transposon-based vectors for genome editing may be developed that similarly combine adenoviral or AAV delivery and transposases.

7.5 *Improving Nuclease Specificity*

A number of methods have been developed to measure (Box 9.3) and improve the specificity of gene editing nucleases. The most straightforward is the careful choice of target sites. Higher off-target cleavage is seen with nucleases targeting sites with similar sites located elsewhere in the genome (Tsai et al. 2014a; Hsu et al. 2013; Cradick et al. 2013; Fu et al. 2014). Conversely, targeting unique sites improves specificity, Therefore using bioinformatics to vet target sites remains a straightforward in silico means to improve the specificity of all types of nucleases and aid the choice of nucleases and target sites (Fine et al. 2014; Cradick et al. 2014; Sander et al. 2010; Cradick et al. 2011; Xiao et al. 2014; Bae et al. 2014).

Alternative nuclease systems may also improve specificity. Early off-target studies often located ZFN cleavage events at genomic locations bound by homodimerization of two "left" or two "right" nucleases. This was especially important, as one nuclease can have much lower specificity (Fine et al. 2014). To avoid cleavage at these types of off-target sites, several groups developed heterodimer-requiring versions of the FokI domain (Miller et al. 2007; Szczepek et al. 2007; Doyon et al. 2011; Lee et al. 2012). The same FokI catalytic dimerization domain and variants

Box 9.3. Specificity Assays

Integrations site mapping

Virus (or vector) insertions site (VIS) mapping has allowed high-throughput study of a major risk in treatment, the possible outcome of integration into regulatory sites, such as those that led to activation of proto-oncogenes with retrovirus[19,38,39]. Although integration into many noncoding sites may not be deleterious, integration near or within cancer-related genes poses a much greater threat. Assays have been developed to measure the level and location of insertional mutagenesis that produce genomic insertion profiles of gene therapy vectors, and provide a means for measuring and discovering safer vectors. In addition to explaining the mutagenic effects of dysregulation due to viral insertion, the integration mapping can help explain the malfunction of inserted transgenes, especially their silencing. VIS can be mapped using methods to capture and amplify the junctions between vector and genomic DNA. One method involves restriction digestion of the chromosome, ligation of adapters with primer sites and PCR amplification using primers in the viral sequence and/or the adapters. A number of amplification methods exist including inverse PCR, linear amplification-mediated (LAM) PCR or ligation-mediated (LM) PCR[40]. Each of the resulting amplification products contains the genomic sequence flanking the insertion site. The amplification products are often reamplified with primers adding barcodes and sequencing primer sites. Next generation sequencing (NGS) of these PCR products produces a large number of reads that can then be mapped to the genome. This method is widely used for identifying the junctions between integrated proviral and host genomic sequences, but the requirement for flanking restrictions site has been reported to introduce selection bias, not fully explained by restriction enzyme-related factors[41]. Once the sites are mapped to unique genome loci, further processing determines the proximity to genes or regulatory regions. Mapping programs can also list annotations, such as if the location in an intron, exon, transcription start site, etc. There are other databases, such as the cancer-related genes that can be compared (described below). VIS data on the local genomic and/or chromatin context must be controlled by comparison to randomly chosen loci[25,42].

There are an increasing number of sequencing platforms that enable integration site mapping and bioinformatics pipelines for genome mapping[43–45]. These type of methods were used to determine the differences between vectors for targeting gene coding regions, CpG islands, and/or transcriptional start sites[16,17]. One database of this type, Retroviral Tagged Cancer Gene Database (RTCGD; http://RTCGD.ncifcrf.gov) contains the genomic position of each retroviral integration site cloned from a mouse tumor, the distance and orientation between it and the nearest candidate disease gene(s). QuickMap (gtsg.org) is one program that analyzes human and murine vector-

(continued)

Box 9.3. (continued)
flanking sequences, providing insertion frequencies and their adjacency to genes, cancer genes, pseudogenes, and other features[46]. Human viral integration sites (VIS) have similarly been logged in an online database to aid identification of potential oncogenes and asses the probability of malignant transformation in gene therapy (Dr.VIS v2.0 http://bioinfo.org/drvis)[47]. This updated database of human disease-related VIS includes chromosomal mapping of the VIS, the viral–host junction sequence, and characteristics of the malignant disease. The database includes 25 diseases and 3340 integration sites of eight oncogenic viruses. The VISA—Vector Integration Site Analysis tool maps VIS from NGS[48]. An assortment of methods were used to generate lists of cancer related genes (http://bushmanlab.org/links/genelists) that were further compiled into a single database.

High-throughput mapping of integration sites can observe the proximity of insertions sites to oncogenes or other coding regions and can also allow tracking of clonally expanded cells[49]. Mapping can therefore be used to follow affected cells in an animal. Analyses of vector integration sites allows follow-up of the gene-corrected cell pool. In addition, such clonal analyses may uncover potential progression or over expansion of individual cell clones, which is a major safety concern in gene therapy studies.

The TRIP (short for Thousands of Reporters Integrated in Parallel) technology studies high-throughput studies of integration and the effects of chromatin position[15,50]. Each barcoded reporter is used for independent and integration site mapping and expression analysis to probe the influence of chromatin context. The dual readout may be particularly relevant to gene therapy applications, but determining the bias out of the essentially random nature of integration requires high numbers to deduce trends.

Nuclease Mutation Analysis
Gene editing can assayed using "digital" evaluation of on- and off-target effects; the amount of editing can be determined using NGS with very high precision, based on the number of cells and sequencing reads. As genome editing with engineered nuclease has the potential to lead to off-target cleavage, there has been increased use of assays monitoring these effects. A straightforward practice is to determine the most likely sites to test for the presence of misrepair, which is indicative of cleavage followed by the introduction of insertions, deletions, and/or mutations (indels) through NHEJ.

A number of programs exist that can scan genomes for sites similar to the target site of ZFNs, TALENs and/or CRISPR nucleases[51–55]. These programs may return few or many genomic sites that match the user-supplied criteria, such as number of mismatches. When there are many sites output, the program must rank them to narrow the list of those to test, generally the top

(continued)

Box 9.3. (continued)
ranked sites. While testing the top 16, 24 or 36 sites might not be exhaustive, it can often be used to rule out nucleases with high off-target cleavage and allow comparison between different treatments.

Cleavage rates are often determined by the indel rate, as correctly repaired breaks cannot currently be measured. The indel rate is observed using several different methods, based on PCR amplification of the sites in question. Once the genomic loci are identified and PCR-amplified, the PCR products can be cloned and individually Sanger-sequenced, which is hard to scale above a very small number of samples. Alternatively, the amplification products can be quickly tested using enzymatic mutation detection assays, such as the Surveyor Assay[56,57]. These assays have been very extensively used, though the detection limit is several percent, assumptions must be made about the diversity of the mutation pool, and the assays are confounded by nearby SNPs. The amplified loci can also be Sanger-sequenced, as a bulk pool without cloning, and the indel and mutation percentage determined using TIDE, which deconvolutes these mixed chromatogram signals[58]. Many sites and samples can be amplified and pooled and sequenced using NGS, which has become more widely used as prices drop and methods improve.

Other methods have been used to look for off-target sites without using bioinformatics to prescan the genome, with the hope that more sites may be identified, even if less similar to the target site. The results of these methods often overlap the sites validated through bioinformatics searches (Lee et al. 2016), but these "unbiased" methods can additionally locate sites that have a greater number of mismatches between the target and the cut site (ZFN data compared in reference 53). These methods include identifying cleavage sites using the insertion of virus, insertion of oligonucleotides, observing translocations, or by measuring the proteins bound to the cut DNA ends[59–62]. While a single off-target analysis method allows effective screening for sites, especially with high off-target cleavage, a series of complementary off-target methods, including these or newer methods, will likely allow more comprehensive testing.

While these off-target analysis methods have begun to be widely used in gene therapy experiments, their use in cellular therapy, such as with CAR T, is being established. A recent study of engineered CAR-T cells used NGS to query for TALEN off-target cleavage by amplifying and sequencing the top 15 in silico predicted putative off-target sites[53]. The amplified PCR products were sequenced: two sites had one sequencing read each with a mutation detected. More reads at these or other sites may determine if these were significant all better understanding of the specificity of these or other nucleases.

(continued)

Box 9.3. (continued)

Another recent study compared cleavage frequencies of different nucleases with nearby target sites[63].

Translocation Analysis

In addition to the correct repair of chromosomal DNA breaks or the mutations, insertions, deletions, described above, there is also the chance that two DNA breaks can lead to chromosomal rearrangements, such as deletions, chromosomal inversions or translocations. There are editing applications where these are wanted, particularly for knockouts[64–66], but they can also result in unintended rearrangements between pairs of on-target sites and between an on- and off-target site[67]. Chromosomal rearrangements are generally only observed in assays specific for their occurrence, such as detecting the different possible chromosomal rearrangements between two loci using amplification primer flanking the combined sites[68]. The risk of unwanted translocations increases greatly when multiple sites are edited, as chromosomal rearrangements can occur between both on- and off-target sites. In a recent study that created CAR-T cells using two pairs of TALENs, possible translocation events between their two on-target sites, CD52 and TRAC, were measured by quantitative PCR (qPCR). Translocation frequencies for the four possible rearrangements ranged from 10^{-4} to 2×10^{-2} of the copy number[69].

Translocations can also be detected by anchoring with a given loci, such as the on-target site and linear amplification and high-throughput, genome-wide, translocation sequencing (HTGTS)[70,71]. Identified translocation and off-target sites can be directly observed using ddPCR and NGS, respectively, to rule out any biases that might present through the requirement for LAM-PCR flanking restrictions sites or other selection bias[41].

Box References

15. Akhtar, W., et al.: Chromatin position effects assayed by thousands of reporters integrated in parallel. Cell **154**, 914–927 (2013)
16. Mitchell, R.S., et al.: Retroviral DNA integration: ASLV, HIV, and MLV show distinct target site preferences. PLoS Biol. **2**, E234 (2004)
17. Schröder, A.R., et al.: HIV-1 integration in the human genome favors active genes and local hotspots. Cell **110**, 521–529 (2002)
19. Hacein-Bey-Abina, S., et al.: Insertional oncogenesis in 4 patients after retrovirus-mediated gene therapy of SCID-X1. J. Clin. Invest. **118**, 3132–3142 (2008)
25. Santoni, F.A., Hartley, O., Luban, J.: Deciphering the code for retroviral integration target site selection. PLoS Comput. Biol. **6**, e1001008 (2010)
38. Hacein-Bey-Abina, S., et al.: LMO2-associated clonal T cell proliferation in two patients after gene therapy for SCID-X1. Science **302**, 415–419 (2003)

(continued)

Box 9.3. (continued)

39. Stein, S., et al.: Genomic instability and myelodysplasia with monosomy 7 consequent to EVI1 activation after gene therapy for chronic granulomatous disease. Nat. Med. **16**, 198–204 (2010)
40. Wang, G.P., et al.: DNA bar coding and pyrosequencing to analyze adverse events in therapeutic gene transfer. Nucleic Acids Res. **36**, e49 (2008)
41. Wu, C., et al.: High efficiency restriction enzyme-free linear amplification-mediated polymerase chain reaction approach for tracking lentiviral integration sites does not abrogate retrieval bias. Hum. Gene Ther. **24**, 38–47 (2013)
42. Li, M.A., et al.: The piggyBac transposon displays local and distant reintegration preferences and can cause mutations at noncanonical integration sites. Mol. Cell. Biol. **33**, 1317–1330 (2013)
43. Jiang, H., Wong, W.H.: SeqMap: mapping massive amount of oligonucleotides to the genome. Bioinformatics **24**, 2395–2396 (2008)
44. LaFave, M.C., Varshney, G.K., Burgess, S.M. GeIST: a pipeline for mapping integrated DNA elements. Bioinformatics **31**, 3219–3221 (2015).
45. Arens, A., et al.: Bioinformatic clonality analysis of next-generation sequencing-derived viral vector integration sites. Hum Gene Ther. Methods **23**, 111–118 (2012)
46. Appelt, J.U., et al.: QuickMap: a public tool for large-scale gene therapy vector insertion site mapping and analysis. Gene Ther **16**, 885–893 (2009)
47. Yang, X., et al.: Dr.VIS v2.0: an updated database of human disease-related viral integration sites in the era of high-throughput deep sequencing. Nucleic Acids Res. **43**, D887–D892 (2015)
48. Hocum, J.D., et al.: VISA—Vector Integration Site Analysis server: a web-based server to rapidly identify retroviral integration sites from next-generation sequencing. BMC Bioinformatics **16**, 212 (2015)
49. Wang, G.P., et al.: Dynamics of gene-modified progenitor cells analyzed by tracking retroviral integration sites in a human SCID-X1 gene therapy trial. Blood **115**, 4356–4366 (2010)
50. Akhtar, W., et al.: Using TRIP for genome-wide position effect analysis in cultured cells. Nat. Protoc. **9**, 1255–1281 (2014)
51. Sander, J.D., et al.: ZiFiT (Zinc Finger Targeter): an updated zinc finger engineering tool. Nucleic Acids Res. **38**(Suppl), W462–W468 (2010)
52. Cradick, T.J., Ambrosini, G., Iseli, C., Bucher, P., McCaffrey, A.P.: ZFN-Site searches genomes for zinc finger nuclease target sites and off-target sites. BMC Bioinformatics **12**, 152 (2011)

(continued)

Box 9.3. (continued)

53. Fine, E.J., Cradick, T.J., Zhao, C.L., Lin, Y., Bao, G.: An online bioinformatics tool predicts zinc finger and TALE nuclease off-target cleavage. Nucleic Acids Res. **42**, e42 (2014)
54. Grau, J., Boch, J., Posch, S.: TALENoffer: genome-wide TALEN off-target prediction. Bioinformatics **29**, 2931–2932 (2013)
55. Naito, Y., Hino, K., Bono, H., Ui-Tei, K.: CRISPRdirect: software for designing CRISPR/Cas guide RNA with reduced off-target sites. Bioinformatics **31**, 1120–1123 (2015)
56. Cradick, T.J.: PhD thesis, vol. PhD thesis 140. University of Iowa, Iowa City, IA (2009)
57. Guschin, D.Y., et al.: A rapid and general assay for monitoring endogenous gene modification. Methods Mol. Biol. **649**, 247–256 (2010)
58. Brinkman, E.K., Chen, T., Amendola, M., van Steensel, B.: Easy quantitative assessment of genome editing by sequence trace decomposition. Nucleic Acids Res. **42**, e168 (2014)
59. Tsai, S.Q., et al.: GUIDE-seq enables genome-wide profiling of off-target cleavage by CRISPR-Cas nucleases. Nat. Biotechnol. **33**, 187–197 (2014)
60. Kuscu, C., Arslan, S., Singh, R., Thorpe, J., Adli, M.: Genome-wide analysis reveals characteristics of off-target sites bound by the Cas9 endonuclease. Nat. Biotechnol. **32**, 677–683 (2014)
61. Kim, D., et al.: Digenome-seq: genome-wide profiling of CRISPR-Cas9 off-target effects in human cells. Nat. Methods **12**, 237–243, 231 p following 243 (2015)
62. Wang, X., et al.: Unbiased detection of off-target cleavage by CRISPR-Cas9 and TALENs using integrase-defective lentiviral vectors. Nat. Biotechnol. **33**, 175–178 (2015)
63. Osborn, M.J.: et al. Evaluation of TCR Gene Editing achieved by TALENs, CRISPR/Cas9 and megaTAL nucleases. Mol. Ther. (2015)
64. Gupta, A., et al.: Targeted chromosomal deletions and inversions in zebrafish. Genome Res **23**, 1008–1017 (2013)
65. Xiao, A., et al.: Chromosomal deletions and inversions mediated by TALENs and CRISPR/Cas in zebrafish. Nucleic Acids Res. **41**, e141 (2013)
66. Lee, H.J., Kweon, J., Kim, E., Kim, S., Kim, J.S. Targeted chromosomal duplications and inversions in the human genome using zinc finger nucleases. Genome Res. **22**, 539–548 (2012)
67. Cradick, T.J., Fine, E.J., Antico, C.J., Bao, G.: CRISPR/Cas9 systems targeting β-globin and CCR5 genes have substantial off-target activity. Nucleic Acids Res. **41**, 9584–9592 (2013)

(continued)

Box 9.3. (continued)

68. Shuga, J., et al.: Single molecule quantitation and sequencing of rare translocations using microfluidic nested digital PCR. Nucleic Acids Res. **41**, e159 (2013)
69. Poirot, L., et al.: Multiplex genome edited T-cell manufacturing platform for "off-the-shelf" adoptive T-cell immunotherapies. Cancer Res. **75**, 3853–3864 (2015)
70. Frock, R.L., et al.: Genome-wide detection of DNA double-stranded breaks induced by engineered nucleases. Nat. Biotechnol. **33**, 179–186 (2015)
71. Klein, I.A., et al.: Translocation-capture sequencing reveals the extent and nature of chromosomal rearrangements in B lymphocytes. Cell **147**, 95–106 (2011)

has also been used to link pairs of TALENs and dCas domains (Guilinger et al. 2014; Tsai et al. 2014b; Aouida et al. 2015; Cermak et al. 2011). The increased binding requirement for this dimerization, though often appears to decrease on-target activity with each type of nuclease.

In another approach to limit off-target mutations, nuclease variants were constructed that resulted in single-stranded DNA breaks per nuclease, instead of double stranded DNA breaks. Pairs of single strand cuts may be created in hope of minimizing off-target double strand breaks. This innovation was first developed for ZFNs, generating ZFNickases by using a pair of ZFNs, one FokI domain with an active catalytic domain and one FokI with a nonfunctional domain (Ramirez et al. 2012; Wang et al. 2012). Treating cells with ZFNickases resulted in less NHEJ than with ZFNs, and therefore a higher ratio of HDR to NHEJ. ZFNickases, though, had a much lower HDR activity than ZFNs. This method of using one active and one inactive nuclease was also used with TAL effectors (Wu et al. 2014). "Nickase" variants of Cas9 were similarly generated by knocking out one of two nuclease domains in the protein. The RuvC or HNH nuclease domains were inactivated, resulting in a Cas9 protein that cleaves only the target strand or nontarget DNA strand, respectively (Mali et al. 2013; Ran et al. 2013b; Shen et al. 2014). The individual half-active Cas9 proteins can be used to drive a form of HDR after cleaving one strand (Davis and Maizels 2014). Two Cas9 that each cleave one strand can be used in pairs to generate a staggered DSB at the on-target locus, with less chance for off-target cleavage unless there are two nearby off-target sites (Mali et al. 2013; Lin et al. 2014c; Frock et al. 2015). Dead Cas9 (dCas9) fused to the FokI nuclease domains functions analogously to the ZFNs and TALENs pairs that require two correctly spaced and oriented binding sites for cleavage of the intervening sequence (Guilinger et al. 2014; Tsai et al. 2014b; Aouida et al. 2015). This method required targeting two sites, and therefore requires delivery of two different proteins for ZFNs or TALENs or two gRNAs for CRISPR/Cas.

A number of strategies have been shown to further improve CRISPR specificity, including modification of the guide strand and changing the nuclease protein. The optimal modifications may be sequence specific, as both gRNA truncation (Fu et al. 2014) and gRNA elongation (Kim et al. 2015) have increased specificity in some situations. The Streptococcus pyogenes Cas9 (SpCas9) protein was modified, resulting in a preference for alternative PAM sequences, thereby changing the binding specificity (Kleinstiver et al. 2015). A range of orthologous Cas9 proteins from other species have been found, which are beginning to be characterized and optimized (Chylinski et al. 2013; Esvelt et al. 2013; Hou et al. 2013; Fonfara et al. 2014). Staphylococcus aureus Cas9 (Ran et al. 2015; Kleinstiver et al. 2015), Neisseria meningitidis (Lee et al. 2016) and Streptococcus thermophilus (Müller et al. 2015) have reduced off-target activity, likely due to their requirement for a longer PAM sequence that should occur at a much lower frequency in genome. Less common PAMs limit the number of off-target sites, but also limits the likelihood that this individual PAM may be near the intended cleavage site. This disadvantage will be mitigated once more orthologs have been developed, giving users a range of available PAMs. Theses Cas9 proteins also have the advantage of being smaller, and therefore fitting within the packaging limits of adeno-associated virus (AAV). The methods listed above for improving specificity can likely be combined if needed, such as using the orthogonal Cas proteins fused with FokI, or fused with inactivated FokI to make nickases. Similarly, it is likely that changing the gRNA may affect their activity and specificity, as with Sp Cas9. Each of these systems will still rely on bioinformatics searches to determine how unique a gRNA is in the genome and if these methods are likely to avoid putative off-target sites.

These and newer strategies can be combined to provide even high activity and specificity as the field improves. These combinations may include changes in the nuclease protein, such as using Cas9 orthologs and/or single-strand cutting nickases. These may be used with one or more guide strands modified in length and composition, designed with improved bioinformatics that can better predict and optimize on and off-target activity.

8 Conclusions

Gene editing will be increasingly useful for cancer research, drug development, and modeling. Developments continue for each family of nuclease for gene editing, particularly CRISPR/Cas. The intersection of gene editing and cellular immunotherapy presents exciting new avenues for treatment. The advances in genome editing and CAR T cell therapy increase the effectiveness of cancer therapy and may allow effective targeting of a range of tumor types. The efficient ability to simultaneous perform multiple editing steps may greatly increase the success of anticancer therapy.

Novel delivery methods continue to be presented and will increase the effectiveness of genome editing and therapeutic outcome. Increased awareness about the importance of targeting specificity, the use of specificity assays, and improved methods are increasing and ensuring specificity. Improved targeting, activation, and persistence of the modified T cells may result from increasing the gene editing steps, raising the importance of optimizing editing activity and specificity. Improvement will likely continue in many aspects of CRISPR/Cas and other nuclease design and the use of combinations of these improvements may provide dramatic increases in therapeutic activity.

References

Almåsbak, H., et al.: Inclusion of an IgG1-Fc spacer abrogates efficacy of CD19 CAR T cells in a xenograft mouse model. Gene Ther. **22**, 391–403 (2015)

Amado, R.G., Chen, I.S.: Lentiviral vectors—the promise of gene therapy within reach? Science **285**, 674–676 (1999)

Ammar, I., et al.: Retargeting transposon insertions by the adeno-associated virus Rep protein. Nucleic Acids Res. **40**, 6693–6712 (2012)

Ankri, C., Cohen, C.J.: Out of the bitter came forth sweet: Activating CD28-dependent co-stimulation via PD-1 ligands. Oncoimmunology **3**, e27399 (2014)

Aouida, M., et al.: Efficient fdCas9 synthetic endonuclease with improved specificity for precise genome engineering. PLoS One **10**, e0133373 (2015)

Aronovich, E.L., McIvor, R.S., Hackett, P.B.: The Sleeping Beauty transposon system: a non-viral vector for gene therapy. Hum. Mol. Genet. **20**, R14–R20 (2011)

Bae, S., Park, J., Kim, J.S.: Cas-OFFinder: a fast and versatile algorithm that searches for potential off-target sites of Cas9 RNA-guided endonucleases. Bioinformatics **30**, 1473–1475 (2014)

Beane, J.D., et al.: Clinical scale zinc finger nuclease-mediated gene editing of PD-1 in tumor infiltrating lymphocytes for the treatment of metastatic melanoma. Mol. Ther. (2015)

Berdien, B., Mock, U., Atanackovic, D., Fehse, B.: TALEN-mediated editing of endogenous T-cell receptors facilitates efficient reprogramming of T lymphocytes by lentiviral gene transfer. Gene Ther. **21**, 539–548 (2014)

Bitinaite, J., Wah, D.A., Aggarwal, A.K., Schildkraut, I.: FokI dimerization is required for DNA cleavage. Proc. Natl. Acad. Sci. U. S. A. **95**, 10570–10575 (1998)

Boissel, S., et al.: megaTALs: a rare-cleaving nuclease architecture for therapeutic genome engineering. Nucleic Acids Res. **42**, 2591–2601 (2014)

Bolotin, A., Quinquis, B., Sorokin, A., Ehrlich, S.D.: Clustered regularly interspaced short palindrome repeats (CRISPRs) have spacers of extrachromosomal origin. Microbiology **151**, 2551–2561 (2005)

Brentjens, R.J., et al.: CD19-targeted T cells rapidly induce molecular remissions in adults with chemotherapy-refractory acute lymphoblastic leukemia. Sci. Transl. Med. **5**, 177ra138 (2013)

Budde, L.E., et al.: Combining a CD20 chimeric antigen receptor and an inducible caspase 9 suicide switch to improve the efficacy and safety of T cell adoptive immunotherapy for lymphoma. PLoS One **8**, e82742 (2013)

Cai, Y., Bak, R.O., Mikkelsen, J.G.: Targeted genome editing by lentiviral protein transduction of zinc-finger and TAL-effector nucleases. Elife **3**, e01911 (2014)

Carroll, D., Morton, J.J., Beumer, K.J., Segal, D.J.: Design, construction and in vitro testing of zinc finger nucleases. Nat. Protoc. **1**, 1329–1341 (2006)

Casucci, M., Bondanza, A.: Suicide gene therapy to increase the safety of chimeric antigen receptor-redirected T lymphocytes. J. Cancer **2**, 378–382 (2011)

Cermak, T., et al.: Efficient design and assembly of custom TALEN and other TAL effector-based constructs for DNA targeting. Nucleic Acids Res. **39**, e82 (2011)

Chen, Z., et al.: Receptor-mediated delivery of engineered nucleases for genome modification. Nucleic Acids Res. **41**, e182 (2013)
Chen, S., et al.: Genome-wide CRISPR screen in a mouse model of tumor growth and metastasis. Cell **160**, 1246–1260 (2015)
Choi, P.S., Meyerson, M.: Targeted genomic rearrangements using CRISPR/Cas technology. Nat. Commun. **5**, 3728 (2014)
Choi, Y., et al.: A high throughput microelectroporation device to introduce a chimeric antigen receptor to redirect the specificity of human T cells. Biomed. Microdevices **12**, 855–863 (2010)
Chylinski, K. et al.: The tracrRNA and Cas9 families of type II CRISPR-Cas immunity systems. RNA Biol **10**, 726–737 (2013)
Cong, L., et al.: Multiplex genome engineering using CRISPR/Cas systems. Science **339**, 819–823 (2013)
Cooney, A.L., Singh, B.K., Sinn, P.L.: Hybrid nonviral/viral vector systems for improved piggyBac DNA transposon in vivo delivery. Mol. Ther. **23**, 667–674 (2015)
Cooper, L.J., et al.: Manufacturing of gene-modified cytotoxic T lymphocytes for autologous cellular therapy for lymphoma. Cytotherapy **8**, 105–117 (2006)
Cradick, T.J., Keck, K., Bradshaw, S., Jamieson, A.C., McCaffrey, A.P.: Zinc-finger nucleases as a novel therapeutic strategy for targeting hepatitis B virus DNAs. Mol. Ther. **18**, 947–954 (2010)
Cradick, T.J., Ambrosini, G., Iseli, C., Bucher, P., McCaffrey, A.P.: ZFN-Site searches genomes for zinc finger nuclease target sites and off-target sites. BMC Bioinformatics **12**, 152 (2011)
Cradick, T.J., Fine, E.J., Antico, C.J., Bao, G.: CRISPR/Cas9 systems targeting β-globin and CCR5 genes have substantial off-target activity. Nucleic Acids Res. **41**, 9584–9592 (2013)
Cradick, T.J., Qui, P., Lee, C.M., Fine, E.J., Bao, G.: COSMID: a web-based tool for identifying and validating CRISPR/Cas off-target sites. Mol. Ther. Nucleic Acids **3**, e214 (2014)
Curran, K.J., Pegram, H.J., Brentjens, R.J.: Chimeric antigen receptors for T cell immunotherapy: current understanding and future directions. J. Gene Med. **14**, 405–415 (2012)
Daniels, T.R., et al.: The transferrin receptor and the targeted delivery of therapeutic agents against cancer. Biochim. Biophys. Acta **1820**, 291–317 (2012)
Davis, L., Maizels, N.: Homology-directed repair of DNA nicks via pathways distinct from canonical double-strand break repair. Proc. Natl. Acad. Sci. U. S. A. **111**, E924–E932 (2014)
de Jong, J., et al.: Chromatin landscapes of retroviral and transposon integration profiles. PLoS Genet. **10**, e1004250 (2014)
Deltcheva, E., et al.: CRISPR RNA maturation by trans-encoded small RNA and host factor RNase III. Nature **471**, 602–607 (2011)
Derniame, S. et al.: American Society of Hematology, San Francisco, CA (2014)
Devaud, C., John, L.B., Westwood, J.A., Darcy, P.K., Kershaw, M.H.: Immune modulation of the tumor microenvironment for enhancing cancer immunotherapy. Oncoimmunology **2**, e25961 (2013)
Ding, L., et al.: Somatic mutations affect key pathways in lung adenocarcinoma. Nature **455**, 1069–1075 (2008)
Doyon, Y., et al.: Enhancing zinc-finger-nuclease activity with improved obligate heterodimeric architectures. Nat. Methods **8**, 74–79 (2011)
Durai, S., et al.: Zinc finger nucleases: custom-designed molecular scissors for genome engineering of plant and mammalian cells. Nucleic Acids Res. **33**, 5978–5990 (2005)
Ellis, B.L., Hirsch, M.L., Porter, S.N., Samulski, R.J., Porteus, M.H.: Zinc-finger nuclease-mediated gene correction using single AAV vector transduction and enhancement by Food and Drug Administration-approved drugs. Gene Ther. **20**, 35–42 (2013)
Eroshenko, N., Church, G.M.: Mutants of Cre recombinase with improved accuracy. Nat. Commun. **4**, 2509 (2013)
Eshhar, Z., Waks, T., Bendavid, A., Schindler, D.G.: Functional expression of chimeric receptor genes in human T cells. J. Immunol. Methods **248**, 67–76 (2001)
Esvelt, K.M., et al.: Orthogonal Cas9 proteins for RNA-guided gene regulation and editing. Nat. Methods **10**, 1116–1121 (2013)

Fedorov, V.D., Themeli, M., Sadelain, M.: PD-1- and CTLA-4-based inhibitory chimeric antigen receptors (iCARs) divert off-target immunotherapy responses. Sci. Transl. Med. **5**, 215ra172 (2013)
Fine, E.J., Cradick, T.J., Zhao, C.L., Lin, Y., Bao, G.: An online bioinformatics tool predicts zinc finger and TALE nuclease off-target cleavage. Nucleic Acids Res. **42**, e42 (2014)
Fonfara, I., et al.: Phylogeny of Cas9 determines functional exchangeability of dual-RNA and Cas9 among orthologous type II CRISPR-Cas systems. Nucleic Acids Res. **42**, 2577–2590 (2014)
Frock, R.L., et al.: Genome-wide detection of DNA double-stranded breaks induced by engineered nucleases. Nat. Biotechnol. **33**, 179–186 (2015)
Fu, Y., et al.: High-frequency off-target mutagenesis induced by CRISPR-Cas nucleases in human cells. Nat. Biotechnol. **31**, 822–826 (2013)
Fu, Y., Sander, J.D., Reyon, D., Cascio, V.M., Joung, J.K.: Improving CRISPR-Cas nuclease specificity using truncated guide RNAs. Nat. Biotechnol. **32**, 279–284 (2014)
Gabriel, R., et al.: An unbiased genome-wide analysis of zinc-finger nuclease specificity. Nat. Biotechnol. **29**, 816–823 (2011)
Gaj, T., Guo, J., Kato, Y., Sirk, S.J., Barbas, C.F.: Targeted gene knockout by direct delivery of zinc-finger nuclease proteins. Nat. Methods **9**, 805–807 (2012)
Gaj, T., Gersbach, C.A., Barbas, C.F.: ZFN, TALEN, and CRISPR/Cas-based methods for genome engineering. Trends Biotechnol. **31**, 397–405 (2013)
Gaj, T., et al.: Enhancing the specificity of recombinase-mediated genome engineering through dimer interface redesign. J. Am. Chem. Soc. **136**, 5047–5056 (2014)
Garneau, J.E., et al.: The CRISPR/Cas bacterial immune system cleaves bacteriophage and plasmid DNA. Nature **468**, 67–71 (2010)
Gasiunas, G., Barrangou, R., Horvath, P., Siksnys, V.: Cas9-crRNA ribonucleoprotein complex mediates specific DNA cleavage for adaptive immunity in bacteria. Proc. Natl. Acad. Sci. U. S. A. **109**, E2579–E2586 (2012)
Gattinoni, L., et al.: Acquisition of full effector function in vitro paradoxically impairs the in vivo antitumor efficacy of adoptively transferred CD8+ T cells. J. Clin. Invest. **115**, 1616–1626 (2005)
Geurts, A.M., et al.: Knockout rats via embryo microinjection of zinc-finger nucleases. Science **325**, 433 (2009)
Gilbert, L.A., et al.: Genome-scale CRISPR-mediated control of gene repression and activation. Cell **159**, 647–661 (2014)
Grupp, S.A., et al.: Chimeric antigen receptor-modified T cells for acute lymphoid leukemia. N. Engl. J. Med. **368**, 1509–1518 (2013)
Guilinger, J.P., Thompson, D.B., Liu, D.R.: Fusion of catalytically inactive Cas9 to FokI nuclease improves the specificity of genome modification. Nat. Biotechnol. **32**, 577–582 (2014)
Hackett, P.B., Largaespada, D.A., Cooper, L.J.: A transposon and transposase system for human application. Mol. Ther. **18**, 674–683 (2010)
Hale, C.R., et al.: RNA-guided RNA cleavage by a CRISPR RNA-Cas protein complex. Cell **139**, 945–956 (2009)
Hale, M., et al.: American Society of Gene & Cell Therapy, New Orleans, LA (2015)
Heckl, D., et al.: Generation of mouse models of myeloid malignancy with combinatorial genetic lesions using CRISPR-Cas9 genome editing. Nat. Biotechnol. **32**, 941–946 (2014)
Hendel, A., et al.: Quantifying genome-editing outcomes at endogenous loci with SMRT sequencing. Cell Rep. **7**, 293–305 (2014)
Hendel, A., et al.: Chemically modified guide RNAs enhance CRISPR-Cas genome editing in human primary cells. Nat. Biotechnol. **33**, 985–989 (2015)
Holkers, M., et al.: Differential integrity of TALE nuclease genes following adenoviral and lentiviral vector gene transfer into human cells. Nucleic Acids Res. **41**, e63 (2013)
Horvath, P., Barrangou, R.: CRISPR/Cas, the immune system of bacteria and archaea. Science **327**, 167–170 (2010)
Hou, Z., et al.: Efficient genome engineering in human pluripotent stem cells using Cas9 from Neisseria meningitidis. Proc. Natl. Acad. Sci. U. S. A. **110**, 15644–15649 (2013)
Hsu, P.D., et al.: DNA targeting specificity of RNA-guided Cas9 nucleases. Nat. Biotechnol. **31**, 827–832 (2013)

Huls, M.H., et al.: Clinical application of Sleeping Beauty and artificial antigen presenting cells to genetically modify T cells from peripheral and umbilical cord blood. J. Vis. Exp., e50070 (2013)
Irving, B.A., Weiss, A.: The cytoplasmic domain of the T cell receptor zeta chain is sufficient to couple to receptor-associated signal transduction pathways. Cell **64**, 891–901 (1991)
Jasin, M.: Genetic manipulation of genomes with rare-cutting endonucleases. Trends Genet. **12**, 224–228 (1996)
Jena, B., Moyes, J.S., Huls, H., Cooper, L.J.: Driving CAR-based T-cell therapy to success. Curr. Hematol. Malig. Rep. **9**, 50–56 (2014)
Jensen, M.C., et al.: Antitransgene rejection responses contribute to attenuated persistence of adoptively transferred CD20/CD19-specific chimeric antigen receptor redirected T cells in humans. Biol. Blood Marrow Transplant. **16**, 1245–1256 (2010)
Jiang, W., Bikard, D., Cox, D., Zhang, F., Marraffini, L.A.: RNA-guided editing of bacterial genomes using CRISPR-Cas systems. Nat. Biotechnol. **31**, 233–239 (2013)
Jiangtao, R., et al.: American Society of Hematology Annual Meeting, Orlando, FL (2015)
Jinek, M., et al.: A programmable dual-RNA-guided DNA endonuclease in adaptive bacterial immunity. Science **337**, 816–821 (2012)
Jinek, M., et al.: RNA-programmed genome editing in human cells. Elife **2**, e00471 (2013)
Joglekar, A.V., et al.: Integrase-defective lentiviral vectors as a delivery platform for targeted modification of adenosine deaminase locus. Mol. Ther. **21**, 1705–1717 (2013)
Kasap, C., Elemento, O., Kapoor, T.M.: DrugTargetSeqR: a genomics- and CRISPR-Cas9-based method to analyze drug targets. Nat. Chem. Biol. **10**, 626–628 (2014)
Kay, M.A.: State-of-the-art gene-based therapies: the road ahead. Nat. Rev. Genet. **12**, 316–328 (2011)
Keswani, R., Su, K., Pack, D.W.: Efficient in vitro gene delivery by hybrid biopolymer/virus nanobiovectors. J. Control. Release **192**, 40–46 (2014)
Kettlun, C., Galvan, D.L., George, A.L., Kaja, A., Wilson, M.H.: Manipulating piggyBac transposon chromosomal integration site selection in human cells. Mol. Ther. **19**, 1636–1644 (2011)
Kim, Y.G., Li, L., Chandrasegaran, S.: Insertion and deletion mutants of FokI restriction endonuclease. J. Biol. Chem. **269**, 31978–31982 (1994)
Kim, S., Kim, D., Cho, S.W., Kim, J., Kim, J.S.: Highly efficient RNA-guided genome editing in human cells via delivery of purified Cas9 ribonucleoproteins. Genome Res. **24**, 1012–1019 (2014)
Kim, D., et al.: Digenome-seq: genome-wide profiling of CRISPR-Cas9 off-target effects in human cells. Nat. Methods **12**, 237–243 (2015). 231 p following 243
Kleinstiver, B.P., et al.: Engineered CRISPR-Cas9 nucleases with altered PAM specificities. Nature **523**, 481–485 (2015)
Kohn, D.B., et al.: CARs on track in the clinic. Mol. Ther. **19**, 432–438 (2011)
Koike-Yusa, H., Li, Y., Tan, E.P., Velasco-Herrera, M.C., Yusa, K.: Genome-wide recessive genetic screening in mammalian cells with a lentiviral CRISPR-guide RNA library. Nat. Biotechnol. **32**, 267–273 (2014)
Konermann, S., et al.: Genome-scale transcriptional activation by an engineered CRISPR-Cas9 complex. Nature **517**, 583–588 (2015)
Kowolik, C.M., et al.: CD28 costimulation provided through a CD19-specific chimeric antigen receptor enhances in vivo persistence and antitumor efficacy of adoptively transferred T cells. Cancer Res. **66**, 10995–11004 (2006)
La Russa, M.F., Qi, L.S.: The new state of the art: Cas9 for gene activation and repression. Mol. Cell. Biol. **35**, 3800–3809 (2015)
Larson, M.H., et al.: CRISPR interference (CRISPRi) for sequence-specific control of gene expression. Nat. Protoc. **8**, 2180–2196 (2013)
Lee, C.M., Flynn, R., Hollywood, J.A., Scallan, M.F., Harrison, P.T.: Correction of the ΔF508 mutation in the cystic fibrosis transmembrane conductance regulator gene by zinc-finger nuclease homology-directed repair. Biores. Open Access **1**, 99–108 (2012)
Levine, B.L.: Performance-enhancing drugs: design and production of redirected chimeric antigen receptor (CAR) T cells. Cancer Gene Ther. **22**, 79–84 (2015)

Li, M.A., et al.: The piggyBac transposon displays local and distant reintegration preferences and can cause mutations at noncanonical integration sites. Mol. Cell. Biol. **33**, 1317–1330 (2013a)

Li, X., et al.: piggyBac transposase tools for genome engineering. Proc. Natl. Acad. Sci. U. S. A. **110**, E2279–E2287 (2013b)

Lim, K.I., Klimczak, R., Yu, J.H., Schaffer, D.V.: Specific insertions of zinc finger domains into Gag-Pol yield engineered retroviral vectors with selective integration properties. Proc. Natl. Acad. Sci. U. S. A. **107**, 12475–12480 (2010)

Lin, Y., et al.: SAPTA: a new design tool for improving TALE nuclease activity. Nucleic Acids Res. **42**, e47 (2014a)

Lin, S.R., et al.: The CRISPR/Cas9 system facilitates clearance of the intrahepatic HBV templates in vivo. Mol. Ther. Nucleic Acids **3**, e186 (2014b)

Lin, Y., et al.: CRISPR/Cas9 systems have off-target activity with insertions or deletions between target DNA and guide RNA sequences. Nucleic Acids Res. **42**, 7473–7485 (2014c)

Lindsay, C.R., Roth, D.B.: An unbiased method for detection of genome-wide off-target effects in cell lines treated with zinc finger nucleases. Methods Mol. Biol. **1114**, 353–369 (2014)

Lipowska-Bhalla, G., Gilham, D.E., Hawkins, R.E., Rothwell, D.G.: Targeted immunotherapy of cancer with CAR T cells: achievements and challenges. Cancer Immunol. Immunother. **61**, 953–962 (2012)

Liu, Y., et al.: Synthesizing AND gate genetic circuits based on CRISPR-Cas9 for identification of bladder cancer cells. Nat. Commun. **5**, 5393 (2014a)

Liu, J., Gaj, T., Patterson, J.T., Sirk, S.J., Barbas, C.F.: Cell-penetrating peptide-mediated delivery of TALEN proteins via bioconjugation for genome engineering. PLoS One **9**, e85755 (2014b)

Liu, J., Gaj, T., Wallen, M.C., Barbas, C.F.: Improved cell-penetrating zinc-finger nuclease proteins for precision genome engineering. Mo.l Ther. Nucleic Acids **4**, e232 (2015)

Lombardo, A., et al.: Gene editing in human stem cells using zinc finger nucleases and integrase-defective lentiviral vector delivery. Nat. Biotechnol. **25**, 1298–1306 (2007)

Maeder, M.L., et al.: CRISPR RNA-guided activation of endogenous human genes. Nat. Methods **10**, 977–979 (2013)

Mahoney, K.M., Rennert, P.D., Freeman, G.J.: Combination cancer immunotherapy and new immunomodulatory targets. Nat. Rev. Drug Discov. **14**, 561–584 (2015)

Mali, P., et al.: CAS9 transcriptional activators for target specificity screening and paired nickases for cooperative genome engineering. Nat. Biotechnol. **31**, 833–838 (2013)

Marraffini, L.A., Sontheimer, E.J.: CRISPR interference: RNA-directed adaptive immunity in bacteria and archaea. Nat. Rev. Genet. **11**, 181–190 (2010)

Miller, J.C., et al.: An improved zinc-finger nuclease architecture for highly specific genome editing. Nat. Biotechnol. **25**, 778–785 (2007)

Miller, J.C., et al.: A TALE nuclease architecture for efficient genome editing. Nat. Biotechnol. **29**, 143–148 (2011)

Moon, R.T., Kohn, A.D., De Ferrari, G.V., Kaykas, A.: WNT and beta-catenin signalling: diseases and therapies. Nat. Rev. Genet. **5**, 691–701 (2004)

Moore, J.D.: The impact of CRISPR-Cas9 on target identification and validation. Drug Discov. Today **20**, 450–457 (2015)

Mou, H., Kennedy, Z., Anderson, D.G., Yin, H., Xue, W.: Precision cancer mouse models through genome editing with CRISPR-Cas9. Genome Med. **7**, 53 (2015)

Mussolino, C., et al.: A novel TALE nuclease scaffold enables high genome editing activity in combination with low toxicity. Nucleic Acids Res. **39**, 9283–9293 (2011)

Mussolino, C., et al.: TALENs facilitate targeted genome editing in human cells with high specificity and low cytotoxicity. Nucleic Acids Res. **42**, 6762–6773 (2014)

Osborn, M.J., et al.: Evaluation of TCR Gene Editing achieved by TALENs, CRISPR/Cas9 and megaTAL nucleases. Mol. Ther. (2015). doi:10.1038/mt.2015.197

Pattanayak, V., Ramirez, C.L., Joung, J.K., Liu, D.R.: Revealing off-target cleavage specificities of zinc-finger nucleases by in vitro selection. Nat. Methods **8**, 765–770 (2011)

Pegram, H.J., Park, J.H., Brentjens, R.J.: CD28z CARs and armored CARs. Cancer J. **20**, 127–133 (2014)

Perez, E.E., et al.: Establishment of HIV-1 resistance in CD4+ T cells by genome editing using zinc-finger nucleases. Nat. Biotechnol. **26**, 808–816 (2008)

Perez-Pinera, P., et al.: RNA-guided gene activation by CRISPR-Cas9-based transcription factors. Nat. Methods **10**, 973–976 (2013)

Philip, B., et al.: A highly compact epitope-based marker/suicide gene for easier and safer T-cell therapy. Blood **124**, 1277–1287 (2014)

Platt, R.J., et al.: CRISPR-Cas9 knockin mice for genome editing and cancer modeling. Cell **159**, 440–455 (2014)

Poirot, L., et al.: Multiplex genome edited T-cell manufacturing platform for "off-the-shelf" adoptive T-cell immunotherapies. Cancer Res. **75**, 3853–3864 (2015)

Porteus, M.H., Baltimore, D.: Chimeric nucleases stimulate gene targeting in human cells. Science **300**, 763 (2003)

Porteus, M.H., Carroll, D.: Gene targeting using zinc finger nucleases. Nat. Biotechnol. **23**, 967–973 (2005)

Pule, M.A., et al.: Virus-specific T cells engineered to coexpress tumor-specific receptors: persistence and antitumor activity in individuals with neuroblastoma. Nat. Med. **14**, 1264–1270 (2008)

Qi, L.S., et al.: Repurposing CRISPR as an RNA-guided platform for sequence-specific control of gene expression. Cell **152**, 1173–1183 (2013)

Rabinovich, P.M., et al.: Chimeric receptor mRNA transfection as a tool to generate antineoplastic lymphocytes. Hum. Gene Ther. **20**, 51–61 (2009)

Ramakrishna, S., et al.: Gene disruption by cell-penetrating peptide-mediated delivery of Cas9 protein and guide RNA. Genome Res. **24**, 1020–1027 (2014)

Ramirez, C.L., et al.: Engineered zinc finger nickases induce homology-directed repair with reduced mutagenic effects. Nucleic Acids Res. **40**, 5560–5568 (2012)

Ran, F.A., et al.: Genome engineering using the CRISPR-Cas9 system. Nat. Protoc. **8**, 2281–2308 (2013a)

Ran, F.A., et al.: Double nicking by RNA-guided CRISPR Cas9 for enhanced genome editing specificity. Cell **154**, 1380–1389 (2013b)

Ran, F.A., et al.: In vivo genome editing using Staphylococcus aureus Cas9. Nature **520**, 186–191 (2015)

Restifo, N.P., Dudley, M.E., Rosenberg, S.A.: Adoptive immunotherapy for cancer: harnessing the T cell response. Nat. Rev. Immunol. **12**, 269–281 (2012)

Reyon, D., et al.: FLASH assembly of TALENs for high-throughput genome editing. Nat. Biotechnol. **30**, 460–465 (2012)

Ru, R., et al.: Targeted genome engineering in human induced pluripotent stem cells by penetrating TALENs. Cell Regen. (Lond.) **2**, 5 (2013)

Sánchez-Rivera, F.J., Jacks, T.: Applications of the CRISPR-Cas9 system in cancer biology. Nat. Rev. Cancer **15**, 387–395 (2015)

Sander, J.D., Joung, J.K.: CRISPR-Cas systems for editing, regulating and targeting genomes. Nat. Biotechnol. **32**, 347–355 (2014)

Sander, J.D., et al.: ZiFiT (Zinc Finger Targeter): an updated zinc finger engineering tool. Nucleic Acids Res. **38**(Suppl), W462–W468 (2010)

Sander, J.D., et al.: In silico abstraction of zinc finger nuclease cleavage profiles reveals an expanded landscape of off-target sites. Nucleic Acids Res. **41**, e181 (2013)

Schiller, J.T., Lowy, D.R.: Virus infection and human cancer: an overview. Recent Results Cancer Res. **193**, 1–10 (2014)

Scholl, C., et al.: Synthetic lethal interaction between oncogenic KRAS dependency and STK33 suppression in human cancer cells. Cell **137**, 821–834 (2009)

Scholler, J., et al.: Decade-long safety and function of retroviral-modified chimeric antigen receptor T cells. Sci Transl Med **4**, 132ra153 (2012)

Scrace, S.F., et al.: Abstract 700: investigating KRAS synthetic lethal/co-dependency interactions using siRNA and CRISPR. Cancer Res. **75**, 700 (2015)

Shalem, O., et al.: Genome-scale CRISPR-Cas9 knockout screening in human cells. Science **343**, 84–87 (2014)

Shalem, O., Sanjana, N.E., Zhang, F.: High-throughput functional genomics using CRISPR-Cas9. Nat. Rev. Genet. **16**, 299–311 (2015)

Shi, J., et al.: Discovery of cancer drug targets by CRISPR-Cas9 screening of protein domains. Nat. Biotechnol. **33**, 661–667 (2015)
Shen, B., et al.: Efficient genome modification by CRISPR-Cas9 nickase with minimal off-target effects. Nat. Methods **11**, 399–402 (2014)
Shuvalov, O., Barlev, N.A.: Current genome editing tools in gene therapy: new approaches to treat cancer. Curr. Gene Ther. **15**, 511–529 (2015)
Singh, H., et al.: Redirecting specificity of T-cell populations for CD19 using the Sleeping Beauty system. Cancer Res. **68**, 2961–2971 (2008)
Springer, C.J., Niculescu-Duvaz, I.: Prodrug-activating systems in suicide gene therapy. J. Clin. Invest. **105**, 1161–1167 (2000)
Srivastava, S., Riddell, S.R.: Engineering CAR-T cells: design concepts. Trends Immunol. **36**, 494–502 (2015)
Stratton, M.R.: Exploring the genomes of cancer cells: progress and promise. Science **331**, 1553–1558 (2011)
Streubel, J., Blücher, C., Landgraf, A., Boch, J.: TAL effector RVD specificities and efficiencies. Nat. Biotechnol. **30**, 593–595 (2012)
Szczepek, M., et al.: Structure-based redesign of the dimerization interface reduces the toxicity of zinc-finger nucleases. Nat. Biotechnol. **25**, 786–793 (2007)
Tan, W., Dong, Z., Wilkinson, T.A., Barbas, C.F., Chow, S.A.: Human immunodeficiency virus type 1 incorporated with fusion proteins consisting of integrase and the designed polydactyl zinc finger protein E2C can bias integration of viral DNA into a predetermined chromosomal region in human cells. J. Virol. **80**, 1939–1948 (2006)
Teachey, D.T., et al.: Cytokine release syndrome after blinatumomab treatment related to abnormal macrophage activation and ameliorated with cytokine-directed therapy. Blood **121**, 5154–5157 (2013)
Tebas, P., et al.: Gene editing of CCR5 in autologous CD4 T cells of persons infected with HIV. N. Engl. J. Med. **370**, 901–910 (2014)
Thompson, J.M., Nguyen, Q.H., Singh, M., Razorenova, O.V.: Approaches to identifying synthetic lethal interactions in cancer. Yale J. Biol. Med. **88**, 145–155 (2015)
Torikai, H., et al.: A foundation for universal T-cell based immunotherapy: T cells engineered to express a CD19-specific chimeric-antigen-receptor and eliminate expression of endogenous TCR. Blood **119**, 5697–5705 (2012)
Tsai, S.Q., et al.: GUIDE-seq enables genome-wide profiling of off-target cleavage by CRISPR-Cas nucleases. Nat. Biotechnol. **33**, 187–197 (2014a)
Tsai, S.Q., et al.: Dimeric CRISPR RNA-guided FokI nucleases for highly specific genome editing. Nat. Biotechnol. **32**, 569–576 (2014b)
Urnov, F.D., et al.: Highly efficient endogenous human gene correction using designed zinc-finger nucleases. Nature **435**, 646–651 (2005)
Urnov, F.D., Rebar, E.J., Holmes, M.C., Zhang, H.S., Gregory, P.D.: Genome editing with engineered zinc finger nucleases. Nat. Rev. Genet. **11**, 636–646 (2010)
Valton, J., et al.: A multidrug-resistant engineered CAR T cell for allogeneic combination immunotherapy. Mol. Ther. **23**, 1507–1518 (2015)
Voigt, K., et al.: Retargeting sleeping beauty transposon insertions by engineered zinc finger DNA-binding domains. Mol. Ther. **20**, 1852–1862 (2012)
Wang, J., et al.: Targeted gene addition to a predetermined site in the human genome using a ZFN-based nicking enzyme. Genome Res. **22**, 1316–1326 (2012)
Wang, H., et al.: One-step generation of mice carrying mutations in multiple genes by CRISPR/Cas-mediated genome engineering. Cell **153**, 910–918 (2013)
Wang, T., Wei, J.J., Sabatini, D.M., Lander, E.S.: Genetic screens in human cells using the CRISPR-Cas9 system. Science **343**, 80–84 (2014)
Wang, X., et al.: Unbiased detection of off-target cleavage by CRISPR-Cas9 and TALENs using integrase-defective lentiviral vectors. Nat. Biotechnol. **33**, 175–178 (2015a)
Wang, D., et al.: Adenovirus-mediated somatic genome editing of Pten by CRISPR/Cas9 in mouse liver in spite of Cas9-specific immune responses. Hum. Gene Ther. **26**, 432–442 (2015b)

Weber, E., Gruetzner, R., Werner, S., Engler, C., Marillonnet, S.: Assembly of designer TAL effectors by Golden Gate cloning. PLoS One **6**, e19722 (2011)
Weber, J., et al.: CRISPR/Cas9 somatic multiplex-mutagenesis for high-throughput functional cancer genomics in mice. Proc. Natl. Acad. Sci. U. S. A. **112**, 13982–13987 (2015)
Wright, A.V., et al.: Rational design of a split-Cas9 enzyme complex. Proc. Natl. Acad. Sci. U. S. A. **112**, 2984–2989 (2015)
Wu, Y., et al.: TALE nickase mediates high efficient targeted transgene integration at the human multi-copy ribosomal DNA locus. Biochem. Biophys. Res. Commun. **446**, 261–266 (2014)
Xiao, A., et al:. CasOT: a genome-wide Cas9/gRNA off-target searching tool. Bioinformatics (2014)
Xue, W., et al.: CRISPR-mediated direct mutation of cancer genes in the mouse liver. Nature **514**, 380–384 (2014)
Yant, S.R., Huang, Y., Akache, B., Kay, M.A.: Site-directed transposon integration in human cells. Nucleic Acids Res. **35**, e50 (2007)
Yin, H., et al.: Genome editing with Cas9 in adult mice corrects a disease mutation and phenotype. Nat. Biotechnol. **32**, 551–553 (2014)
Yoon, S.H., et al.: Adoptive immunotherapy using human peripheral blood lymphocytes transferred with RNA encoding Her-2/neu-specific chimeric immune receptor in ovarian cancer xenograft model. Cancer Gene Ther. **16**, 489–497 (2009)
Zhang, F., et al.: Efficient construction of sequence-specific TAL effectors for modulating mammalian transcription. Nat. Biotechnol. **29**, 149–153 (2011)
Zhao, Y., et al.: Sequence-specific inhibition of microRNA via CRISPR/CRISPRi system. Sci. Rep. **4**, 3943 (2014)
Zhou, Y., et al.: High-throughput screening of a CRISPR/Cas9 library for functional genomics in human cells. Nature **509**, 487–491 (2014)
Zhu, Y., et al.: Anti-CD19 chimeric antigen receptor-modified T cells for B-cell malignancies: a systematic review of efficacy and safety in clinical trials. Eur. J. Haematol. (2015). doi:10.1111/ejh.12602

Chapter 10
Targeting the Physicochemical, Cellular, and Immunosuppressive Properties of the Tumor Microenvironment by Depletion of Hyaluronan to Treat Cancer

Christopher D. Thanos

Abbreviations

CDx	Companion diagnostic
ECM	Extracellular matrix
EMT	Epithelial-mesenchymal transition
HA	Hyaluronan
HABP	Hyaluronan-binding protein
IFP	Interstitial fluid pressure
KPC	$Kras^{LSL\text{-}G12D/+}$;$Trp53^{LSL\text{-}R172H/+}$;Cre
ORR	Objective response rate
PDA	Pancreatic ductal adenocarcinoma
PFS	Progression-free survival
TME	Tumor microenvironment
TSG-6	Tumor necrosis factor-stimulated gene 6 protein

1 Introduction

A large portion of the volume in vertebrate tissue corresponds to the space between cells, or extracellular matrix (ECM). The macromolecular composition of the ECM is comprised of a complex organization of glycosaminoglycans and structural proteins that influence tissue shape and function. Glycosaminoglycans are polysaccharide chains of two sugars of a repeating disaccharide subunit (Alberts et al.). Hyaluronan (HA) is a glycosaminoglycan with repeating disaccharide subunits of glucuronic acid and n-acetylglucosamine (Fig. 10.1). HA is highly hydrophilic and anionic (Laurent

C.D. Thanos, Ph.D. (✉)
Halozyme Therapeutics, Inc., 11388 Sorrento Valley Road, San Diego, CA 92121, USA
e-mail: cthanos@halozyme.com

P.D. Rennert (ed.), *Novel Immunotherapeutic Approaches to the Treatment of Cancer*, DOI 10.1007/978-3-319-29827-6_10

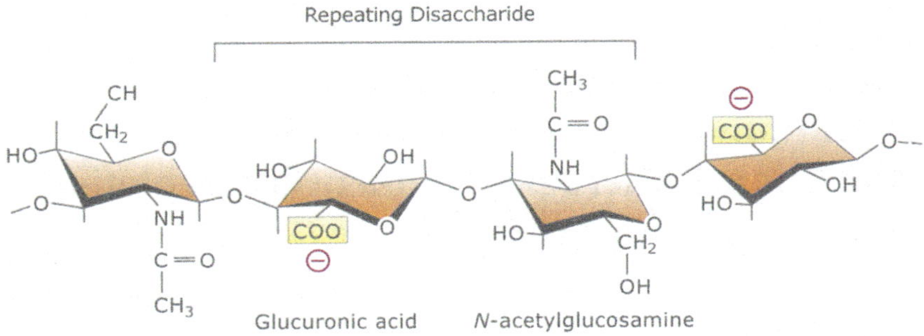

Fig. 10.1 Hyaluronan is an anionic, polymeric, glycosaminoglycan composed of repeating subunits of glucuronic acid and *N*-acetylglucosamine. Figure adopted with permission from *Molecular Biology of the Cell*

and Fraser 1992), and can swell to many times its size when fully hydrated, forming a highly viscous solution (Necas et al. 2008). A single molecule of HA can form highly extended, random conformations, occupying large volumes, despite possessing a low overall mass (Alberts et al.) (Fig. 10.2). The physical properties of HA promote turgor, allowing tissue to withstand significant compressive and shear forces, and promote water homeostasis. Therefore it is no surprise that megadalton polymers of HA play a key structural role and are found in large quantities in skin and connective tissue, where they help to maintain tissue viscoelasticity, and in joint fluid, where they serve as a lubricant, space filler, and shock absorber (Laurent and Fraser 1992; Necaṣ et al. 2008). However, a significant body of work has described the abnormal accumulation of HA in some solid tumors which usurp the special properties of HA to promote a more aggressive tumor pathology (Stern 2008). This chapter focuses on HA-mediated alterations of the physicochemical, cellular, and immunosuppressive properties of the TME and highlights an emerging therapeutic option, based on the use of PEGPH20 (Thompson et al. 2010), which is currently in clinical development.

2 Hyaluronan Content in Tumors Is Correlated with Poor Prognosis and More Aggressive Tumor Growth

Early publications in the 1930s described the HA found in tissue as acid mucopolysaccharides (Meyer et al. 1934, 1936). Soon after in 1939, Kabat characterized the properties of a highly concentrated, viscous polysaccharide in fluid drawn from avian sarcoma tumors (Kabat 1939). Since then, a significant body of literature has emerged, describing the accumulation of HA in cancerous tissue (Stern 2008; Ropponen et al. 1998; Auvinen et al. 2000; Anttila et al. 2000). Elevated levels of HA have been observed across a broad range of solid tumor types (Jacobetz et al. 2013; Kultti et al. 2012). Many of these tumor types are associated with a low 5-year mortality, including pancreatic ductal adenocarcinoma, non-small-cell lung, gastric, and breast cancers (Fig. 10.3).

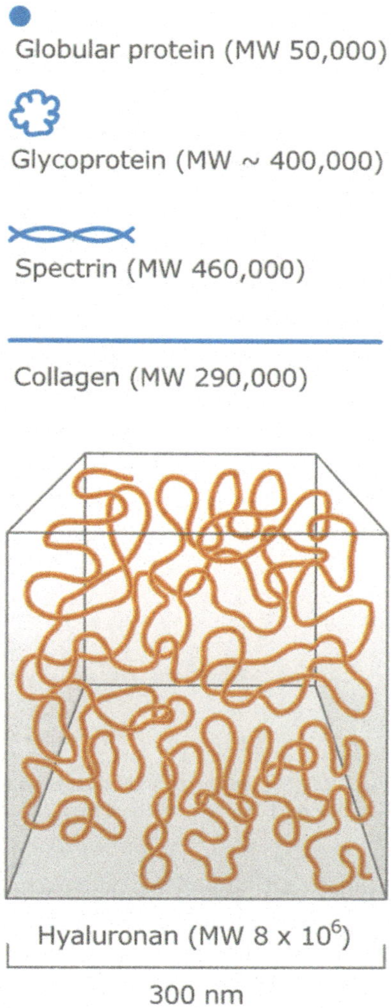

Fig. 10.2 A single hydrated molecule of hyaluronan (MW 8×10^6) adopts a random coil conformation, occupying a significantly larger volume than a 50,000 MW globular protein, a glycogen granule, spectrin, and collagen. Figure adopted with permission from *Molecular Biology of the Cell*

Elevated levels of tumor HA are associated with more aggressive disease states and poor prognoses. A recently published study examined the correlation between structural components of the tumor stroma and patient survival (Whatcott et al. 2015). Fifty patient biopsies were assembled from individuals diagnosed with pancreatic cancer over a range of stages (6 % stage IA, 18 %, stage IB, 18 % stage IIA, 40 % stage IIB, 8 % stage III, 10 % stage IV). Each specimen was assessed for HA status and categorized as HA-low or HA-high, based on specific immunohistochemical staining using biotinylated HA-binding protein (HABP). Kaplan-Meier survival curves were plotted for individuals based on having an HA-low or HA-high status. A separation of 15.0 months in median survival was observed between the two groups (9.3 for the HA-high

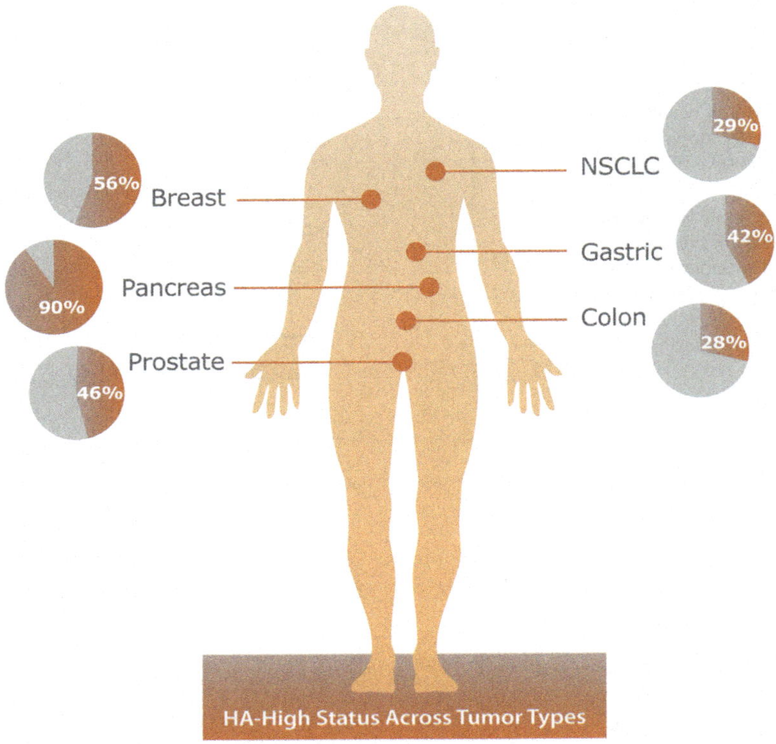

Fig. 10.3 Percentage of solid tumors with elevated HA levels, as assessed by Tissue Microarray Staining for HA. Data obtained from Jacobetz et al., Gut 2013;62:112–120

group, 24.3 months for the HA-low group, Fig. 10.4), demonstrating that in the case of pancreatic cancer, HA-high status is an indicator of poor prognosis. Auvinen and colleagues assessed HA status and survival in 278 breast cancer cases (Auvinen et al. 2000). HA levels in each specimen were designated as weak, mild, moderate, or intense based on stained sections and survival outcomes were then plotted based on those four levels. The level of survival was dependent on the level of HA staining; those with the weakest HA staining had the best prognosis and those with intense HA staining had the worst prognosis. More recent studies have also confirmed that the accumulation of HA in breast cancer is associated with poor prognosis (Auvinen et al. 2013, 2014). In addition, elevated HA levels are associated with poor prognosis in colon (Ropponen et al. 1998), prostate (Lipponen et al. 2001), and ovarian cancers (Anttila et al. 2000), as reviewed in more detail by Tammi et al. (2008).

Evaluation of HA levels in experimental animal tumor models supports the findings observed in patients. HA accumulation is associated with altered structure of tumor stroma and accelerated more aggressive tumor growth. Koyama and colleagues used the mouse mammary tumor virus (MMTV)-Neu transgenic model

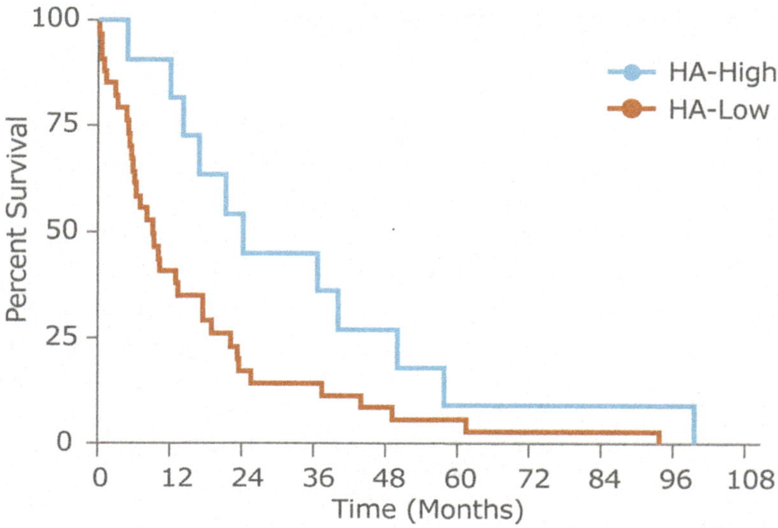

Fig. 10.4 Kaplan–Meier survival curves for patients with high and low levels of hyaluronan (HA) in their primary tumors. Median survival in the "high" HA group was 9.3 months, as opposed to 24.3 months for the "low" HA group. Figure adopted with permission from Clin Cancer Res; 21(15) August 1, 2015, ©2015 American Association for Cancer Research

of spontaneous breast cancer to assess the impact of HA accumulation on tumor growth rate (Koyama et al. 2007). They did this by crossing MMTV-Neu mice with conditional transgenic mice that express *Has2*, a gene that encodes hyaluronan synthetase 2 by Cre-mediated recombination. This enzyme, which catalyzes the synthesis of HA, was added to encourage hyper-production and accumulation of HA into the TME. Immunohistochemical staining demonstrated that *Has2* introduction led to significant deposition of HA in tumors. The *Her2*/*Neu*/*Has2* tumors with the added HA phenotype grew significantly faster, doubling in size when compared to control, parental tumors grown over the same time frame (Fig. 10.5a). In addition, the incidence of measurable mammary tumors was significantly greater in the Has2 transgenic mice with a HA-high tumor status. Mechanistically, HA accumulation from Her2/Neu/Has2 transgenic mouse tumors resulted in significant recruitment of stromal cells to the TME, which will be discussed below.

In a separate line of experimentation, Kultti and colleagues examined the impact of introducing the HA synthetase genes Has2 or Has3 into human BxPC-3 pancreatic tumor cells and assessed the impact on tumor xenografts grown from these cells. Introduction of either enzyme led to significant increases in HA content in tumors grown from these engineered cell lines. HA produced from HAS2 was both intracellular and extracellular, whereas HA produced from Has3 was predominantly extracellular. HA corresponded to 0.034 % of the mass of tumors grown from the parental BxPC-3 cell line (0.344 μg/mg calculated on a weight:weight basis). Introduction of Has3 led to an approximate fivefold increase in HA level in the Bx-PC3^{Has3} tumors

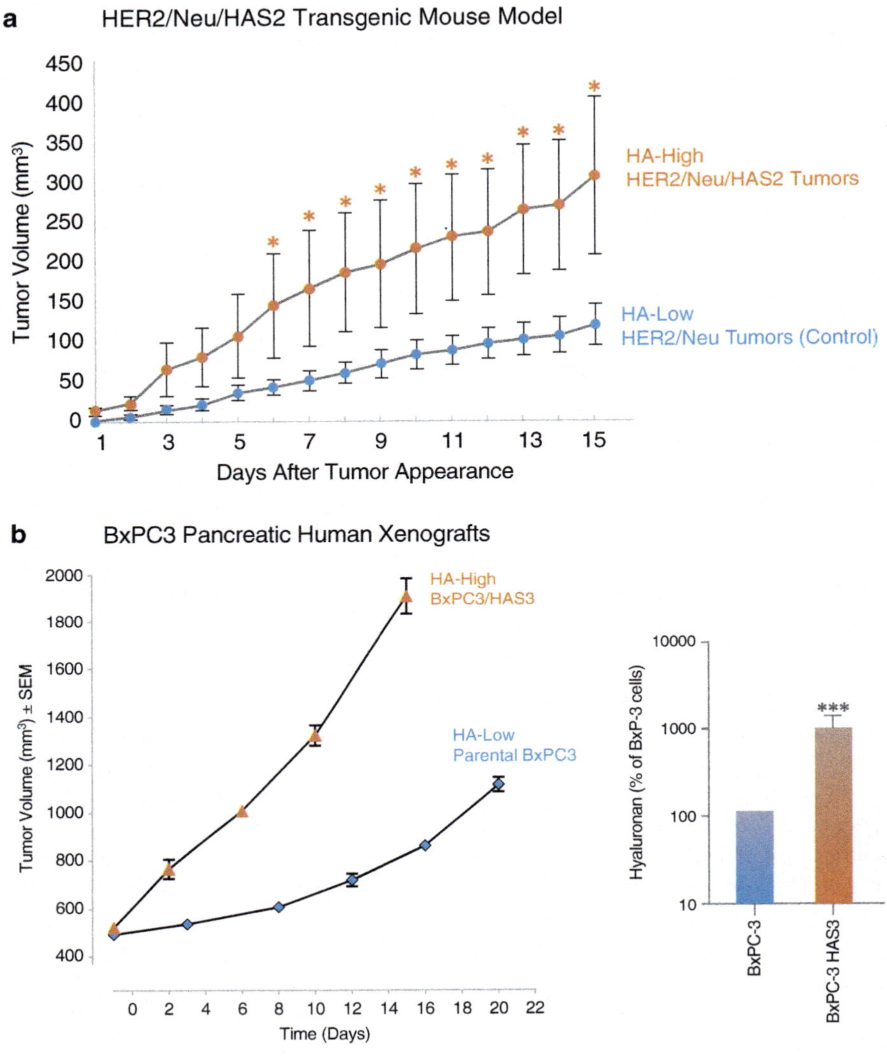

Fig. 10.5 (**a**) Growth acceleration of Neu-initiated mammary tumors by Has2 overexpression and HA accumulation. Figure adopted from *The American Journal of Pathology*, *Vol. 170*, *No. 3*, *p1093*, with permission from *American Society for Investigative Pathology*. (**b**) Pancreatic cancer xenograft tumors overexpressing HAS3 grow faster than parental tumors (*left* panel). An approximate tenfold increase in the accumulation of extracellular HA was observed in tumors that overexpress HAS3 (*right* panel). Figure adopted from Biomed Res Int. 2014;2014:817613

and accounted for approximately 0.18 % of the tumor mass (1.864 μg/mg). As was seen in the Koyama study, the introduction of the HA-synthesizing enzyme resulted in significant acceleration of tumor growth (Fig. 10.5b).

3 Why Does Tumor HA Accumulation Lead to Poor Prognosis and More Aggressive Disease?

HA likely contributes to cancer progression by multiple mechanisms (Fig. 10.6). Experimental models have demonstrated that HA facilitates the recruitment and proliferation of stromal cells, which cooperate with tumor cells to generate an environment that promotes tumor progression. HA accumulation has been shown to promote tumor invasiveness, migration, and malignancy. Furthermore, HA appears to play a key role in EMT through interactions with its receptor, CD44. HA contributes to tumor desmoplasia, significantly increased tumor IFP interstitial fluid pressure, which can lead to hypoxia and to a tumorigenic growth environment. Finally, the presence of HA in the TME could also impact immune system recognition and dysregulation and promote immunosuppression.

3.1 Tumor-Cell/Stromal Cell Interactions

Both clinical evidence and experimental data point to a close coordination between tumor and host stromal cells, which promotes tumor progression (Kalluri and Zeisberg 2006; Bhowmick and Moses 2005). In the TME, precise autocrine and paracrine cross talk between tumor and stromal cells influences cellular composition and

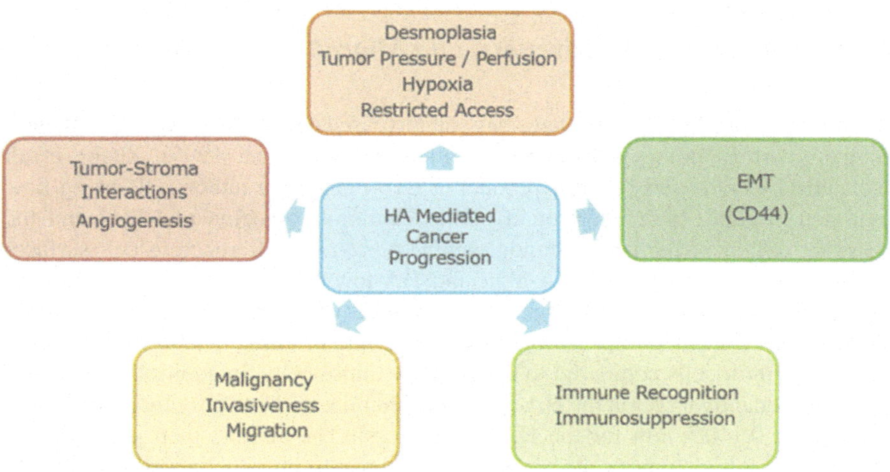

Fig. 10.6 HA mediates cancer progression by multiple factors

facilitates tumor proliferation through angiogenesis and spread of the disease through tissue invasion and metastasis (Bhowmick and Moses 2005). HA accumulation from Her2/Neu/Has2 transgenic mouse tumors resulted in significant recruitment of stromal cells which was then followed by the formation of tumor stroma (Koyama et al. 2007). The Neu/Has2 tumors had an increased cellular proliferation status as assessed by PCNA and fivefold slower rate of cell death as assessed by a TUNEL assay when compared to the non-Has2 tumors. The authors also found that an aggressive HA-mediated disease state was supported by the activation of PI3-kinase/AKT signaling pathway, which is involved in fundamental cellular processes including proliferation, protein translation, and survival. However, an increase in tumor VEGF levels was not observed. Instead, the HA-rich TME strongly induced stromal cell infiltration in the TME, and two markers for stromal cell-induced hyper-neovascularization, bFGF and CXCL12, were elevated in these tumors. In addition, there was a sixfold increase in versican, an HA-binding proteoglycan, which may promote the infiltration of stromal myofibroblasts. Cells that were stained with α-SMA and vimentin were typically characteristic of myofibroblasts and consistently had a strong pericellular HA staining, prompting the authors to suggest that HA accumulation in the TME was possibly derived primarily from those stromal cells that had infiltrated the tumor parenchyma. Earlier in vitro studies suggest that tumor and stromal cells can cooperate to produce HA. Co-cultures between lung tissue-derived tumor cells and fibroblasts resulted in a synergistic increase in HA synthesis when the cells were grown together in the same vessel (Knudson et al. 1984). In a separate study (Merrilees and Finlay 1985), conditioned growth media from the human tumor cell lines MM-96 and HT-29 stimulated greater than eight- to tenfold increase in HA synthesis from human skin fibroblasts. Thus, tumor cells appeared to secrete a factor that was responsible for the increased HA synthesis by fibroblasts.

3.2 Malignancy, Invasiveness, and Migration

Tumor cells with an HA-high status have an increased metastatic potential compared to their corresponding HA-low counterparts (Zhang et al. 1995). Zhang et al. isolated HA-high- and HA-low-producing B16 melanoma tumor cells using flow cytometry against a fusion protein of the HA-binding region of CD44 and the constant region of human immunoglobulin. A 32-fold difference in cell surface-associated HA between the HA-high and HA-low B16 cell types was reported. When cells were injected into the tail vein of mice, there was a greater than 50-fold increase in the mean number of metastatic lung nodules/lung ($p < 0.01$) induced by HA-high tumor cells compared to the HA-low tumor cells. In addition, metastases were significantly larger in the HA-high-injected mice (0.1–8.0 mm for the HA-high tumors vs. 0.1–0.5 mm for the HA-low tumors). The authors then proceeded to show that HA-high tumor cells bound to CD44-positive endothelial cells to a greater extent than HA-low cells, suggesting that a possible mechanism for the enhanced metastatic phenotype of the HA-high tumor cells is due to HA-mediated tumor cell adhesion to endothelial cells. Interestingly, a separate study revealed that breast cancer primary lesions which stained positive for HA also stained positive for HA in paired metastatic brain lesions (Jadin et al. 2015), similar to the findings of Whatcott et al., who compared HA levels between the primary tumor and unmatched metastases in specimens from pancreatic cancer patients (Whatcott et al. 2015).

An early study demonstrated that HA deposition overlapped with tumor invasiveness in an experimental model. Toole and colleagues (1979) observed that the HA content in highly invasive rabbit V2 tumors was 3–4 times greater than when the same tumor is grown in the nude mouse, where it is noninvasive. The HA content was highest in areas at the interface between the tumor mass and connective tissue. Moreover, the concentration of HA in the tumor parenchyma or connective tissue was independent of the site of tumor implantation—similar HA levels were observed in tumors that were grown in muscle or in subcutaneous tissue.

In a separate set of in vitro experiments, cells engineered to overproduce HA showed decreased contact-mediated cell growth inhibition and increased migration (Itano et al. 2002). Itano et al. engineered non-transformed rat 3Y1 cells to express the HA synthases (three isoforms—HAS1, HAS2, or HAS3) in an ectopic manner. Transfectants demonstrated multiple phenotypic changes, due to the significant deposition of HA in the extracellular matrix. Each of the three HAS transfectants was able to significantly increase its confluent cell densities (forming overlapping cell layers) and demonstrated a change in cell morphology to a fibroblastic shape, losing contact-mediated inhibition of migration and cell growth. In addition, each of the three HA-producing transfectants demonstrated increased motility using a scratch-wound assay.

3.3 HA Accumulation Promotes the Epithelial-Mesenchymal Transition

The epithelial-mesenchymal transition (EMT) (Kalluri and Weinberg 2009) is a process that normally occurs during the development of healthy tissue. A polarized epithelial cell undergoes multiple changes in its biochemistry to assume a mesenchymal phenotype, which leads to greatly enhanced production of extracellular matrix components, increased ability to migrate, invasiveness, and increased resistance to apoptosis. Unfortunately cancer cells usurp the EMT mechanism to increase migration and ability to form metastases. A number of studies have pointed to a role for HA in cancer progression when EMT-like changes occur (Camenisch et al. 2000; Zoltan-Jones et al. 2003; Porsch et al. 2013). First, Zolton-Jones et al. (2003) demonstrated that recombinant adenoviral expression of the HA-synthesizing enzyme HAS2 in normal canine kidney and in MCF-10 human mammary epithelial cells promoted the EMT in both cell types through increased production of HA. Second, HAS2 was identified as a likely source of HA during embryonic development. Has2(–/–) embryos were found to lack HA and died during mid-gestation due to severe cardiac and vascular abnormalities (Camenisch et al. 2000). Explanted heart cells from *Has2(−/−)* embryos lacked the ability to transition into mesenchyme; however that phenotype could be reversed through the addition of exogenous HA (Camenisch et al. 2000). Third, an early indication of EMT is acknowledged to be loss of plasma membrane E-cadherin and β-catenin, which leads to disruption of cell-cell junctions (Kalluri and Weinberg 2009). HA accumulation in the TME of BxPC-3 tumors that were lentivirally transduced with *Has3* resulted in loss of plasma membrane E-cadherin and accumulation of cytoplasmic β-catenin, suggesting disruption of cell-cell junctions that is HA dependent (Kultti et al. 2014).

3.4 HA Accumulation Promotes Significant Increases in Tumor Pressure, Decreased Perfusion, and Hypoxia

The impact of HA accumulation on the biophysical properties of tumors (in particular, the examination of IFP using a piezoelectric pressure transducer) was first investigated in human PC3 tumor xenograft models by Thompson et al. in 2010 (discussed below) followed by more recent work using a genetically engineered mouse model of pancreatic ductal adenocarcinoma (PDA) (Jacobetz et al. 2013; Provenzano et al. 2012). Work from the Hingorani laboratory (Provenzano et al. 2012) examined the dynamic changes in both molecular and cellular components of the TME that lead to desmoplasia in PDA using both biopsied human specimens and the murine KPC ($Kras^{LSL\text{-}G12D/+}$;$Trp53^{LSL\text{-}R172H/+}$;Cre) model of PDA, a genetically engineered mouse model that recapitulates both the molecular progression and clinical pathology of the disease (Hingorani et al. 2005). Immunohistochemical analysis was performed to identify preinvasive, invasive, and metastatic disease in tumor specimens from both species. HA accumulation appeared to increase upon disease progression, becoming especially abundant during advanced and metastatic stages of disease. The staining and pathological assessment was closely matched between human and murine PDA samples, reinforcing the previously accumulated data that murine KPC tumors highly resemble human PDA. Using a piezoelectric pressure transducer directly inserted into tumors of KPC mice, the authors measured abnormally high tumor interstitial pressures, suggesting that the desmoplastic reaction requires significant remodeling of the structural architecture of the TME compared to healthy tissue. These data were consistent with earlier findings which showed that HA-high PC3 tumor xenografts have abnormally high tumor IFP (Thompson et al. 2010). Treatment of KPC tumor-bearing mice with PEGPH20 reversed the high IFP and significantly increased perfusion into the tumor (measured by multiphoton laser scanning microscopy), suggesting that HA plays a key role in the desmoplastic reaction and that HA accumulation directly contributes to elevated tumor pressure and decreased perfusion. Jacobetz et al. (2013) also observed that treatment with PEGPH20 significantly increased vascular patency in murine KPC tumors. In addition, enzymatic depletion of HA by administration of PEGPH20 to

KPC tumor-bearing mice resulted in significantly increased macromolecular permeability into tumors, but not into healthy tissue. Scanning electron microscopy revealed a significant increase in fenestration in tumor blood vessels after treatment with PEGPH20 which was not observed within PEGPH20-treated blood vessels of healthy tissue, suggesting that HA plays a role in maintaining junctional integrity in the vascular endothelium of PDA tumors. As mentioned above, early work demonstrated that human PC3 tumor xenografts, which are high in HA (Thompson et al. 2010), have abnormally high IFP. A dose-dependent decrease in IFP was observed as the dose of PEGPH20 was increased (Fig. 10.7), suggesting that there is a highly dynamic correlation between tumor HA levels and tumor IFP. A significant vascular decompression was observed in the same tumors after treatment with PEGPH20, by measuring expanded blood vessels that were stained with an anti-CD31 probe. Increased tumor blood flow was observed after PEGPH20 treatment, using imaging of hyperechoic microbubbles to measure perfusion, consistent with the Provenzano and Jacobetz findings described above that were reported more recently (Thompson et al. 2010). Finally, Kultti and colleagues (2014) noticed a decrease in the nuclear levels of hypoxia-related proteins, HIF-1a and Snail in HA-high status tumors after treatment with PEGPH20. Their data suggests that HA appears to play a role in promoting or maintaining a hypoxic TME, consistent with previous observations that HA levels modulate hypoxia in the synovial fluid (Chou et al. 2011).

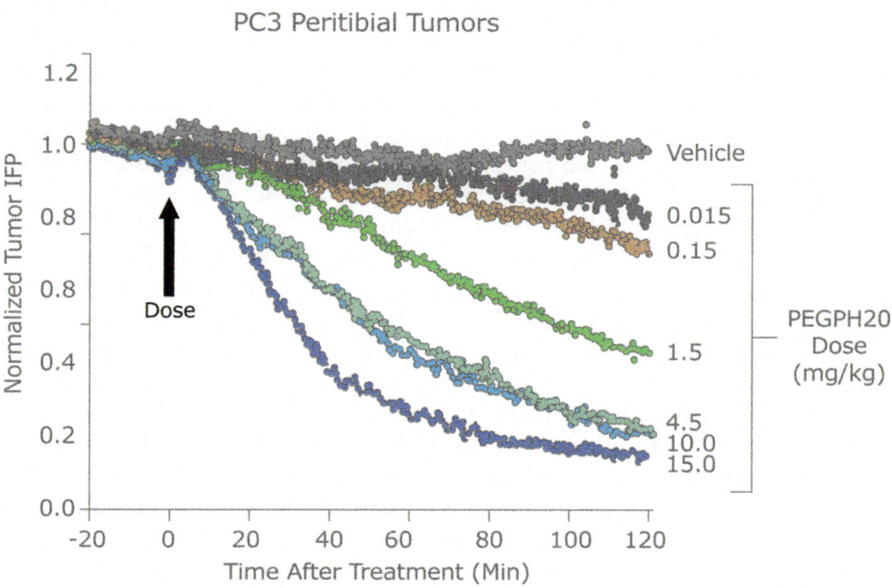

Fig. 10.7 A dose-dependent effect of PEGPH20 (0, 0.015, 0.15, 1.5, 4.5, 10, and 15 mg/kg) on tumor IFP was observed in HA-high PC3 tumors over a 2-h period following i.v. administration. Figure adopted by permission from Mol Cancer Ther; 9(11) November 2010, © 2010 American Association for Cancer Research

3.5 Impact of HA Accumulation on Immune System Recognition, Dysregulation, and Immunosuppression

Multiple lines of evidence suggest that high tumor HA levels could both limit the ability of the immune system to fight cancer and contribute to usurping immune system programs involved in wound repair and resolution to promote tumor growth. First, HA is capable of directly obstructing the ability of immune cells to contact and destroy tumor cells. Kultti et al. engineered MCF-7 breast cancer cells to overproduce HA by transfection of DNA gene encoding the HAS3 gene. The MCF-7-HAS3 cells secreted high levels of HA into the tissue culture medium and formed significant microvillus-like protrusions which emanated outward from the cell and were composed of HA, CD44, and actin filaments. Added particles such as red blood cells were unable to come into direct contact with the MCF-7-HAS3 tumor cells due to the presence of a pericellular HA coat on the surface of the tumor cells. However, control MCF-7 cells lacking pericellular HA were able to directly contact adjacent red blood cells. Singha et al. hypothesized that the presence of pericellular HA could shield tumor cells from recognition and destruction by NK cells (Singha et al. 2015). They mixed HA-overproducing SKBR3-HAS2 and MDA-MB-231-HAS2 tumor cells with human NK cells. In both experiments, the pericellular accumulation of HA prevented NK cells from forming the prerequisite immunological synapse with tumor cells and from commensurate tumor cell destruction. Treatment of the pericellular HA matrix with PEGPH20 broke down the HA barrier and allowed for direct NK cell contact with the tumor cells, which enabled NK cell-mediated cytotoxicity. In the context of a solid tumor, the authors also showed that PEGPH20 treatment significantly improved the access of peripherally administered NK cells into the tumor. This cloaking mechanism does not appear to be limited to tumor cells: interestingly, pathogenic Streptococcal bacteria also use pericellular HA to shield themselves from immune cell destruction (Laurent and Fraser 1992). Second, HA helps to contribute to the function and persistence of regulatory T cells (Bollyky et al. 2007, 2009), a subset of T cells that inhibit activation of helper and cytotoxic T cells (Beyer and Schultze 2009). It is tempting to speculate that abnormal accumulation of HA in the TME, in conjunction with other extracellular matrix components, contributes to a tumorigenic growth environment by inhibiting the ability of immune cells to proceed with their normal differentiation process, a theory discussed in more detail by Lu et al. (2012). Third, macrophages appear to exploit HA to penetrate and invade tumor tissue, and both M2 (immune-suppressive) and M1 (pro-inflammatory) macrophages can be involved, depending on the cancer type, stage, level of initiation, and progression. A recent study identified a strong correlation between HA levels and M2-like ($CD163^+$) tumor-associated macrophages in 273 biopsied specimens assembled from breast cancer patients, which was also associated with poor prognosis (Tiainen et al. 2015). On the other hand, HA is known to induce the expression of the pro-inflammatory cytokine IL-1β, characteristic of M1 macrophages, in a process mediated through its receptor, CD44 (Noble et al. 1993), which is upregulated in tumor-associated macrophages. Thus interactions between HA and macrophages in the TME appear to be highly dynamic and based on precise determinants, and whether the cancerous tissue is exploiting the pro-inflammatory wound healing or anti-inflammatory, wound resolution properties of the immune system. This concept is discussed in more detail in a recent review article by Schwertfeger et al. (2015).

4 Therapeutic Targeting of HA to Treat Cancer

Baumgartner first hypothesized that a hyaluronidase could be used to break down extracellular HA to improve delivery of chemotherapeutics to a tumor (Baumgartner et al. 1998; Pillwein et al. 1998; Klocker et al. 1998). Early tests using a hyaluronidase partially purified from animal tissue showed promise during initial clinical trials in malignant pediatric brain tumors and patients with advanced head and neck tumors, but later testing in a randomized trial failed to show benefit over chemotherapy alone (Baumgartner et al. 1998). However, since then, the significance of HA in solid tumor biology has gained a better understanding, and new therapeutic and diagnostic options for addressing HA-high tumors have become available. Subsequently, clinical interest in the original Baumgartner hypothesis has risen significantly.

A new potential therapeutic option is PEGPH20, which is a pegylated version of recombinant human PH20 (rHuPH20). Early experiments demonstrated that the HA-associated matrix resynthesis following hyaluronidase treatment is quite rapid (approximately 24 h in vitro) (Thompson et al. 2010). In mice, the serum half-life of rHuPH20 was found to be only 2.3 min; however pegylation improved the pharmacokinetic profile approximately 270-fold, with the PEGPH20 having an in vivo half-life of approximately 10.3 h (Thompson et al. 2010). PEGPH20 has therefore been used in a number of preclinical studies to evaluate whether HA depletion can improve therapeutic access to the tumor, and tested in combination with a variety of different therapeutic agents in experimental HA-high tumor models, including chemotherapeutic small molecules (Thompson et al. 2010; Jacobetz et al. 2013; Provenzano et al. 2012), monoclonal antibodies (Singha et al. 2015), and cellular immunotherapies (Manuel et al. 2015). In each case, concomitant administration of PEGPH20 depleted HA and improved the antitumor activity of those agents, regardless of the therapeutic modality that was combined with PEGPH20.

Two studies have demonstrated that combination PEGPH20 treatment with gemcitabine significantly increased overall survival in the KPC mouse model (Jacobetz et al. 2013; Provenzano et al. 2012). In the Provenzano study, an 83 % increase in the median overall survival (55.5 days for gemcitabine + placebo to 91.5 days for gemcitabine + PEGPH20) was reported. However, repeated injections resulted in sclerosing of the tail vein, limiting the treatment course to 3 months. Hence, the study did not likely reflect the maximal achievable benefit from combination therapy. In addition, a significant decrease in metastatic burden was observed for the gemcitabine + PEGPH20 combination arm of the study vs. gemcitabine + placebo arm. The decrease in metastases was observed across multiple tissues, including liver, lungs, diaphragm, mesenteric lymph nodes, and malignant ascites. In the Jacobetz study, KPC tumor-bearing mice receiving combination therapy with PEGPH20 also had significantly improved median survival outcomes vs. mice given gemcitabine monotherapy (28.5 days vs. 15 days). They measured a significant increase in uptake of gemcitabine into the tumor, consistent with a mechanism of action by HA depletion that includes reduction of tumor IFP, leading to increased vascular patency, and increased perfusion of the tumor. In addition, tumor-specific vascular fenestrations were observed, as mentioned above, which could lead to increased therapeutic access to the tumor. They also examined the ability of PEGPH20 treatment to mediate fluorescently labeled dextran uptake into murine KPC tumors. Interestingly, PEGPH20 treatment mediated significant increase of dextran into the tumor, but not healthy tissue, suggesting that in the absence of a PEGPH20-mediated decrease in high IFP, HA depletion does not increase access of therapies to healthy tissue. Finally, PEGPH20 has been shown to significantly improve the tumor growth inhibition of chemotherapy in murine tumor xenografts with a HA-high status (Thompson et al. 2010). A significant increase in intra-tumoral chemotherapy was observed as a result of PEGPH20 treatment. In addition, as a monotherapy, PEGPH20 at a high dose was effective at inhibiting tumor growth for HA-high tumors; however that effect was restricted to tumors with a HA-high status (Thompson et al. 2010).

In addition to chemotherapy, PEGPH20 treatment could be used to improve the accessibility of therapeutic mAbs to solid tumors with high HA levels. It is generally recognized that only a small percentage of dosed therapeutic mAbs penetrate deep into solid tumors and recognize their targets (Beckman et al. 2007). For example, a study using radiolabeled antibodies demonstrated that only 0.01 % of the injected dose per gram of tumor was able to penetrate the tumor (Sedlacek 1992). This is due in part due to high tumor IFP, vasculature composition, high cell density, target affinity, solid tumor tissue structure, and extracellular matrix (ECM) components (Beckman et al. 2007). This phenomenon may be exacerbated in tumors that have accumulated high amounts of HA, as it is now known that HA contributes to increases in tumor IFP, resulting in collapsed vasculature and decreased perfusion (Thompson et al. 2010; Jacobetz et al. 2013; Provenzano et al. 2012) (discussed above). In a HA-high tumor xenograft model, concomitant PEGPH20 treatment resulted in a significant increase in fluorescently labeled trastuzumab accumulation in the tumor, as well as improved tumor growth inhibition (Singha et al. 2015). Interestingly, an added benefit was observed when peripherally administered NK cells were given with trastuzumab, suggesting that HA depletion also improves antibody effector function (Singha et al. 2015).

Next-generation immuno-oncology therapeutics such as checkpoint inhibitors and adoptive T cell therapy are showing great promise in their ability to treat cancer. It is tempting to speculate that concomitant PEGPH20 treatment status could improve the efficacy of these agents for tumors with high HA levels; a recent published study supports this hypothesis (Manuel et al. 2015). Manuel and colleagues at City of Hope have engineered a cellular immunotherapy based on an attenuated strain *Salmonella typhimurium* (Manuel et al. 2015) that carries a short hairpin RNA-based inhibitor to the gene that encodes indoleamine 2,3 dioxygenase (IDO). The therapeutic candidate, called shIDO-ST, failed to demonstrate significant antitumor activity as a single-agent treatment in an orthotopic KPC-derived pancreatic tumor model. However, when co-administered with PEGPH20, complete tumor responses were observed

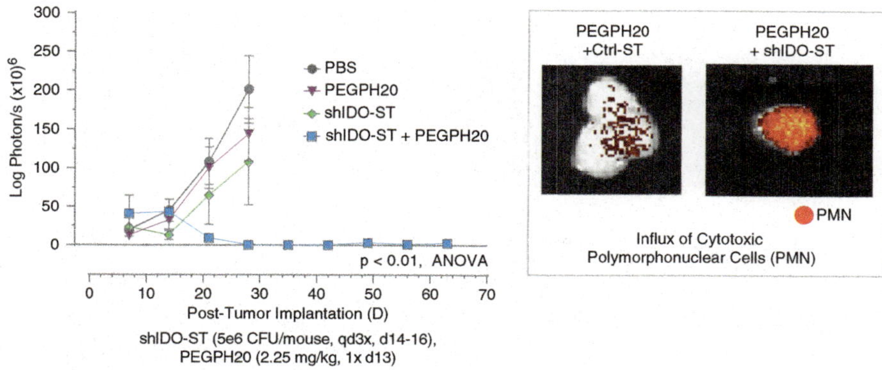

Fig. 10.8 Combination therapy with PEGPH20/shIDO-ST controls KPC-derived tumor growth. Adopted with permission from *Cancer Immunol Res September 2015 3:1096-1107*; *© 2015 American Association for Cancer Research*

(Fig. 10.8). Treatment with PEGPH20 allowed for significantly increased trafficking of polymorphonuclear cells (Fig. 10.8), followed by significant infiltration of CD8+ T cells to the tumor (Manuel et al. 2015). These data suggest that it might be possible to combine PEGPH20 with immunotherapies to treat HA-high status tumors that are considered impregnable by these agents.

4.1 Determining HA Levels in Tumors

A companion diagnostic (CDx) must be generated that can prospectively stratify patients with an HA-high status that will most likely respond to treatment with regimens that include PEGPH20. Significant improvements have been made in the ability to measure HA levels in tumors. A first-generation probe that was derived from bovine cartilage tissue HABP was initially used for this purpose (Jacobetz et al. 2013). However, while this probe has proven quite useful for staining HA in the context of research studies (Jacobetz et al. 2013), the nature of the HABP was suboptimal for use as a CDx. First, HABP protein preparations were heterogeneous mixtures purified from bovine tissue, making it a challenge to obtain desired purity and consistency from batch to batch. Second, HABP also binds to aggrecan-cartilage link protein, which makes it difficult to obtain accurate and quantitative binding constants to HA. Thus, alternative probes for binding to HA were pursued. Tumor necrosis factor-stimulated gene 6 protein (TSG-6) contains a link module that binds HA (Jadin et al. 2014). TSG-6 has several qualities that lend itself to being developed as a CDx, including small size, a well-defined structure, and defined HA binding properties. TSG-6 was further engineered through structure-based rational design to eliminate its affinity for heparin, another glycosaminoglycan, in order to narrow the

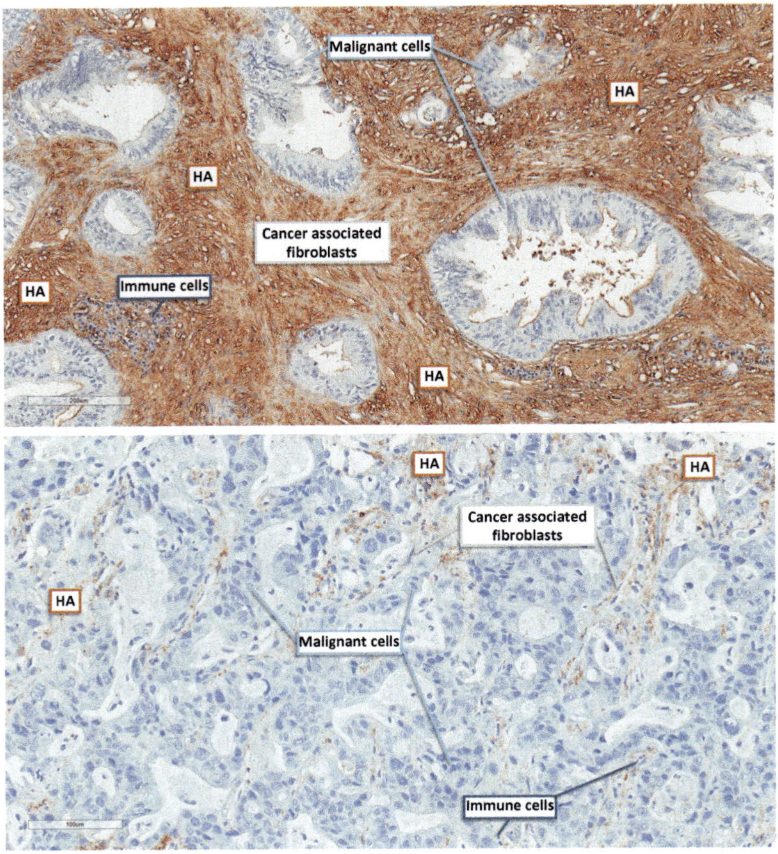

Fig. 10.9 Human pancreatic adenocarcinoma tissue sections were stained with a biotinylated version of Halozyme's recombinant human-Fc-TSG6 (named HTI-601) using a Leica autostainer. Here DAB (3,3′ Diaminobenzidine) was used as chromogen generating *brown* colored staining where HA was present. The tissue sections were counterstained with Gill's hematoxilin staining cell nuclei in *blue*. An HA-high tumor is shown on the *top* and an HA-low tumor is shown on the *bottom*

substrate specificity of TSG-6 solely to HA (Jadin et al. 2014). The engineered TSG6 was then constructed as a genetic fusion to the region encoding the Fc domain of IgG1, which assists in protein expression, purification, stability, and readout of stained specimens (Jadin et al. 2014). Formalin-fixed and paraffin-embedded tissue microarrays from both healthy and malignant tissue were stained using the engineered TSG-6-Fc probe and showed a strong degree of specificity for HA (Jadin et al. 2014). An example of two specimens from human PDA that were stained with the engineered TSG-6-Fc probe and determined to have either a low or a high HA status is shown in Fig. 10.9.

4.2 Evidence of Clinical Efficacy with PEGPH20

Data from early clinical studies that examine the effects of PEGPH20 in combination with chemotherapy have been encouraging. Promising signs of efficacy were observed in a Phase Ib study examining the effects of PEGPH20 plus gemcitabine in pancreatic cancer patients (Hingorani et al. 2013). More recently, PEGPH20 has shown promise of efficacy in an ongoing Phase II, open-label, randomized study of PEGPH20 + nab-paclitaxel + gemcitabine (PAG) vs. nab-paclitaxel + gemcitabine (AG) in previously untreated patients with stage IV pancreatic ductal adenocarcinoma (Hingorani et al. 2015). In the HA-high patient population, 71 % of patients being treated with PAG (12/17) had improved objective response rate (ORR) compared to only 29 % of patients being treated with AG (5/17), with a *p*-value of 0.02. The progression-free survival (PFS) was 9.2 months for PAG-receiving patients (12/25) comparing to 4.3 months for the AG group (15/23), with a *p*-value of 0.03. In contrast, the ORR and PFS were indistinguishable between the PAG and AG treatment groups for subjects with HA-low tumors. This suggests that in the future, prospective identification of HA-high status patients using the engineered TSG-6-Fc probe could likely define patient populations that best respond to PEGPH20 treatment.

5 Summary

Tremendous knowledge has been gained since Kabat first described a highly concentrated, viscous polysaccharide in fluid drawn from avian sarcoma tumors over 75 years ago. Healthy tissue dynamics are supported by HA, a megadalton, polymeric glycosaminoglycan. It is now well established that HA can also accumulate in many types of solid tumors, which is linked to poor prognosis in cancer patients. This is most likely due to multiple factors, including facilitation of tumor-stroma interactions leading to tumor progression, promotion of the EMT, physicochemical alterations of TME (desmoplasia, increased tumor IFP, reduced perfusion, and increased hypoxia), enhanced metastasis, and finally tumor cloaking from the immune system and immune dysregulation. Experimental studies with PEGPH20, which enzymatically degrades HA, have demonstrated significant improvement in the access of therapeutics to a tumor, through reduction of tumor IFP, decreased vascular compression, and improved blood flow to the tumor, as outlined in the illustration shown in Fig. 10.10. As a result of this mechanism of action, PEGPH20 holds promise as a future treatment strategy, not just for chemotherapeutics, but also for targeted therapies, immune checkpoint inhibitors, and next-generation cellular immunotherapies.

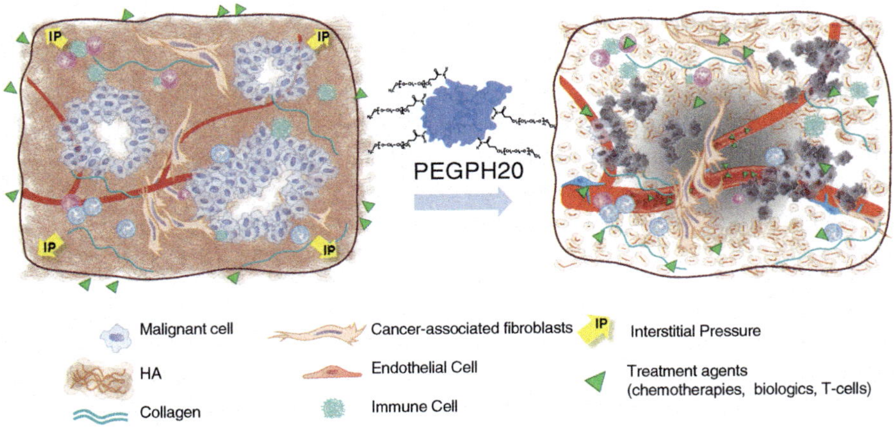

Fig. 10.10 Illustration of the impact of PEGPH20 treatment on the tumor microenvironment. PEGPH20 enzymatically degrades HA which results in significantly decreased tumor interstitial fluid pressure. This results in vascular expansion and increased perfusion into the tumor. Therapeutics have increased access to HA-high tumor with concomitant HA administration

Acknowledgements The author would like to thank Dr. Chunmei Zhao, Dr. Sanna Rosengren, Dr. Curtis Thompson, Dr. H. Michael Shepard, and Dr. Mike LaBarre for thoughtful comments and critical review during manuscript preparation. Special thanks to Dr. Mathieu Marella for assistance with Fig 10.9.

Conflict of Interest Dr. Thanos is an employee of Halozyme Therapeutics, Inc.

References

Alberts, B., Johnson, A., Lewis, J., et al. Mol. Biol. Cell. 804–805 (1989). Second Edition

Anttila, M.A., et al.: High levels of stromal hyaluronan predict poor disease outcome in epithelial ovarian cancer. Cancer Res. **60**, 150–155 (2000)

Auvinen, P., et al.: Hyaluronan in peritumoral stroma and malignant cells associates with breast cancer spreading and predicts survival. Am. J. Pathol. **156**, 529–536 (2000)

Auvinen, P., et al.: Increased hyaluronan content and stromal cell CD44 associate with HER2 positivity and poor prognosis in human breast cancer. Int. J. Cancer **132**, 531–539 (2013)

Auvinen, P., et al.: Hyaluronan synthases (HAS1-3) in stromal and malignant cells correlate with breast cancer grade and predict patient survival. Breast Cancer Res. Treat. **143**, 277–286 (2014)

Baumgartner, G., Gomar-Höss, C., Sakr, L., Ulsperger, E., Wogritsch, C.: The impact of extracellular matrix on the chemoresistance of solid tumors—experimental and clinical results of hyaluronidase as additive to cytostatic chemotherapy. Cancer Lett. **131**, 85–99 (1998)

Beckman, R.A., Weiner, L.M., Davis, H.M.: Antibody constructs in cancer therapy: protein engineering strategies to improve exposure in solid tumors. Cancer **109**, 170–179 (2007)

Beyer, M., Schultze, J.L.: Regulatory T cells: major players in the tumor microenvironment. Curr. Pharm. Des. **15**, 1879–1892 (2009)

Bhowmick, N.A., Moses, H.L.: Tumor-stroma interactions. Curr. Opin. Genet. Dev. **15**, 97–101 (2005)

Bollyky, P.L., et al.: Cutting edge: high molecular weight hyaluronan promotes the suppressive effects of CD4 + CD25+ regulatory T cells. J. Immunol. **179**, 744–747 (2007)

Bollyky, P.L., et al.: Intact extracellular matrix and the maintenance of immune tolerance: high molecular weight hyaluronan promotes persistence of induced CD4 + CD25+ regulatory T cells. J. Leukoc. Biol. **86**, 567–572 (2009)

Camenisch, T.D., et al.: Disruption of hyaluronan synthase-2 abrogates normal cardiac morphogenesis and hyaluronan-mediated transformation of epithelium to mesenchyme. J. Clin. Invest. **106**, 349–360 (2000)

Chou, L.-W., Wang, J., Chang, P.-L., Hsieh, Y.-L.: Hyaluronan modulates accumulation of hypoxia-inducible factor-1 alpha, inducible nitric oxide synthase, and matrix metalloproteinase-3 in the synovium of rat adjuvant-induced arthritis model. Arthritis Res. Ther. **13**, R90 (2011)

Hingorani, S.R., et al.: Trp53R172H and KrasG12D cooperate to promote chromosomal instability and widely metastatic pancreatic ductal adenocarcinoma in mice. Cancer Cell **7**, 469–483 (2005)

Hingorani, S.R., et al.: A phase Ib study of gemcitabine plus PEGPH20 (pegylated recombinant human hyaluronidase) in patients with stage IV previously untreated pancreatic cancer. ASCO Meet. Abstr. **31**, 4010 (2013)

Hingorani, S.R., et al.: High response rate and PFS with PEGPH20 added to nab-paclitaxel/gemcitabine in stage IV previously untreated pancreatic cancer patients with high-HA tumors: interim results of a randomized phase II study. ASCO Meet. Abstr. **33**, 4006 (2015)

Itano, N., et al.: Abnormal accumulation of hyaluronan matrix diminishes contact inhibition of cell growth and promotes cell migration. Proc. Natl. Acad. Sci. U. S. A. **99**, 3609–3614 (2002)

Jacobetz, M.A., et al.: Hyaluronan impairs vascular function and drug delivery in a mouse model of pancreatic cancer. Gut **62**, 112–120 (2013)

Jadin, L., et al.: Characterization of a novel recombinant hyaluronan binding protein for tissue hyaluronan detection. J. Histochem. Cytochem. **62**, 672–683 (2014)

Jadin, L., et al.: Hyaluronan expression in primary and secondary brain tumors. Ann. Transl. Med. **3**, 80 (2015)

Kabat, E.W.: A polysaccharide in tumors due to a virus of leucosis and sarcoma of fowls. J. Biol. Chem. **130**, 143–147 (1939)

Kalluri, R., Weinberg, R.A.: The basics of epithelial-mesenchymal transition. J. Clin. Invest. **119**, 1420–1428 (2009)

Kalluri, R., Zeisberg, M.: Fibroblasts in cancer. Nat. Rev. Cancer **6**, 392–401 (2006)

Klocker, J., Sabitzer, H., Raunik, W., Wieser, S., Schumer, J.: Hyaluronidase as additive to induction chemotherapy in advanced squamous cell carcinoma of the head and neck. Cancer Lett. **131**, 113–115 (1998)

Knudson, W., Biswas, C., Toole, B.P.: Interactions between human tumor cells and fibroblasts stimulate hyaluronate synthesis. Proc. Natl. Acad. Sci. U. S. A. **81**, 6767–6771 (1984)

Koyama, H., et al.: Hyperproduction of hyaluronan in neu-induced mammary tumor accelerates angiogenesis through stromal cell recruitment: possible involvement of versican/PG-M. Am. J. Pathol. **170**, 1086–1099 (2007)

Kultti, A., et al.: Therapeutic targeting of hyaluronan in the tumor stroma. Cancers **4**, 873–903 (2012)

Kultti, A., et al.: Accumulation of extracellular hyaluronan by hyaluronan synthase 3 promotes tumor growth and modulates the pancreatic cancer microenvironment. Biomed Res. Int. **2014**, 817613 (2014)

Laurent, T.C., Fraser, J.R.: Hyaluronan. FASEB J. **6**, 2397–2404 (1992)

Lipponen, P., et al.: High stromal hyaluronan level is associated with poor differentiation and metastasis in prostate cancer. Eur. J. Cancer **37**, 849–856 (2001)

Lu, P., Weaver, V.M., Werb, Z.: The extracellular matrix: a dynamic niche in cancer progression. J. Cell Biol. **196**, 395–406 (2012)

Manuel, E.R., et al.: Salmonella-based therapy targeting indoleamine 2,3-dioxygenase coupled with enzymatic depletion of tumor hyaluronan induces complete regression of aggressive pancreatic tumors. Cancer Immunol. Res. **3**, 1096–1107 (2015)

Merrilees, M.J., Finlay, G.J.: Human tumor cells in culture stimulate glycosaminoglycan synthesis by human skin fibroblasts. Lab. Invest. **53**, 30–36 (1985)

Meyer, K., et al.: The polysaccharide of the vitreous humor. J. Biol. Chem. **107**, 629–634 (1934)

Meyer, K., et al.: On glycoproteins: II. The polysaccharides of vitreous humor and of umbilical cord. J. Biol. Chem. **114**, 689–703 (1936)

Necas, J., Bartosikova, L., Brauner, P., Kolar, J.: Hyaluronic acid (hyaluronan): a review. Vet. Med. (Praha) **53**, 397–411 (2008)

Noble, P.W., Lake, F.R., Henson, P.M., Riches, D.W.: Hyaluronate activation of CD44 induces insulin-like growth factor-1 expression by a tumor necrosis factor-alpha-dependent mechanism in murine macrophages. J. Clin. Invest. **91**, 2368–2377 (1993)

Pillwein, K., et al.: Hyaluronidase additional to standard chemotherapy improves outcome for children with malignant brain tumors. Cancer Lett. **131**, 101–108 (1998)

Porsch, H., et al.: Efficient TGFβ-induced epithelial-mesenchymal transition depends on hyaluronan synthase HAS2. Oncogene **32**, 4355–4365 (2013)

Provenzano, P.P., et al.: Enzymatic targeting of the stroma ablates physical barriers to treatment of pancreatic ductal adenocarcinoma. Cancer Cell **21**, 418–429 (2012)

Ropponen, K., et al.: Tumor cell-associated hyaluronan as an unfavorable prognostic factor in colorectal cancer. Cancer Res. **58**, 342–347 (1998)

Schwertfeger, K.L., Cowman, M.K., Telmer, P.G., Turley, E.A., McCarthy, J.B.: Hyaluronan, inflammation, and breast cancer progression. Front. Immunol. **6**, 236 (2015)

Sedlacek, H.H.: Antibodies as Carriers of Cytotoxicity. Karger, Basel (1992)

Singha, N.C., et al.: Tumor-associated hyaluronan limits efficacy of monoclonal antibody therapy. Mol. Cancer Ther. **14**, 523–532 (2015)

Stern, R.: Association between cancer and 'acid mucopolysaccharides': an old concept comes of age, finally. Semin. Cancer Biol. **18**, 238–243 (2008)

Tammi, R.H., et al.: Hyaluronan in human tumors: pathobiological and prognostic messages from cell-associated and stromal hyaluronan. Semin. Cancer Biol. **18**, 288–295 (2008)

Thompson, C.B., et al.: Enzymatic depletion of tumor hyaluronan induces antitumor responses in preclinical animal models. Mol. Cancer Ther. **9**, 3052–3064 (2010)

Tiainen, S., et al.: High numbers of macrophages, especially M2-like (CD163-positive), correlate with hyaluronan accumulation and poor outcome in breast cancer. Histopathology **66**, 873–883 (2015)

Toole, B.P., Biswas, C., Gross, J.: Hyaluronate and invasiveness of the rabbit V2 carcinoma. Proc. Natl. Acad. Sci. U. S. A. **76**, 6299–6303 (1979)

Whatcott, C.J., et al.: Desmoplasia in primary tumors and metastatic lesions of pancreatic cancer. Clin. Cancer Res. **21**, 3561–3568 (2015). doi:10.1158/1078-0432.CCR-14-1051

Zhang, L., Underhill, C.B., Chen, L.: Hyaluronan on the surface of tumor cells is correlated with metastatic behavior. Cancer Res. **55**, 428–433 (1995)

Zoltan-Jones, A., Huang, L., Ghatak, S., Toole, B.P.: Elevated hyaluronan production induces mesenchymal and transformed properties in epithelial cells. J. Biol. Chem. **278**, 45801–45810 (2003)

Index

P.D. Rennert (ed.), *Novel Immunotherapeutic Approaches to the Treatment of Cancer*, DOI 10.1007/978-3-319-29827-6

D

E

CPSIA information can be obtained
at www.ICGtesting.com
Printed in the USA
LVOW02*1115100716
495763LV00002B/39/P